D1493121

THE
HARRIET LANE
HANDBOOK
A Manual for Pediatric House Officers

THE
HARRIET LANE
HANDBOOK

A Manual for Pediatric House Officers

TENTH EDITION

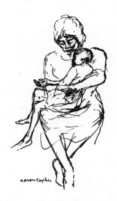

The Harriet Lane Service,
Children's Medical and Surgical Center
of the
Johns Hopkins Hospital

Editor
Cynthia H. Cole, M.D.

YEAR BOOK MEDICAL PUBLISHERS, INC.
CHICAGO

LIBRARY OF CONGRESS CATALOGING IN PUBLICATION DATA

Main entry under title:

The Harriet Lane handbook.

Includes index.
1. Pediatrics—Handbooks, manuals, etc. I. Cole, Cynthia H.
II. Johns Hopkins Hospital. Children's Medical and Surgical
Center.   [DNLM: 1. Pediatrics—handbooks. WS 29 H297]
RJ48.H35   1984   618.92   84—11902
ISBN 0—8151—4923—9

NOTICE

Every effort has been made to ensure that the drug dosage schedules herein are accurate and in accord with the standards accepted at the time of publication. However, as new research and experience broaden our knowledge, changes in treatment and drug therapy occur. Therefore, the reader is advised to check the product information sheet included in the package of each drug he plans to administer to be certain that changes have not been made in the recommended dose or in the contraindications. This is of particular importance in regard to new or infrequently used drugs.

Thirty-four years have passed since the original conception of the Harriet Lane Handbook by the house staff of 1950-1953. In revising the handbook for the tenth edition, one is continually reminded of the heritage of knowledge and wisdom that has been imparted so freely to each of us by our predecessors. This present edition is written in the spirit of providing pertinent, practical information to those who advocate for and serve the needs of children. As indicated in the first edition, the assumption exists throughout this text that, in the words of Dr. Francis Schwentker, ''There is no substitute for brains.''

The information collected over the years in our pocket ''pearl book'' has of necessity required updating existing information, and eliminating the obsolete. Virtually every section of this new edition has undergone revision and more thorough documentation of references.

The Formulary has been extensively revised to provide the most recent dosage recommendations for pediatric patients who span the range of neonates to adult-size teenagers. New drugs have been added, seldom recommended drugs deleted, and commonly prescribed oral theophylline preparations updated.

The Hematology, Endocrinology, Nephrology, Cardiology, Radiology, Poisoning, Burns, Perinatology, Pulmonary, Infectious Diseases, and Procedures sections have each been expanded, reorganized, or clarified where necessary. The Reference Data, Fluid and Electrolyte Therapy, and Nutrition sections have been corrected and updated. A Pediatric Neurology section has been added to provide information on seizures, anticonvulsants, head trauma, and coma. The index has been liberally cross-referenced in the hope that it will clarify what is indeed included.

All fourteen Senior Assistant Residents served as contributing editors and deserve special credit. Their enthusiasm and endurance have made editing this handbook a pleasurable experience. I am most appreciative to them for their help and suggestions.

Procedures, Metabolic Tests, Ketogenic Diet—
    Dr. Lawrence M. Nogee
Hematology—Dr. David M. Virshup
Nephrology—Dr. Miriam J. Behar
Infectious Diseases and Microbiologic Diagnostic Tests—
    Dr. Yvonne A. Maldonado
Cardiology—Dr. Anne M. Murphy

Endocrinology—Dr. Karen D. Crissinger
Developmental, Radiology, and Neurology—
    Dr. Barry S. Schonwetter
Formulary—Dr. Daniel A. Goldstein and Dr. David C. Goodman
Fluid and Electrolyte Therapy—Dr. Daniel A. Goldstein
Poisoning—Dr. Peter C. Rowe
Burns—Dr. Stuart A. Rowe
Perinatology—Dr. S. Lee Marban
Respiratory Care and Pulmonary Function—
    Dr. Karen D. Crissinger and Dr. Quan C. Nguyen
Nutrition—Dr. David C. Goodman
All other Reference Data—Dr. Quan C. Nguyen
Index—Dr. Pamela J. Stone

I am indebted to the faculty members of the Department of
Pediatrics for their advice, assistance, and constructive criti-
cism, and to our chairman, Dr. John W. Littlefield, for his support in this new edition.

This edition, of course, would not be possible without the
cumulative efforts of house staff and chief residents who pains-
takingly compiled earlier editions of the Harriet Lane Handbook.
A special word of appreciation is due to previous editors, Drs.
Henry Seidel, Harrison Spencer, Herbert Swick, William Friedman,
Robert Haslaam, Jerry Winkelstein, Dennis Headings, Kenneth
Schuberth, Basil Zitelli, Jeffrey Biller, and Andrew Yeager. Ms.
Diana McAninch and Mr. Joe Frank from Year Book Medical Publish-
ers, Inc. have been particularly helpful with their advice and
understanding. It has been a pleasure to work with them.

I want to sincerely thank Ms. Cindy Dean who has efficiently
and cheerfully transcribed illegible medical script into a well-
prepared manuscript.

Finally, I am appreciative to my family and to my husband,
George, who has been most patient, understanding, and supportive
throughout the years and especially during the editing of this
tenth edition.

Cynthia H. Cole, M.D.
Chief Resident
Editor

Baltimore, 1984

Preface ... v

PART I—DIAGNOSTIC TESTS

PART II—FORMULARY

PART III—THERAPEUTIC DATA

PART IV—REFERENCE DATA

PART I

DIAGNOSTIC TESTS

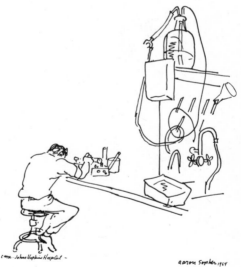

P R O C E D U R E S

The following are guidelines for common pediatric procedures. For a more detailed description see: Hughes, WT and Buescher, ES: Pediatric Procedures, 2nd Edition Philadelphia: W.B. Saunders, 1980; Fletcher, MA, et al.: Atlas of Procedures in Neonatology, Philadelphia: J. B. Lippincott Co., 1983.

1. Obtaining Blood

    A. Capillary Blood
       The extremity should first be warmed in order to provide optimal blood flow and more accurate samples. Care should be used not to use too warm (>40°C) a towel, as burns may result.
       1) The lateral or medial side of the heel may be used; avoid heel pad. For digital artery sampling use the lateral surface of the distal phalanx of second, third, or fourth finger.
       2) Use a 2.5 mm lancet for optimal skin penetration.
       3) Wipe away first drop of blood with dry gauze. Alcohol used in sterilizing skin may produce hemolysis.
       4) Massage extremity but avoid squeezing finger or heel.
       5) Samples may be inaccurate with poor perfusion or polycythemia.

       Ref: Blumenfeld, TA, et al.: Lancet 1:230, 1979; Morgan, EJ: Am Rev Resp Dis 120:795, 1979.

    B. External Jugular Puncture
       1) Wrap infant in mummified manner.
       2) Turn head to one side and extend.
       3) Prepare area carefully with iodine and alcohol.
       4) Provoke child to cry in order to distend external jugular vein, which runs from angle of mandible to posterior border of lower third of sternocleidomastoid muscle.

    C. Femoral Puncture

       NOTE: Reported complications of septic arthritis demand careful and efficient skin antisepsis. Femoral puncture is particularly hazardous in neonates and is not recommended in this age group. Avoid femoral punctures in children with thrombocytopenia, coagulation disorders, and those scheduled for cardiac catheterization.

       Ref: Asnes, RS and Arendar, GM: Pediatrics 38:837, 1966.

       1) An assistant should hold the child securely.

    2) The assistant stands behind the infant, leans over the head and trunk, and holds the legs in "semi-frogleg" position. The assistant also holds the infant's arms down by use of the upper arms and elbows.

    3) Prepare area carefully as for blood culture.

    4) After locating the femoral pulse just below the inguinal ligament, insert needle, aiming slightly medial to the pulse beat.

    5) Insert needle slowly to a depth of approximately 0.5 to 0.75 cm.

    6) While exerting suction, slowly withdraw needle until a small amount of blood enters syringe.

    7) If flow ceases, push needle deeper and withdraw as before.

    8) Hold both syringe and legs stationary to insure drawing maximum amount of blood.

D. Internal Jugular Puncture

    1) Wrap infant securely in sheet.

    2) Place child on table and adjust position so that head falls over the side. With the neck extended, turn head slightly to one side. This makes the posterior margin of the sternocleidomastoid muscle on the opposite side stand out.

    3) Sterilize area.

    4) Insert needle just deep to and behind posterior margin of sternocleidomastoid muscle, approximately halfway between its origin and insertion. Then advance needle under the muscle, parallel to skin surface and in direction of suprasternal notch, for a distance equal to width of sternocleidomastoid.

    5) Slowly withdraw needle while keeping a negative pressure on syringe, until the point is reached at which blood enters syringe.

    6) After obtaining blood, hold child upright and apply pressure.

2. Bone Marrow Aspiration

A. General Comments and Warnings

    1) Always use sterile surgical technique for bone marrow aspirations.

    2) In children from birth to 3 months of age, the tibia is the preferred site for aspiration.

    3) Posterior iliac crest is technically superior in children over 3 months of age.

    4) Anesthetize skin, soft tissue, and periosteum with local anesthetic.

    5) Insert needle with a boring motion and steady but not excessive pressure.

    6) The classical description of a "give" when the marrow cavity is entered not only is unreliable, but also indicates loss of control.

7)   Do not aspirate more than 0.2 ml of marrow due to dilution with sinusoidal blood.

B.   Iliac Marrow Technique
1)   With patient lying on side, locate and sterilize iliac crest area and posterior iliac crest.
2)   Enter the ilium 2 cm below the outer lip, perpendicular to the outer table.

C.   Tibial Marrow Technique
Best obtained from medial aspect of the head of the tibia, below medial condyle and tibial tuberosity. Insert needle perpendicular to outer table.

D.   Spinous Process
1)   May be performed with patient in sitting position, leaning slightly forward.
2)   Third or fourth lumbar vertebra is preferred as it is likely to present broadest spinous process.
3)   Push needle through skin and insert with rotary motion into the spinous process.
4)   Instead of puncturing tip of spinous process directly, operator can introduce needle into one side of it.

E.   Smear Technique
1)   Eject marrow from syringe onto clean slide.
2)   With another syringe and needle, aspirate excessive blood and plasma from marrow to concentrate it.
3)   Use remaining marrow to make multiple smears in usual way.

3.   Suprapubic Aspiration of Urine
Used for obtaining urine for culture in suspected urinary tract infection or sepsis. Avoid in children with genito-urinary tract anomalies.

A.   The infant's diaper should be dry and the infant should not have voided in the 30-60 minutes before the procedure. Anterior rectal pressure in females, or gentle penile pressure in males may be used to prevent urination during the procedure.

B.   Restrain the infant in the supine, frog-leg position. Clean the lower abdomen suprapubic area with iodine and alcohol.

C.   The site for puncture is just above the symphysis pubis (0.5-1 cm) in the midline. Use a syringe with a 22 gauge 1½ inch needle and puncture at 10-20° to the perpendicular aiming slightly caudad. Exert suction gently as the needle is advanced until urine enters syringe. Aspirate the urine with gentle suction.

4. Tympanocentesis
   A. Restrain patient in standard fashion.

   B. Sedation is not usually necessary in infants and toddlers. Sedation may be used with the larger child, more for the allaying of fear than for analgesia.

   C. Gently remove cerumen with a wire curette.

   D. Swab the tympanic membrane and canal with alcohol for 1 minute.

   E. Attach 2½ ml plastic syringe (containing approximately 1 ml nonbacteriostatic saline) to an 18 gauge, 3½ inch spinal needle that has a double bend to permit visualization of needle point.

   F. Visualize the posterior inferior quadrant of tympanic membrane using an otoscope with operating head.

   G. Perforate the tympanic membrane and apply negative pressure for 1-2 seconds.

   H. The first drop is sent for culture. The next drop is used for the Gram stain. One drop each on blood and chocolate agar plates and the rest into thioglycolate broth.

   NOTE: A culture of the canal after cleaning with alcohol, but before puncturing, allows comparison with organisms obtained from aspirate.

5. Paracentesis
   Valuable as a diagnostic or therapeutic test for abnormal collection of fluid within the peritoneal cavity.

   A. Precautions
      1) In performing a paracentesis for therapeutic measures, do not remove a large amount of fluid too rapidly because hypovolemia and hypotension may result from rapid fluid shifts.
      2) Avoid scars from previous surgery; localized bowel adhesions increase the chances of entering a viscus in these areas.

   B. Technique
      Prepare and drape the abdomen as for a surgical procedure.
      1) With patient in supine position, perform needle aspiration just lateral to the rectus muscle in either the right or left lower quadrants.
      2) With patient in semi-Fowler or cardiac position, employ a midline subumbilical aspiration technique.

3) The use of an intravenous catheter is preferable in this procedure. Apply negative pressure as catheter is inserted into the peritoneal cavity. Use a "Z" tract technique in most instances.

4) Once fluid appears in the syringe, remove introducer needle and leave catheter in place. Continue aspiration slowly with negative pressure until an adequate amount of fluid has been obtained for diagnostic studies.

5) If upon entering the peritoneal cavity air is aspirated, withdraw the needle immediately. Aspirated air indicates entrance into a hollow viscus. (In general, penetration of a hollow viscus during paracentesis does not lead to complications.) Then repeat paracentesis with sterile equipment.

6) Send fluid for lab studies, including: electrolytes, glucose, protein, cell count, differential, Gram stain, culture (AFB, if suspected), and cytospin (if malignancy suspected).

6. Thoracentesis
Valuable as a diagnostic or therapeutic test for an abnormal collection of fluid within the pleural space.

Ideally, perform procedure with the patient sitting on the side of the bed, and with an assistant standing in front to support the patient. Select the interspace to be tapped on the basis of dullness to percussion and the level of effusion on the erect chest x-ray. In the event of a small effusion the patient may be tilted laterally toward the affected side to maximize yield.

A. Technique
1) Carry out surgical preparation and draping of the chest.

2) Use a local anesthetic for the interspace to be entered.

3) A large bore needle or intravenous catheter attached to a 3-way stopcock and syringe are the necessary equipment. With needle bevel down, insert into skin at lower edge of the selected rib and "walk" needle over superior edge into the pleural space.

4) Upon entering the pleural space, apply negative pressure on the syringe and slowly withdraw the desired amount of fluid.

5) At the end of the procedure, withdraw the needle or catheter and place dressing over the thoracentesis site.

6) Obtain follow-up chest x-ray after thoracentesis to rule out pneumothorax.

NOTE: Send the fluid obtained for routine lab studies (see above, Paracentesis).

7. Venous Cutdown
    Readily accessible veins are the external jugular as it crosses
    the sternocleidomastoid muscle below the angle of the man-
    dible, and the long saphenous just anterior and superior to
    the medial malleolus. A venous cutdown should be performed
    under careful aseptic conditions and thereafter treated as a
    potential source of local and/or systemic infections.

    NOTE: In small premature infants bilateral jugular vein cut-
    downs have been associated with superior vena cava syndrome
    and chylothoraces, and should be avoided if possible.

    Prepare the skin for surgical procedure and make a trans-
    verse incision directly over the vein selected. Isolate the
    vein by blunt dissection and place two 4-0 silk sutures
    around the vein. Tie the distal ligature and use for traction.
    Make an oblique incision in the vein and insert the appropri-
    ate beveled Silastic catheter (previously filled with saline) to
    the desired length and tie the proximal ligature snugly about
    the vein and catheter. Close the skin incision with fine silk
    and an additional silk ligature about the catheter in the skin
    to secure the catheter externally. Place an antibiotic oint-
    ment over the wound and apply a dressing.

8. Exchange Transfusion in Newborns

    NOTE: Hct, reticulocyte count, peripheral smear, bilirubin,
    total protein, infant blood type, and Coombs test should be
    performed on pre-exchange sample of blood since they can no
    longer be of diagnostic value on post-exchange blood. If
    indicated, also save pre-exchange serum for serologic or
    chromosome studies.

    A. Routine Exchange: for removal of sensitized cells or
        bilirubin.
        1) Cross match donor blood against maternal serum for
            first exchange and against post-exchange blood for
            subsequent exchanges.
        2) Blood:
            a) Type: 0 negative (low titer) anytime; infant's
                type if no chance of maternal-infant incompat-
                ibility.
            b) Anticoagulant: ACD or CPD unless infant is
                acidotic or hypocalcemic.
            c) Temperature: room temperature.
            d) Age: fresh up to 48 hours old.
        3) Infant feeding: N.P.O. during exchange. Empty
            stomach if infant was fed within 4 hours of
            exchange. Maintain infant N.P.O. for 4 hours after
            exchange.
        4) Procedure: (using Umbilical Vein Catheterization)
            a) Provide for: cardiorespiratory monitoring and
                frequent temperatures. Have resuscitation
                equipment ready.

b) Prep and drape patient for sterile procedure.

c) Cut umbilical cord 1 cm or less from skin margin and find thin-walled vein.

d) Clear thrombi with forceps and insert catheter: Minimum - until blood returns; maximum - 1/2 to 2/3 of vertical distance from shoulder-tip to umbilicus. (See chart on page 281.)

NOTE: Obtain x-ray confirmation if maximum insertion is performed to avoid portal vein.

e) Prewarm blood in quality-controlled blood warmer if available; do not improvise with a water bath!

f) Use 15 ml increments in vigorous full-term infants, smaller volumes for smaller, less stable infants. Do not allow cells in donor unit to sediment.

g) Rate: 2-3 ml/kg/min avoiding mechanical trauma to patient and donor cells.

h) Calcium gluconate 10% solution: 1-2 ml slowly IV for EKG evidence of hypocalcemia. (i.e. prolonged Q-T$_c$ intervals see page 59).

Flush tubing with NaCl before and after calcium infusion. Observe for bradycardia during infusion.

i) Total volume exchanged should be 160 ml/kg (up to one donor unit). (double volume exchange)

j) Use last withdrawal for: Hct, smear, glucose, potassium, Ca^{++}, and future cross-matching.

Ref: Kitterman, JA, et al.: Ped Clin North Am 17:895, 1970.

B. Exchange Transfusion for Anemic Heart Failure in Newborns

Have O-negative concentrated RBCs in the delivery room. Perform a partial exchange with packed RBCs to correct anemia and failure (30-50 ml/kg). Allow infant to stabilize if possible before attempting a full two volume exchange.

C. Complications of Exchange Transfusion

1) Cardiovascular: thrombo- or air emboli, thromboses, arrhythmias, volume overload, and cardiorespiratory arrest.

2) Chemical: hyperkalemia, hypernatremia, hypocalcemia, hypoglycemia, and acidosis.

3) Hematologic: decreased platelets, over-heparinization (may use 3 micrograms protamine for each unit of heparin in donor unit), and transfusion reaction.
4) Infectious: hepatitis and bacteremia.
5) Physical: injury to donor cells (especially from overheating), vascular or cardiac perforation, and blood loss.

9. Umbilical Artery Catheterization

A. Restrain infant appropriately. Prepare and drape umbilical cord and adjacent skin in sterile fashion. Place sterile drapes sparingly so as to avoid unnecessary cooling of small infants. Make exterior measurements needed to determine length of catheter insertion for either high (T7-T9) or low (below L3) position. Place marker (sterile bandage or tape) on catheter at desired length (see page 278). Flush catheter with sterile saline solution prior to insertion.

NOTE: Catheter length is approximately 1/3 of crown-heel length.

B. Place sterile umbilical tape around base of cord. Cut through cord horizontally approximately 1.5-2.0 cm from skin; tighten umbilical tape so as to prevent bleeding.

C. Identify large, thin-walled umbilical vein and smaller, thick-walled arteries. Use one tip of open curved iris forceps to gently probe and dilate one artery. Then gently probe with both points of closed forceps and dilate artery by allowing forceps to open gently. Grasp catheter 1 cm from tip with toothless forceps and insert catheter into lumen of artery. Gently feed catheter in to desired distance. DO NOT FORCE. (If resistance is encountered, try loosening umbilical tape, steady gentle pressure, or manipulating angle of umbilical cord to skin.)

D. The catheter should be secured by means of a suture through the cord and marker tape, and a tape bridge. The position of the catheter tip should be confirmed radiologically. An antibiotic ointment and sterile dressing are used to cover the umbilical stump.

COMPLICATIONS: blanching or cyanosis of lower extremities, perforation, thrombosis, embolism, and infection.

Ref: Mokrohisky, ST, et al.: New Engl J Med 299:561, 1978.

10. Percutaneous Catheterization of the Radial Artery

A. Use the right radial artery because it is more representative of preductal blood flow. Perform a modified Allen test to assess adequate ulnar blood flow to the entire hand: passively clench the hand and simultaneously compress the ulnar and radial arteries. Release the ulnar artery and note the degree of flushing of the blanched hand. Catheterization may be performed if the entire hand flushes while the radial artery is still compressed. Avoid inadvertent compression of the ulnar artery while compressing the radial vessel.

B. Secure the hand to an armboard with the wrist extended. Leave the fingers exposed to observe any color changes. Under sterile conditions, palpate the radial artery at the wrist and note the point of maximum impulse. Use a 20 gauge needle to make a small skin puncture at the point of maximal impulse.

C. Place a 22 gauge intravenous catheter through the puncture site at a 30° angle to horizontal and pass the needle through the artery to transfix it. Withdraw the inner needle. Very slowly withdraw the catheter until free flow of blood is noted, then advance the catheter. Apply an antibiotic ointment and pressure dressing over the puncture site and secure the catheter with adhesive tape.

D. Firmly attach the catheter to a T-connector to permit a continuous infusion of heparinized isotonic saline (1 unit heparin/ml saline) at a rate of 1 ml/hour via a constant infusion pump. A pressure transducer may be connected in order to monitor blood pressure.

E. To obtain samples, occlude the distal end of the T-connector with the attached clamp. Clean the rubber end of the T-connector with an antiseptic solution and insert a 22 or 25 gauge needle. Allow 3 to 4 drops of blood and fluid (0.3 - 0.5 ml) to drip out to clear line. Attach a 1 ml syringe and withdraw 0.3 - 0.5 ml of blood.

NOTE: Do not infuse any fluids (other than the flushing fluid), medications, or blood products through the arterial line.

Ref: Todres, ID, et al.: J Pediatr 87:273, 1975.

11. Chest Tube Placement in the Neonate for Pneumothorax

A. Position the infant with the affected side up. The desired location for chest tube insertion is in the third or fourth intercostal space in the midaxillary line. Avoid breast tissue.

B. Temporary decompression may be obtained by using a "butterfly" or angiocath in the same location or in the ipsilateral anterior 2nd intercostal space.

C. After anesthetizing the area locally with 0.5% lidocaine, make an 0.5 cm incision directly over the rib below the desired interspace. Then use the trocar or a small curved clamp to bluntly dissect a track over the superior margin of the higher rib through the intercostal muscles and into the pleural cavity.

D. Place clamp 0.5-1.0 cm from tip of chest tube and pass through previously punctured space into pleural cavity. Angle tube anteriorly and superiorly and insert tube desired distance.

E. Secure tube to chest wall with suture through skin incision and then around tube. (Cover incision with petroleum gauze and a sterile dressing.)

F. Connect tube to 15-20 cm water suction for decompression via one-way valve.

G. Confirm position and function with chest x-ray.

COMPLICATIONS: lung perforation, hemorrhage, scarring, and malpositioning of tube.

Ref: Henderson, R: Pediatrics 58:861, 1976.

12. Endotracheal Intubation

A. The patient should be well oxygenated and lying on his back on a firm surface with the head midline prior to intubation.

B. Holding the laryngoscope blade in the left hand, and with the patient's head extended, insert the blade on the right side of the mouth and sweep the tongue to the left out of the line of vision.

C. Advance the blade to the vallecula and gently raise the epiglottis by lifting the laryngoscope straight up. The cords can now be visualized.

D. Advance the endotracheal tube from the right corner of the mouth and pass it through the cords while maintaining direct visualization. In infants, the tip of the tube may be palpated in the suprasternal notch after it passes through the cords.

13. Sweat Electrolyte Test Using Pilocarpine Iontophoresis

A. Purpose
Test for increased sweat chloride content in cystic fibrosis.

B.   Procedure for Quantitative Pilocarpine Iontophoresis Sweat Test

   1)   Wash arm with distilled water and dry with salt-free gauze.
   2)   Place filter paper or gauze moistened with 0.2% pilocarpine on forearm and iontophorese with a current 2-4 mAmps for 5 minutes. Decrease current if patient is uncomfortable.
   3)   Clean stimulated area with distilled water and wipe dry.
   4)   Place pre-weighed gauze or filter paper (from pre-weighed bottle) over stimulated area and cover with airtight seal of parafilm and adhesive.
   5)   Collect sweat for 30-60 minutes.
   6)   Lift seal, grasp gauze or filter paper with forceps and quickly return to pre-weighed bottle.
   7)   Weigh bottle and record weight of sweat sample.
   8)   Determine sodium and/or chloride concentrations by accepted laboratory procedures.

C.   Interpretation
   Cystic fibrosis is associated with values of >60 mEq/L. Addison's Disease and panhypopituitarism may also give abnormally high values.

   NOTE: The amount of chloride in the sweat test may be falsely low in children with cystic fibrosis in the face of significant edema.

   Ref: Cooke, RE and Gibson, LE: Pediatrics 23:545, 1959; Elian, E, et al.: New Engl J Med 264:13, 1961.

14. Lumbar Puncture

   Indications
      Examination of spinal fluid for suspected infection or malignancy, or installation of intrathecal chemotherapy.

   Contraindications
      Bleeding diathesis, infection in skin overlying site, cerebral mass lesion, or increased intracranial pressure.

   A.   Position the child in either the sitting position or lateral recumbent position with hips, knees, and neck flexed. Have the patient's head on the nondominant side of the person performing the technique. Care should be taken to ensure that small infants' cardiorespiratory status is not compromised by positioning.

   B.   Locate the desired interspace (either L3-L4 or L4-L5) by drawing a line between the top of the iliac crests.

C. Prepare the skin by cleaning with iodophor and draping conservatively so as to be able to monitor the infant. Use a spinal needle with stylet (epidermoid tumors from introduced epithelial tissue have been reported).

D. Anesthetize overlying skin with 0.5% lidocaine.

E. Puncture skin in midline just below palpated spinous process, angling slightly cephalad. Use two fingers to guide needle and thumbs to slowly advance. Advance several mm at a time and withdraw stylet frequently to check for CSF flow. In small infants, one may not feel a change in resistance or "pop" as the dura is penetrated.

F. If resistance is met, withdraw needle to skin surface and redirect angle slightly.

G. Send CSF for appropriate cultures, glucose, protein, cell count and differential, antigen detection tests, and cytospin (if suspected malignancy).

HEMATOLOGY

1. Routine Hematology (methods adapted from Williams, WJ, et al. (ed.): Hematology, New York: McGraw-Hill Book Company, 1983. For normal values see pages 359-360.

   A. Microhematocrit Determinations
   Fill standard microhematocrit tube with blood and seal one end with clay. Centrifuge (12,000 g) for 5 minutes. Falsely high hematocrits with increased plasma trapping occur with inadequate centrifugation time and disorders with decreased red cell deformability (e.g., sickle cell anemia, thalassemia, spherocytosis).

   Electronic cell counters calculate hematocrit as the product of cell volume and red cell number, and are calibrated to agree with centrifuged hematocrits.

   B. Wright's Staining Technique
   1) Place air-dried blood smears, film side up, on a staining rack.
   2) Cover smear with undiluted Wright's stain and leave for 1 to 2 minutes.
   3) Add equal volume of distilled water and blow gently on the surface until a greenish metallic sheen appears. Leave diluted stain on smear for 2 to 6 minutes. Without disturbing the slide, flood with water and wash until stained smear is pinkish-red.

   NOTE: Staining times must be adjusted for each batch of stain.

   C. Hematologic Indices
   1) Mean Corpuscular Volume (MCV): average RBC volume. Usually measured directly by electronic counters. Expressed in femtoliters (fl, 10^{-12}L).

   $$MCV = \frac{Hct~(\%)~x~10}{RBC~count~(millions/mm^3)}$$
   Normals vary with age; see pages 359-360.

   2) Mean Corpuscular Hemoglobin (MCH): average amount of Hb per red cell expressed in picograms per cell.

   $$MCH = \frac{Hb~(gm~\%)~x~10}{RBC~count~(millions/mm^3)}$$

   3) Mean Corpuscular Hemoglobin Concentration (MCHC): grams of Hb per 100 ml packed cells.

   $$MCHC = \frac{Hb~(gm\%)~x~100}{Hematocrit~(percent)}$$
   High in spherocytosis, low in iron deficiency

4) Coefficient of Variation (CV) or Red Cell Distribution: statistical description of heterogeneity of red cell size, generated by electronic cell counters. Increases with increasing anisocytosis. In adults, normal 11.5-14.5%. Increased in reticulocytosis, iron deficiency, newborns. Normal in thalassemia trait.

D. Reticulocyte Count
Technique: Mix equal amounts new methylene blue or brilliant cresyl blue with whole blood. Let stand 10-20 minutes then prepare thin smears. Count the number of reticulocytes (cells containing reticulum or blue granules) per 1000 red cells and report as % of RBCs. For normal values see page 359. Corrected reticulocyte count = retic count X $\frac{\text{obs Hct}}{45\%}$.

Corrects for variation in hematocrit, providing a better estimate of red cell production.

E. Platelet Estimation
Approximation of platelet count may be made by examination of Wright's stained blood smear. Presence of platelets on a smear usually excludes severe thrombocytopenia. Always examine periphery of smear or coverslip as platelet clumps may be deposited there.

NOTE: For rough approximation, 1 platelet/oil immersion field corresponds to 10,000-15,000 platelets/mm³.

2. Approach to the Anemic Patient

A. Evaluation of Anemia
Is the patient anemic? Anemia is defined by age specific norms (see pages 359-360). These data are derived from white children. Black children's Hb levels average 0.5 gm/dl lower.

1) Is the Hb alone depressed or are other cell lines (plts, wbc) also affected? (Pancytopenia suggests bone marrow failure or general immune-mediated destruction.)

2) Are the red cells large or small? (See pages 359-360 for appropriate norms.)
a) Microcytosis suggests iron deficiency, thalassemia, and lead poisoning.
b) Normocytic anemias include congenital hemolytic anemias (hemoglobinopathies, enzyme deficiencies), acquired hemolytic anemias, acute blood loss, bone marrow dysfunction, and the anemia of chronic disease.

      c)   Macrocytic anemias occur with reticulo-
cytosis, bone marrow dysfunction, hypothyroidism, folate and B_{12} deficiency.

3)   Is red cell production increased or decreased?
Increased reticulocyte count occurs with blood
loss or hemolysis (reticulocyte count >10%
suggests hemolysis). Inappropriately low reticulocyte count suggests bone marrow dysfunction,
and/or nutritional anemia (e.g., iron deficiency).

4)   Are there characteristic red cell morphologic
changes? e.g., spherocytes in immune hemolysis
and hereditary spherocytosis; sickled cells in the
sickle hemoglobinopathies; fragmented cells in
DIC; or target cells in HbC, thalassemias.

B.   Specific Tests of Value in the Evaluation of the Anemic
Patient

1)   Therapeutic trial of iron
Adequate iron therapy should result in reticulocytosis peaking between seventh and tenth day of
therapy. Significant increase in Hb concentration
should be evident after 3-4 weeks of therapy.

2)   Ferritin
Measurement is accurate reflection of total body
iron stores after 6 months of age; it is more reliable than serum iron and total iron binding
capacity. Normal values, 6mo-15yr: 10-150
ng/ml.

NOTE: Ferritin may rise to falsely normal levels with
infection or inflammation.

Ref: Siimes, MA, et al.: Blood 43:581, 1974.

3)   Serum iron/total iron binding capacity
Generally replaced by ferritin because of diurnal
variability, poor reproducibility, and poor predictive value. Normal serum iron; age 6mo-17yr >20
µg/dl (adults >50). Normal transferrin saturation, >7% (adults >16%).

Ref: Koerper, MA and Dallman, PR: J Pediatr 91:870,
1977.

4)   Free erythrocyte protoporphyrin (FEP)
Accumulates when the conversion of protoporphyrin to heme is blocked by elevated lead levels
or iron deficiency. Normal values: <3 µg/gm
Hb, <50 µg/dl whole blood, <130 µg/dl PRBC's.
Elevated in iron deficiency, plumbism, and
erythropoietic protoporphyria (rare). Levels >300
µg/dl PRBC generally found only with lead intoxication.

5) Screening tests for sickle hemoglobin
   a) Sulfite solution: Mix one or two drops of 2% sodium metabisulfite or sodium hyposulfite on a slide with one drop of blood; apply coverslip. Read preparation at 30 minutes and again at 3 hours. Positive test: presence of sickled cells.

   NOTE: Sulfite solutions should be prepared fresh daily; sodium metabisulfite capsules are available (one 200 mg capsule in 10 ml distilled water yields 2% solution).

   b) "Sickledex": a solubility test using dithionate reduction of HbS. Used in many commercial and hospital diagnostic laboratories.

   NOTE: Venous blood will sickle more readily than capillary blood. False negatives may be obtained with either test in neonates.

   c) Principle: any substance which reduces O_2 tension will cause HbS containing red cells to sickle. A positive "sickle prep" is found in the sickle hemoglobinopathies (SS, SC, Sβthal, and others) as well as in sickle trait. All positive tests should be confirmed with cellulose acetate electrophoresis.

6) Note on electrophoresis terminology: the initials of the hemoglobins found are listed in order of relative abundance in the sample; e.g., sickle cell trait is ASA_2, sickle cell disease SFA_2.

7) Indicators of hemolysis
   a) Haptoglobin: binds free hemoglobin. Normal levels: 100-300 mg/dl (after 6 weeks of age) Interpretation: Decreased with intravascular and extravascular hemolysis, hepatocellular disease. Falsely normal or increased levels may occur in association with inflammation, infection or malignancy.

   b) Hemopexin: binds free heme groups.
      Normal levels: premature   2-26 mg/dl
                      newborn   8-42 mg/dl
                      ages 1-12yr 40-70 mg/dl
                      >12yr   50-100 mg/dl
      Interpretation: decreased with intravascular hemolysis. Low levels also seen with renal disease and hepatocellular disease. Hemopexin is usually not increased in states of inflammation, infection, or malignancy.

8) Differentiating features of microcytic anemias

	Hb	MCV	Ferritin	FEP	Pb	Trial of Iron
Iron deficiency	↓ or nml	↓	↓	↑	nml	↑ Hb
Thalassemia trait	↓ or nml	↓↓	nml	nml	nml	–
Lead intoxication	nml or ↓	nml or ↓	nml	↑	↑	–

NOTE: Iron deficiency often accompanies lead intoxication.

3. Coagulation (See coagulation cascade page 21.)

    A. Normal clotting depends on adequate platelet number and function as well as intact coagulation cascade.

    B. Platelet function depends on adequate number and adequate function, as measured by bleeding time.
       1) Bleeding time - IVY technique

    NOTE: This is a screening test only.

          a) Blood pressure cuff is placed on upper arm and inflated to 40 mm Hg. The forearm is cleaned with alcohol and allowed to dry.
          b) A standardized incision is made, taking care to avoid a superficial vein, with a nonheparinized long point disposable lancet (3 mm deep) or with a commercially available template. Gently absorb the blood onto filter paper every 30 seconds, without disturbing the wound. The time required for bleeding to cease is the bleeding time. Normal <9 minutes. Aspirin ingestion within past week may prolong bleeding time in normal individuals.

          NOTE: Ear lobe bleeding (Duke Method) may be difficult to control in patients with abnormal hemostasis. Do not perform bleeding time on patients with hemophilia or thrombocytopenia.

          A prolonged bleeding time in a non-hemophiliac patient with normal platelet count indicates Von Willebrand's disease or platelet dysfunction.

    C. Clot observation
       Depends upon adequate platelet number and function, as well as the integrity of coagulation pathways.
       3 ml fresh whole blood is placed in clean non-siliconized glass tube and incubated at 37°C.

At one hour, a firm clot which has retracted from the sides of the tube and occupies ~50% of the original volume should be seen. Marked retraction should be seen at 18-24 hours. Clot retraction is defective in thrombocytopenia, thrombasthenia, erythrocytosis, or decreased fibrinogen. A small ragged clot or rapid clot dissolution suggests low fibrinogen, excessive fibrinolysis, and/or α_2-antiplasmin deficiency.

D. Disseminated Intravascular Coagulation
If DIC is suspected clinically the following laboratory tests should be performed.
1) Rapid evaluation
   a) Peripheral blood smear
      (1) Fragmented RBCs usually present
      (2) Platelet count: low or decreasing
   b) Plasma color: a pink color, indicating hemoglobinemia, may be present
   c) Clot retraction: poor
   d) Clot lysis: accelerated
   e) Prothrombin time (PT): prolonged
   f) Activated partial thromboplastin time (PTT): prolonged
   g) Fibrinogen: low or decreasing
2) Confirmatory tests
   a) Fibrin split products (FSP): present
   b) Factor V assay: decreased
   c) Factor VIII assay: decreased

4. Miscellaneous Hematologic Studies

A. Erythrocyte Sedimentation Rate (ESR)
1) Collect venous blood in EDTA-containing or oxalated tube. Determine ESR within one hour of blood drawing.
2) Place 1 ml in a Wintrobe tube, using long Pasteur pipette. Fill carefully; do not shake tube or allow air bubbles to form in column of blood.
3) Place tube in its special upright rack, which is exactly vertically aligned.
4) Read depth of fall of RBC column at the end of 60 minutes.
5) Normal values (mm/hr):
      Men   0-10
      Women   0-20
      Children 4-20
6) Factors which will artificially increase rate of fall: anemia, tilting, warming, and shaking.
7) Factors associated with decreased rate of fall: hypo- or afibrinogenemia, old or cold blood, excessive anticoagulant, sickle cell anemia (NOTE: Oxygenate sickle cell blood sample before performing ESR), congestive heart failure, polycythemia, trichinosis, pertussis.

COAGULATION SYSTEM

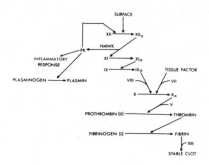

NOTE: PK = prekallikrein; HMWK = high-molecular weight kininogen

Vitamin K Dependent Factors: II, VII, IX, X

Activated Partial Thromboplastin Time (APTT) requires factors XII, XI, IX, VIII, X, V, II, I (the intrinsic system)

Prothrombin Time (PT) requires VII, X, V, II, I (extrinsic system)

Modified from: Montgomery, RR and Hathaway, WE: Ped Clin North Am 27:327, 1980.

8) NOTE: "Correction" of ESR for anemia is no longer recommended. However, simultaneous hematocrit determination should be performed.

B. Cold Agglutinins - Rapid Screening Test
   1) Method:
      a) Collect 4-5 drops of blood in EDTA-containing tube.
      b) Cap tube and place in ice water bath for 30-60 seconds.
      c) Tilt tube and observe blood as it runs down wall of tube.
      d) Definite floccular agglutination (seen with the unaided eye) with disappearance thereof upon warming to 37°C, is considered a positive (3-4+) test. Use of a control sample is useful for interpretation of test.
   2) Interpretation: positive test frequently correlates with cold agglutinin titer of >1:64. 75-85% of patients with atypical pneumonia and a positive rapid screening test will develop serologic evidence of mycoplasma pneumonia infection.

   Ref: Griffin, JP: Ann Intern Med 70:701, 1969; Coradero, L, et al.: J Pediatr 71:1, 1967.

C. Mononucleosis "Spot Test"
   1) Basis of test: Heterophile (mono) antibody, unlike Forssman antibody, is not adsorbed by guinea pig kidney extract. Both antibodies will agglutinate sheep or horse erythrocytes.
   2) Test for heterophile antibodies:
      a) Obtain test card (Monosticon, Organon Laboratories) and place one drop of water onto blue spot (horse erythrocyte antigen). Stir to suspend the antigen.
      b) Add one drop of serum to buff spot (guinea pig kidney antigen). Mix thoroughly and let stand one minute to fully adsorb Forssman antibody.
      c) Mix buff and blue spots together and rock slide gently for 2 minutes. Read results under strong, glare-free light; look for agglutination.
      d) Interpretation of test: Positive "card" test correlates with horse cell titer of >1:244 or a sheep cell titer (Davidsohn) of 1:28 to 1:56.

5. Blood Component Replacement Guidelines

   A. Estimation of Blood Volume

Premature infants	85-100 ml/kg
Term newborns	85 ml/kg
>1 month	75 ml/kg

Ref: Oski, FA, in Nathan, DG and Oski, FA: <u>Hematology</u> <u>of Infancy and Childhood</u>. Philadelphia: W.B. <u>Saunders</u>, 1981, pp. 29, 1507.

B. <u>Quantity of Packed Cells Needed to Raise Hematocrit</u>

$$\text{Vol of cells (ml)} = \frac{\text{Est Bld Vol (ml) x } \Delta\text{Hct desired}}{\text{Hct of packed cells (60-70\%)}}$$

Infused no faster than 2-3 ml/kg/hr or in 10 ml/kg aliquots infused over several hours.

C. <u>Partial Exchange Transfusion for Symptomatic Poly-</u><u>cythemia</u> (e.g., symptomatic newborns, cyanotic con-genital heart disease)

Vol of Exchange (ml) =
$$\frac{\text{Est Blood Vol (ml) x } \Delta\text{Hct desired}}{\text{obs Hct}}$$

Exchange patient's blood for fresh frozen plasma or 5% albumin solution.

D. <u>Partial Exchange Transfusion Formula for Rapid</u> <u>Correction of Severe Anemia</u> (e.g., preoperatively, severe congestive heart failure)

$$\text{Exchange Vol (ml)} = \frac{\text{Bld Vol (ml) x desired rise in Hb}}{22 \text{ gm/dl} - \text{HbR}}$$

Where $\text{HbR} = \dfrac{\text{Hb (initial)} + \text{Hb (desired)}}{2}$

Perform exchange with PRBC (est. Hb 22 gm/dl)

Ref: Nieburg, PI and Stockman, JA: <u>Am J Dis Child</u> 131:60, 1977.

E. <u>Partial Exchange Transfusion to Reduce Load of Sickle</u> <u>Cells</u> (e.g., in stroke, lung infarction, priapism)

Exchange volume = Est Bld Vol x Pt. Hct (%) x 2
Usually reduces sickle cells to <40%

Ref: Zinkham, WH, Personal Communication, 1984.

F. <u>Platelet Transfusions</u>
Usually give 4 units/M². Hemorrhagic complications due to thrombocytopenia are rare with platelet counts >20,000/mm³. Platelet counts >50,000/mm³ are advis-able before performing lumbar punctures. One unit of platelets per M² will raise the platelet count 10,000/mm³ in the absence of platelet destruction or antiplatelet antibodies.

Platelet increment (expected)/mm³ =

$$\frac{3 \times 10^{10} \times \text{(number of units)}}{\text{Est Bld vol (ml)} \times 10^3}$$

G. <u>Coagulation</u> <u>Factor</u> <u>Replacement</u> <u>Guidelines</u>
1 unit Factor activity = amount of activity in 1 ml normal plasma
Factor VIII increase = 2% increase/unit/kg
Factor IX   increase = 1% increase/unit/kg

Type of Hemorrhage	Approximate Level Desired (%)
Hemarthrosis, simple hematoma	20-40%
Simple dental extraction*	50%
Major soft tissue bleeding Serious oral bleeding*	80-100%
Head injuries Major surgery (dental, orthopedic, other)	100+%

*Aminocaproic Acid, 100 mg/kg IV or PO Q6h (up to 24 gm/d) is useful in oral bleeding and prophylactically for dental extractions.

H. <u>Irradiation</u> <u>of</u> <u>Blood</u> <u>Products</u>
Principle: Many blood products (PRBC, platelet preparations, leukocytes, FFP, and others) contain viable lymphocytes capable of sustained survival in recipient. Irradiation of all blood products with >1500 rad prior to transfusion is advisable to prevent graft vs. host disease in children with severe immunosuppression.
Indications include:
1) Intensive chemotherapy
2) Leukemia and lymphoma
3) Bone marrow transplantation
4) Known or suspected T-cell deficiencies e.g. SCIDS, DiGeorge Syndrome, Wiscott-Aldrich Syndrome.
5) Intrauterine transfusions for erythroblastosis fetalis.
6) Possibly, exchange transfusions in neonates

Ref: Von Fliedner, V, et al.: <u>Am</u> <u>J</u> <u>Med</u> <u>72</u>:951, 1982.

NEPHROLOGY

1. Routine Urinalysis - should be done on freshly voided specimen (within 1 hour), ideally the first morning void.

   A. Color
      1) Yellow brown-deep brown: bilirubin, carotene, Vit. B complex.
      2) Red: hemoglobin, RBC's, porphyrins, urates, adriamycin, food coloring, povan, pyridium, phenolphthalein (used in laxatives).
      3) Brown-black: old blood, hemosiderin, myoglobin, homogentisic acid (alkaptonuria), melanin (especially if alkaline).
      4) Purple-brown: porphyrias (after specimen stands a few days).
      5) Deep yellow: riboflavin.
      6) Orange: Rifampin.
      7) Blue-green: Methylene blue; biliverdin (seen in chronic obstructive jaundice); blue diaper syndrome (familial metabolic disease associated with hypercalcemia).

   B. Clarity

   C. Specific Gravity
      1) Hydrometer.
      2) Refractometer (American Optical Company T.S. Meter). Requires only 1 drop of urine. Principle: Refractive index of a solution is related to content of dissolved solids. The presence of glucose or large amounts of protein in the urine elevates the specific gravity.

   D. pH - Nitrazine Paper

   E. Albumin
      1) Sulfosalicylic Acid (SSA) Test:
         a) Add 0.5-0.8 ml (5-8 drops) 20% SSA to 5 ml of urine (pH should be 4.5-6.5) and examine after one minute for turbidity. Barely evident turbidity is ±, increasing amounts of turbidity are graded 1-4+.
         b) False positives: proteoses, tolbutamide, sulfonamides, penicillin and derivatives, IVP dyes, PAS, phosphates.
      2) Heat Coagulation Test: Add 3% acetic acid to 7-10 ml of clear urine until pH is 4.0-4.6 (check with Bromcresol green pH paper). Heat until boiling begins. Any turbidity, cloudiness or precipitate indicates the presence of protein.

Appearance	Reading	Approx. Protein Concentration (mg/100 ml)
No turbidity	negative	0.4
Slight turbidity	±	4-10
Definite turbidity - light print readable	1+	15-30
Light cloud - heavy print readable	2+	40-100
Moderate cloud with slight precipitate	3+	200-500
Heavy cloud with precipitation	4+	over 800 - 1000

3) Albustix (Ames Co.)

Ref: Tietz, NW, <u>Fundamentals of Clinical Chemistry</u>, Philadelphia: W. B. Saunders Co., 1976, pp. 358-359.

F. <u>Reducing Substance</u>
1) Clinitest (Ames Co.) or Tes-Tape (Eli Lilly Co.): specific for glucose; cannot use for quantitation.
2) Clinitest tablets (Ames Co.): not specific for glucose. 5 drops urine, 10 drops water, 1 tablet. Compare with scale supplied. Reducing substances such as glucose, fructose, galactose, pentose (xylulose), lactose, ascorbic acid, chloramphenicol, chloral hydrate, penicillin, PAS, tetracycline, and amino acids all give positive tests with Clinitest. Sucrose is not a reducing sugar and does not react with Clinitest.

Blue	Negative
Greenish blue	Trace
Green	0.5% reducing substance
Greenish brown	1% reducing substance
Yellow	1.5% reducing substance
Brick red	2% reducing substance

3) UGK Chemstrips (Bio-Dynamics Co.): tests for both glucose and ketones

G. <u>Acetone</u>
1) Acetest tablets (Ames Co.): directions from manufacturer - measures acetone but <u>not</u> B-hydroxybutyrate.
2) Ketostix (Ames Co.): directions from manufacturer.

H. <u>Urine Hemoglobin and Myoglobin</u>
1) The reagent found in dipstick methods (Hemastix, Bili-Lab Stix, Ames Co.) reacts positively with intact red blood cells, hemoglobin and myoglobin; can detect as little as 3-4 RBC/hpf.

2) Perform a microscopic examination to differentiate hemoglobinuria or myoglobinuria from hematuria (intact RBC's).

3) Distinguish myoglobinuria from hemoglobinuria.
   a) By history
      Hemoglobinuria - seen with hemolytic states, hematuric urine that has been sitting a long time.
      Myoglobinuria - crush injuries, after vigorous exercise or major motor seizures, hyperthermia, electrocution.
   b) Laboratory methods
      (1) Ammonium sulfate adsorption test - simple and widely used but often erroneous.
      (2) Electrophoresis (on cellulose acetate, or even better, polyacrylamide gel).
      (3) Spectrophotometry.

Ref: Tietz, NW: _Fundamentals of Clinical Chemistry._ Philadelphia: W. B. Saunders Co., 1976, pp. 448-451.

4) If one suspects pigment nephropathy secondary to myoglobinuria, obtain both a CPK and serum urea nitrogen/serum creatinine ratio. This ratio should be very low in myoglobin nephropathy.

Ref: Hamilton, R, et al.: _Ann Int Med_ 77:77, 1972.

5) False Positive Hemastix
   a) Microbial peroxidase associated with urinary tract infections.
   b) Ascorbic acid concentrations >10 mg% (used as a preservative for antibiotics, esp. tetracycline).
   c) Betadine (Povidone - iodine), particularly on the fingers of medical and nursing staff.

Ref: Ames Co.; Rasoulpour, M, et al.: _J Peds_ 92:852, 1978.

I. Urine Bilirubin - Bili Labstix (Ames Co.)

J. Urine Gram Stain
   1) Purpose: to screen for suspected urinary tract infections.
   2) Interpretation: Almost all uncentrifuged urine specimens with bacterial colony counts of 10^5/ml or greater will have positive Gram stains. A urine culture should be taken to confirm these results.

Ref: Greenhill, A and Gruskin, AB: _Ped Clin North Am_ 23:661, 1976.

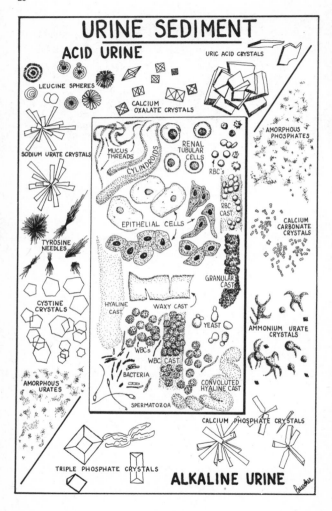

K. Sediment
Examine all fields for red cells, white cells, casts, and
crystals. Area at edge of coverslip should also be
examined as formed elements collect there. See illustration on page 28.

2. Renal Function Tests

A. Endogenous Creatinine Clearance (Ccr)
1) Purpose: This is a good measure of glomerular
filtration rate (GFR) and closely approximates the
inulin clearance in the normal ranges of GFR.
With the low GFR of advanced renal disease, Ccr
is > the inulin clearance. (See section 2A4).
2) Method: Timed collection of urine is made for
any time period, recording the nearest minute.
Draw a single blood specimen during the collection
period unless the patient's renal function is rapidly changing. In the latter condition, draw
specimens at the beginning and end of the period.
3) Calculation:

$$Ccr = \frac{UV}{P} \times \frac{1.73}{S.A.}$$

NOTE: See page 331 for surface area nomogram.

U = urinary concentration of creatinine in mg/dl
V = total volume of urine divided by number of
minutes in the collection period = ml/min
(NOTE: 24 hrs = 1440 mins)
P = serum creatinine level (or average of 2 lev-
els) in mg/dl
S.A. = surface area in square meters

4) With decreased renal function (Ccr <25), creatinine clearance is elevated over true GFR because
of tubular secretion of creatinine. The method of
choice for measuring low GFR is a renal scan with
a GFR study using ^{99M}Technetium-labelled DTPA.

Ref: Chervu, LR, et al.: Semin Nucl Med 121:224,
1982; Rubovsky, EV, et al.: Semin Nucl Med 12:308,
1982, with permission.

5) Normal values:
a) Newborns, 27-43 weeks gestation, first 24
hours of life: mean GFR (measured by
inulin clearance) expressed as a function of
body weight is fairly constant regardless of
gestational age: 1.07 ± 0.12 ml/min/kg.
b) Prematures >24 hours of age - GFR correlates with gestational age; no good reference
values available.

    c)   Term newborns after 24 hours; Ccr = 40-65 ml/min/1.73 M².

    d)   6 months: 75 ml/min/1.73 M².

    e)   1½ Years and Older:
        (1)   Males
              124 ± 25.8 ml/min/1.73 M²
        (2)   Females
              108.8 ± 13.5 ml/min/1.73 M²

    f)   Adults
        (1)   Males
              105 ± 13.9 ml/min/1.73 M²
        (2)   Females
              95.4 ± 18 ml/min/1.73 M²

Ref: Tobias, GJ, et al.: _New Engl J Med_ 266:317, 1962; Winberg, J: _Acta Paediatr Scand_ 48:443, 1959; Avery, GB: _Neonatology_, Toronto: J.B. Lippincott, 1981, p. 1179; Robillard, JE, et al.: _Pediatrics Update - Reviews for Physicians._ New York: Elsevier North Holland, 1980, pp. 168-189.

B.   Estimating Creatinine Clearance with Length and Plasma Creatinine (a useful alternative when a timed urine specimen can not be collected; correlates well with standard creatinine clearance)

    An estimate of the creatinine clearance can be obtained using the formula: 0.55 L/Pcr, where L = length in centimeters; Pcr = plasma creatinine in mg/dl.

    This formula is not accurate <6 months of age and must be used with caution in patients with severe reduction of muscle mass.

Ref: Schwartz, GJ, et al.: _Pediatrics_ 58:259, 1976.

C.   Concentration Test
    1)   Concentration: A random urine S.G. of 1.023 or more indicates intact concentrating ability within the limits of clinical testing and no further tests are indicated. A first-voided specimen following an overnight fast is adequate to test concentrating ability.

Ref: Edelman, CM, et al.: _Am J Dis Child_ 114:639, 1967.

    2)   Technique: See Water Deprivation Test, page 89.

D.   Proteinuria
    1)   24-hour urine protein - normally <100 mg/M²
    2)   Proteinuria by dipstick
        a)   Transient - most common cause in children, associated with exercise, changes in posture,

exposure to cold, fever, emotional stress; not associated with renal disease.

b) Orthostatic - another common cause, also not associated with renal disease.

    (1) Method for diagnosis:

        (a) No fluids after 6 p.m.

        (b) Empty bladder immediately before retiring and discard this urine.

        (c) Remain flat in bed during night. Discard any urine voided during night.

        (d) Collect a voided specimen immediately after waking in bed in the morning. Label #1.

        (e) Drink 2 glasses of water. Stand erect and quietly for 20 minutes, then void and label #2.

        (f) Kneel on a chair for 20 minutes with the back arched backward as much as possible. Then void and label #3.

        (g) Walk about actively for 30 minutes, then void and label #4.

For each specimen record the specific gravity and the protein content (by the sulfosalicylic acid or other simple test).

In orthostatic albuminuria, urine excreted in recumbent position contains no albumin. Urine excreted in upright or lordotic positions contains variable amounts of albumin.

c) Persistent proteinuria - requires evaluation for associated renal disease.

Ref: Rudolf, AM: Pediatrics. Norwalk, Conn.: Appleton-Century-Crofts, 1982, pp. 1165-1166; Dodge, WF, et al.: J Pediatr 88:327, 1976.

E.   Urine Acidification Test

1)   Purpose: In order to evaluate the renal tubular acidification mechanisms when random urine pH values are >6 in the presence of systemic metabolic acidosis, a challenge with ammonium chloride may be required.

2)   Method:

a) Give ammonium chloride 75 mEq/M^2.

b) Over the next 5 hours measure urine pH every hour if possible.

c) Measure plasma bicarbonate concentration 3 hours after ingestion of ammonium chloride.

3) Results: The urine pH should fall below 5.5. If urine pH is not lower than 5.5 and the plasma bicarbonate is not below 17 mEq/L, larger doses (100 mEq/M²) of ammonium chloride may be necessary to produce a plasma bicarbonate concentration below an abnormal renal bicarbonate reabsorption threshold. Extreme care should be taken when using larger doses of ammonium chloride.

4) Interpretation:
    Normal Response

    a) Fall in plasma bicarbonate concentration.
    b) Fall in urine pH to below 5.5.

    Type 1 Renal Tubular Acidosis – Distal – defect in distal tubular excretion of hydrogen ion.

    a) Fall in plasma bicarbonate concentration.
    b) Urine pH remains above 6.0.

    Type 2 Renal Tubular Acidosis – Proximal – defect in proximal tubular reabsorption of bicarbonate.

    a) Fall in plasma bicarbonate concentration (see above).
    b) Fall in urine pH below 5.5.

    Type 3 Renal Tubular Acidosis – the pediatric variant of hereditary Type 1 RTA; a defect in distal tubular hydrogen ion excretion plus massive bicarbonaturia (subsides after adolescence).

    Type 4 Renal Tubular Acidosis – hyperchloremic acidosis, hyperkalemia, and acid urinary pH. Has five subtypes.

    For more detailed information on renal tubular acidosis, the best reference is: McSherry, E: Kidney Int 20:799, 1981, with permission.

3. Acute Peritoneal Dialysis

    A. Procedure (Whenever possible, this procedure should be performed by a surgeon or nephrologist.)
        1) Place patient in supine position, prep and shave appropriate area after the bladder has been emptied by catheterization.
        2) Inject local anesthesia (1% xylocaine) in the midline, down 1/3 of the distance from the umbilicus to the symphysis pubis.
        3) Make a small puncture with a #11 scalpel point in the anesthetized area down to the linea alba but not through the peritoneum.

4) Insert an intracath into the peritoneal cavity and remove the needle.

5) Introduce a quantity of warmed dialysis fluid (37°C) into the peritoneal cavity sufficient to distend the abdomen slightly and allow the intestines to float (approximately 20 ml/kg).

6) Remove the intracath and push the trocar (with the dialysis catheter fitted over it) through the existing perforation. This may require considerable force. Lifting the peritoneal membrane with pickups and making a small incision with a scalpel can make insertion more controlled in difficult cases. One hand should be used to control the depth of the initial entry. Remove the trocar and after making sure all the perforations on the dialysis catheter are within the peritoneal cavity, cut the catheter to an appropriate length. Connect catheter to the warmed dialysis solution, support the entire apparatus by gauze squares and cover with a dressing. The quantity of fluid for each pass varies according to the weight of the child. In a child <2 years of age, 50-80 ml/kg or 1200 ml/M² may be used per pass. In a very small infant, 25-50 ml/kg may be sufficient. In a child age 2-5 years, 500 ml is used. For a child >5 years old, 1 liter passes can be used. Final volume should be limited by abdominal distention.

7) It should take no longer than 10 minutes to run in each pass. The fluid should remain in the peritoneal cavity 30-45 minutes, and run out in 10-15 minutes.

8) 24-36 passes have been used as a standard number. The catheter should not be left in beyond 72 hours because of the danger of peritonitis. Prolonged peritoneal dialysis is an indication for the surgical insertion of a soft subcutaneous catheter (Tenckhoff catheter).

9) All fluid should be warmed and maintained at 37°C.

10) Careful records of vital signs, time and amounts of fluid in and out, and cumulative deficits in either direction, must be kept with each pass. In addition electrolytes, SUN, cultures of the peritoneal fluid, and patient's weight should be determined at least every 12 passes.

11) Major risks – perforation of viscera and/or major vessels, infection.

B. Available Fluids and Additives

1) Solution with 1.5% dextrose: one standard solution (McGaw) whose osmolality is 370 mOsm/L contains (mEq/L): Na 140, Ca 4, Mg 1.5, Cl 100.5, acetate 5.

2) Solution with 4.25% dextrose and the same electrolyte composition as the 1.5% solution. Much higher osmolality (550 mOsm/L) for taking off large quantities of fluid rapidly. Must be used carefully and sparingly due to large fluid shifts and subsequent hypotension. Hypertonic passes should remain in the peritoneal cavity no longer than 30 minutes.

3) Heparin can be added, 500 to 1000 units/L, to avoid fibrin clots on the catheter but this is usually not necessary.

4) If the serum potassium is <3.5 mEq/L and renal function is adequate, K^+ may be given IV or added to the dialysis fluid (4 mEq/L).

5) Some fluids commercially available are prepared with lactate as a bicarbonate precursor. In situations where there is hepatic failure, metabolic acidosis, or lactic acidosis, a solution prepared with acetate is better. If the commercial acetate solution is not available, prepare a lactate free solution in the following manner:
    (Roberts KB, Personal communication, 1978)

905 ml	0.45 N NaCl
15 ml	NaCl (2 mEq/ml)
50 ml	$NaHCO_3$ (1 mEq/ml)
30 ml	$D_{50}W$
1000 ml	($D_{1.5}$; 150 mEq Na; 100 mEq Cl; 50 mEq HCO_3)

Ref: Rubin, M (ed): Pediatric Nephrology. Baltimore: Williams and Wilkins, 1975, p. 833.

CEREBROSPINAL FLUID

Caution: Lumbar puncture may be dangerous in the presence of the following:

Increased intracranial pressure
Prior to lumbar puncture, perform a fundoscopic exam. The presence of papilledema/hemorrhage calls for extreme caution and may be a contraindication to the procedure. A sudden drop in intraspinal pressure by rapid release of CSF may cause fatal herniation.

Bleeding tendency
A platelet count of >50,000/mm³ is desirable prior to L.P. Correct any clotting factor deficiencies.

Overlying skin infections
May result in inoculation of CSF with organisms.

A. Cerebrospinal Fluid Pressure
Accurate measurement of CSF pressure can only be made with the patient lying quietly on his side. Once free flow of spinal fluid is obtained, attach the manometer and measure CSF. (Normal values, see page 358.)

B. Collection of Cerebrospinal Fluid
Collect 3 tubes of spinal fluid under sterile conditions (save a fourth tube if possible for additional studies). The first tube is for culture, the second for chemistry determinations, and the third for cell count. About 1-2 ml in each tube will suffice for routine examinations, but cell count and Gram stain can be done on less than 1 ml. Collect larger amounts of fluid if special studies are contemplated (i.e., IgG, myelin basic protein, antigen studies, cytology).

C. Appearance
Record:
1) Color
2) Clarity
3) Coagula, pellicles, or sediments. Time required for their formation will vary with different diseases; coagula may form in a short time in suppurative meningitis, whereas T.B. meningitis may take 12-24 hours to produce pellicle.

D. Culture
Most microbiology laboratories are open 24 hours a day, seven days a week, and CSF is treated as a major medical emergency.

However, whenever immediate culture is not available through the hospital laboratory, see pages 39-41 for culture techniques.

E. Cell Count, Differential WBC and Cell Morphology
The appropriate CSF tubes should be sent immediately to the hospital laboratories for these studies. (Normal values, see page 358.)

F. Examination for Bacteria
1) If pellicle forms, remove and crush it between 2 clean slides. Pull the slides apart, giving 2 smears. Stain one with Gram stain and the other for acid-fast bacilli (see page 39).
2) Spin uncontaminated CSF, smear the sediment on a slide and Gram stain it.

G. Examination for Fungus
Place one drop of CSF and one of India ink on a slide and mix well. Cover with coverslip and press out excess fluid. Ring with vaseline. Examine for round organisms with large halos. If the index of suspicion for fungi is high, incubate the preparation at 37°C and reexamine at 24 and 48 hours.

H. Chemical Determination
The appropriate CSF tubes should be sent immediately to the hospital laboratories for sugar and protein determinations.

I. Serologic Studies
May be performed in serology laboratory. Normal values see page 356.

S Y N O V I A L   F L U I D

Examination of Synovial Fluid

A. **Appearance**
Note quantity, turbidity, pH, clot formation, viscosity, and icterus.

B. **Microscopic**
Examine undiluted for total RBC and WBC count and crystals. Dilute with saline to obtain WBC if necessary. The use of acidic WBC diluting fluids may produce clotting. Any cell count >50,000/mm³ must be assumed to represent septic arthritis until proven otherwise. Crystal induced synovitis is rare in children. The exception is acute gout in Lesch-Nyhan syndrome or glycogen storage diseases. Please see page 38 for normal values.

C. **Chemical**
Obtain sugar and protein determinations. Sugar should be within 10 mg/dl of blood sugar. Be sure to obtain blood sugar before procedure. Normal joint fluid contains little protein.

D. **Mucin**
A qualitative test for hyaluronic acid. To 1 ml of synovial fluid, from which the cells have been centrifuged, add 4 ml water, then 2-3 drops glacial acetic acid, and stir. A tight rope of mucin is normal. In infection and rheumatoid arthritis no precipitate, or a loose fibrillar precipitate, is formed.

E. **Bacteriologic**
Gram stain sediment; culture aerobically, anaerobically, and for AFB.

F. **Icterus**
May indicate trauma. Send sample to chemistry lab for bilirubin.

NOTE: A portion of the fluid may be placed in a heparinized tube to prevent clotting.

SYNOVIAL FLUID ASSESSMENT

Etiology	Appearance	Leukocytes /mm³	% Neutrophils	Mucin	Blood glucose / Synovial glucose
Normal	clear, straw	<2,000	<40%	good	<2
Inflammatory	clear – turbid	2,000 – 100,000	>50%	loose friable	>2
Infectious	turbid	>50,000	>75%	loose friable	>2

Adapted from: Hoekelman, RA, et al. (eds.): *Principles of Pediatrics.* New York: McGraw Hill, 1978, p. 1099.

M I C R O B I O L O G I C A L   E X A M I N A T I O N S

1. Examination of Fresh Preparations and Stained Smears
    One of the most important steps in the laboratory identifica-
    tion of microorganisms is the staining of slide preparations.
    Staining makes the organisms clearly visible under the micro-
    scope and also differentiates them on the basis of their stain-
    ing characteristics.   The three most important screening
    methods available are:

    A. The Gram stain
    B. The acid-fast stain
    C. India ink stain

    The following guidelines are helpful when performing the
    above stains:
        When making smears for staining, it should be remem-
        bered that thin smears give the best results.
        Always allow the smears to air dry before they are
        fixed. (Heating wet smears will usually distort orga-
        nisms and cells.)
        The smears are fixed in gentle heat by quickly passing
        slide through a bunsen burner flame (no more than four
        times). Test heat by tapping slide on the back of your
        hand. It should feel just warm.
        Allow slide to cool before staining.

    A. Gram Stain (Rapid Method)
        1) Flood slide with gentian violet - 10 seconds.
        2) Wash gentian violet away with Gram's iodine - 10
            seconds
        3) Decolorize until no blue washes out - 5 seconds.
        4) Wash with water immediately
        5) Counterstain with safranin - 10 seconds

    B. Acid Fast Stain
        1) Flood slide with Kenyoun's stain - 5 minutes. Wash
            with water.
        2) Decolorize with acid alcohol - 2 minutes. Wash with
            water.
        3) Counterstain with 1/2% methylene blue - 2 minutes.

    C. India Ink
        A negative stain used mainly for identification of
        Cryptococcus. Mix one drop of test fluid and one drop
        of India ink and examine for presence of organism iden-
        tified as a refractile image against a black background.
        (See technique under CSF examination for fungus, page
        36.)

2. Culture Methods
    When immediate culturing is not available through the hospital
    laboratory, culture as follows:

A. Culture the Following Materials Immediately
    1) Blood: The sample volume should equal 10% of the
        volume of the culture medium. When patient is
        treated with penicillin request that the laboratory
        add penicillinase, if desired. (The use of peni-
        cillinase is of questionable validity).
    2) CSF:
        a) Chocolate blood agar (place in CO_2 jar)
        b) 5% sheep blood agar
        c) MacConkey
        d) Thioglycolate broth
        e) Original fluid
    3) Cavity Fluid:
        a) Culture the same as CSF.
        b) Peritoneal and abscess cultures should be
            placed in special anaerobic containers.

B. To Expedite Cultures the Following Media May Be Used
    Directly
    1) Nasopharynx, eye and ear:
        a) 5% sheep blood agar
        b) MacConkey
        c) Chocolate blood agar
        d) Swab in transport media
        e) Thayer-Martin (in infants)
    2) Throat:
        a) 5% sheep blood agar
        b) MacConkey
        c) Swab in transport media
    3) Vagina and urethra:
        a) Thayer-Martin agar
        b) 5% sheep blood agar
        c) Chocolate blood agar
        d) Thioglycolate broth

        NOTE: Always culture immediately, and always do
        Gram stain as well.

    4) Skin:
        a) 5% sheep blood agar
        b) MacConkey
        c) Inoculate thioglycolate broth
        d) Swab in transport media

C. Fungus Preparation
    Scrape the edges of a lesion in which fungus is suspect-
    ed with a scalpel onto a glass slide. Cover the scrap-
    ings with 10% to 20% KOH or NaOH and apply a coverslip.
    Warm over light bulb for a few minutes. Examine for
    fragments of mycelia and spores.

D. Culture for Chlamydia Trachomatis
    All specimens should be sent in the Chlamydia transport
    media if that is available from the hospital microbiology
    or virology laboratory. If swabs are used to collect the

specimen, they should be immediately extracted into the transport medium and discarded. Extraction is done by pressing and rotating the swab against the wall of the specimen container. Dacron swabs must be used. Cotton-wood swabs and calcium alginate swabs are unacceptable.

1) Specimen
   a) Genital: urethral swab, urethral scrapings, prostatic secretions from males, cervical swabs from females.
   b) Conjunctival: conjunctival scrapings or swab.
   c) Respiratory: throat, NP swabs, lung biopsy.
   d) Other: inner ear secretions, synovial fluid, pus from LGV-suspected lesions and lymph nodes.

2) Specimen storage
   For best results, specimens should be inoculated without delay onto cell cultures. However, the following is done if this is not possible.
   a) If inoculation will take place within 24 hours of collection, the specimen should be refrigerated at 4°C.
   b) If inoculation will take place after 24 hours of collection, the specimen should be frozen at -70°C in the mechanical freezer.

E. Tzanck Test
   This test can be used to identify the multinucleated giant cells that are seen in lesions of herpes simplex, herpes zoster, and varicella infections. The lesions tested must be vesicular or bullous. The vesicle or bulla should be unroofed, the fluid blotted off, and the base curetted gently with the blunt end of a scalpel. The scraping should be spread on a glass slide, fixed in methyl alcohol, then stained with a Giemsa or Wright stain.

STOOL EXAMINATION

1. Parasitology Preparations
   See page 43 for illustrations.

   Direct Smear
   Add small amount of feces to drop of saline, mix and remove feces with applicator stick. Cover. Examine under low power to locate the parasite and high dry for identification. Species identification of protozoan cysts can be made by adding iodine stain (KI 1.0% saturated with crystalline iodine) to smear, or by making an additional prep in a drop of stain.

2. Examination for Pinworms

   A. Parents inspect perianal area at night about an hour after the child retires, looking for thread-like white worms (1/4 to 1/2 inch).

   B. Pinworm Smear (Cellophane Tape Method)
      1) Obtain smear in morning before bath.
      2) Cover one end of a tongue depressor with cellophane tape, sticky side out.
      3) Apply to perianal area with mild pressure.
      4) Put 1 drop xylol on glass slide, then apply tape to slide.
      5) Look for ova under microscope.

   C. Examination of Stool after Purgative and Enema

3. Test for Occult Blood in Stool (Guaiac Method)

   A. Reagents
      1) Glacial acetic acid
      2) Guaiac
      3) Hydrogen peroxide (fresh)

   B. Method
      Make thin stool smear on filter paper. Serially apply 2 drops of each in this order: acetic acid, guaiac, hydrogen peroxide. A royal blue color is 4+; a green color is negative. Other gradations of blue are 1-3+.

      NOTE: Medicinal iron does not give a positive guaiac reaction.

4. Apt Test for Fetal Hemoglobin

   A. Purpose
      To differentiate fetal blood from swallowed maternal blood.

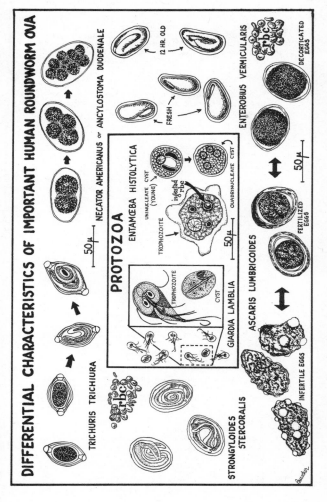

B. Method

Mix specimen (stool, vomitus, etc.) with an equal quantity of tap water. Centrifuge or filter. Supernatant must have pink color to proceed. To 5 parts of supernatant, add 1 part of 0.25 N (1%) NaOH.

C. Interpretation

A pink color persisting over 2 minutes indicates fetal hemoglobin. Adult hemoglobin gives a pink color that becomes yellow in 2 minutes or less indicating denaturation of hemoglobin.

Ref: Apt, L and Downey, WS: J Pediatr 47:6, 1955.

5. Microscopic Stool Fat Test

A. Purpose

Few, if any, neutral fats are found in normal stool. Presence of neutral fats suggests pancreatic insufficiency. Split fats are increased in most patients with steatorrhea due to mucosal disease.

B. Method

Mix specimen thoroughly with applicator stick and place small representative amounts on glass slide.

1) Neutral fats: Add 2 drops H_2O and mix; add 2 drops 95% ethyl alcohol and mix; add few drops of Sudan III and mix; apply coverslip. Examine for yellow or pale orange refractile globules with high lens (x400), noting edges especially since neutral fat tends to float there.

2) Split fats: Add few drops 36% acetic acid and mix; add few drops of Sudan III and mix; heat until boiling starts and repeat x 3. Examine for deep orange fat globules while still warm.

NOTE: Stool fat tests are less reliable in young infants who are consuming formula only, since fat absorption in the newborn may be only 60-70%.

3) In the presence of fecal fat, proceed to a 72 hour fecal fat test. (See pages 53-54.)

6. Test for Sugar in Stool (Reducing Substances)

A. Purpose

Detection of carbohydrate malabsorption by measuring reducing substances in stool. Since sucrose is not a reducing substance modify test as noted.

B. Method

1) Place a small amount of fresh liquid stool in a test tube.

2) Dilute with twice its volume of water. To look for sucrose use 1 N HCl instead of water and boil briefly.

3) Place 15 drops of this suspension in second test tube containing a Clinitest tablet.
4) Compare the resulting color with the chart provided for urine testing.

C. Interpretation
Normally <0.25% reducing substances in the stool. Values of 0.25% to 0.5% are questionable. The finding of ≥0.5% reducing substances in the stool is abnormal and suggests carbohydrate malabsorption. Stool pH will be <6.0 if there are reducing substances in the stool.

7. Fecal Leukocyte Exam

A. Purpose
To aid in the early diagnosis of diarrhea by noting the presence or absence of leukocytes.

B. Method
1) Place a small fleck of stool or mucus (ideally from a rectal swab) on a clean glass slide.
2) Mix thoroughly with 2 drops of 0.5% methylene blue stain.
3) Wait 2-3 minutes for good nuclear staining, cover with coverslip and examine under low power.

C. Interpretation
PMNs are seen with any inflammatory enterocolitis, most commonly shigellosis, salmonellosis, Yersinia, Campylobacter, invasive E. coli infections, and ulcerative or granulomatous colitis. A predominance of mononuclear cells is seen in typhoid fever.

Ref: Harris, JC, et al.: Ann Intern Med 76:697, 1973.

M E T A B O L I C   T E S T S

1. ### Oral Glucose Tolerance Test (OGTT)

   A. **Purpose**
      Tests both absorption and metabolism of glucose.

   B. **Pre-Test Preparation**
      1) Adequate diet required for three days prior to the test, consisting of 50% of total calories as carbohydrate and a minimum caloric intake of:
         1-12 yr old ... 1000 kcal + 100 kcal per year of age

      2) Fast for 12 hours or overnight.

      NOTE: Delay test 2 weeks after period of illness. Discontinue all hyper- or hypoglycemic agents (salicylates, diuretics, oral contraceptives, phenytoin, etc.)

   C. **Test Dosage**
      1.75 gm/kg (max 100 gm) of glucose administered orally after a 12 hour fast allowing up to 5 minutes for ingestion. Mix glucose with water and lemon juice as a 20% solution.

   D. **Samples**
      Sampling method (venous vs. capillary) and analysis method (serum, plasma or whole blood; reducing substance or glucose oxidase) must be consistent throughout the test.

      NOTE: Mutiplying whole blood values by 1.15 and adding the constant 6 mg% converts whole blood to plasma or serum glucose.

   E. **Time**
      Draw blood samples at 0, 30, 60, 120, 180 and 240 minutes. Analyze urine samples for sugar at 0, 60, and 120 minutes.

   F. **Test Milieu**
      Quiet activity is permissible.

   G. **Interpretation**
      (Venous plasma using autoanalyzer ferricyanide method).
      1) Normal: Fasting <110 mg%
                60 min <160 mg%
              120 min <140 mg%
              180 min <130 mg%
              240 min <115 mg%
      2) Two values greater than the above norms or one value above 200 mg% in the absence of overt diabetes mellitus is evidence of chemical diabetes mellitus.

      Ref: Rosenbloom, A: *Metabolism* 22:301, 1973.

2. <u>Screening Test for Genetic Metabolic Diseases</u>

A. <u>Screening Lab Tests Include</u>:
   CBC: neutropenia, thrombocytopenia associated with organic acidemia
   Serum: HCO_3, pH, anion gap, glucose, lactate, ammonia
   Urine: odor, $FeCl_3$, ketones, reducing substances, plasma amino acids, and urine organic acids.

B. <u>Diseases Associated with an Unusual Urine Odor</u>

Disorder	Compound	Odor
Phenylketonuria	Phenylacetic acid	Musty
Maple syrup urine disease	Branched chain alpha-keto acids	Maple syrup, burned sugar
Isovaleric acidemia	Isovaleric acid	Cheesy, or sweaty feet
Methionine malabsorption (Oasthouse Urine Disease)	Alpha-hydroxy-butyric acid	Brewery (dried malt or hops)
Hypermethio-ninemia	Alpha-keto-gamma-methiol-butyric acid	Rancid butter or rotten cabbage
Trimethyl-aminuria	Trimethylamine	Stale fish
Tyrosinemia	Tyrosine	Cabbage-like, fishy
Butyric and hexanic acidemia	Butyric and hexanoic acids	Sweaty feet
Multiple carboxylase deficiency	β-methylcrotonylglycine 3-hydroxyproprionate β-hydroxyisovaleric acid	Cat's urine

C. <u>Ferric Chloride Reactions</u>
   Ferric iron (Fe^{+3}) forms colored derivatives when combined with many organic compounds.
   1) Results depend on methodology.
      a) Use <u>fresh urine</u>.
      b) Standard reagent: 10% ferric chloride
      c) Mix 2 drops of $FeCl_3$ to 1 ml of urine, mix and observe color immediately and upon standing.
   2) The test is relatively insensitive and usually requires high concentrations of the reacting metabolite. Salicylate is an exception.
   3) Phosphate ions yield cloudy precipitates which may mask positive results.

4) Interpretation:
   DUE TO THE INSENSITIVITY, A NEGATIVE TEST
   DOES NOT RULE OUT THE DISEASE

Ref: Buist, NRM: Brit Med J 2:745, 1968; Thomas, GH
and Howell, RR: Selected Screening Tests for Genetic
Metabolic Diseases. Chicago: Year Book Medical Publishers Inc., 1973.

CLINICAL CONDITIONS WITH POSITIVE URINARY FERRIC
CHLORIDE TEST

Disorder	Reacting Compound in Urine	Color with $FeCl_3$
Normal	Phosphates	Brown, Yellow, or White
Phenylketonuria	Phenylpyruvic acid	Green
Maple Syrup Urine Disease	Branched Chain Ketoacids	Gray-Green
Tyrosinemia	p-hydroxyphenyl pyruvic acid	Green, fades rapidly
Histidinemia	Imidazole pyruvic acid	Blue-Green
Methionine Malabsorption (Oasthouse Urine Disease)	α-Hydroxybutyric acid	Purple
Alkaptonuria	Homogentesic acid	Dark Brown
Conjugated Hyperbilirubinemia	Bilirubin	Green
Formiminotransferase Deficiency	Imidazolcarboxamide	Gray-Green
Ketoacidosis	Acetoacetic acid	Cherry Red
Melanoma	Melanin	Black
Pheochromocytoma	Cathecholamines	Blue-Green
Drug Ingestions	Salicylates PAS (p-aminosalicylic acid) Phenothiazines L-Dopa Antipyrine and Acetophenetidine Isoniazid	Deep Purple Red-Brown Blue-Purple Green Cherry Red Yellowish-Green to Gray

D. Phenistix Test of Urine

Positive in	Color
Phenylketonuria	Gray-Green
Histidinemia	Gray
Tyrosinemia	Green
Salicylate, Phenothiazine Ingestion	Purple

E. Dinitrophenylhydrazine (DNPH) - for Keto Acids
    1) Reagent: 100 mg of 2, 4-dinitrophenylhydrazine in
        100 ml of 2 N HCl. Must be refrigerated.
    2) Method: Add 10 drops of reagent to 1 ml of urine
        (urine must not be cold).
    3) Interpretation: Positive reaction is the formation of
        a yellow or chalky white precipitate within 10 min-
        utes. It indicates the presence of keto acids found
        in the following disorders:

Acetonuria   Ketotic Hyperglycinemia
Diabetes Mellitus   Lactic Acidosis
Fructose 1,6 Diphos-   Maple Syrup Urine
   phatase Deficiency   Disease
Glycogen Storage Disease   Methylmalonic Aciduria
Histidinemia   Phenylketonuria*
Isovaleric Acidemia   Tyrosinosis

* May be positive with phenylpyruvic acid levels as low
as 5 mg %.

F. Urine Reducing Substances

NOTE: "Dipsticks" use a glucose oxidase reagent which
will only detect glucosuria. To detect other reducing
sugars, mix 2 drops of urine with 10 drops of water
plus a Clinitest (TM) tablet. The degree of color
change denotes quantity of reducing sugar. Conditions
associated with a positive test include:
galactose - galactosemia, galactokinase deficiency, severe
            liver disease
fructose - hereditary fructose intolerance, essential
           fructosuria
glucose - diabetes mellitus, renal glycosuria, Fanconi's
          type RTA
xylulose - pentosuria
p-hydroxyphenyl pyruvic acid - tyrosinemia

Ref: Burton, BK and Nadler, HL: Pediatrics 61:398, 1978;
Aleck, KA and Shapiro, LJ: PCNA 25:431, 1978.

G. Neonatal Hyperammonemia
    1) with ketoacidosis and increased anion gap suggests
        an organic acidemia such as: proprionic, methyl
        malonic, isolvaleric acidemias, ß-ketothiolase defi-
        ciency, glutaric acidemia type II, and multiple
        carboxylase deficiency.
    2) without ketoacidosis suggests a urea cycle defect or
        transient hyperammonemia of the newborn. Deter-
        mination of plasma citrulline will help determine the
        specific defect.

Ref: Brusilow, SW, et al.: Adv in Pediatr 29:69, 1982.

H. Interpretation of Urine and Serum Amino Acid Screening

1) Inherited disorders with generalized aminoaciduria as part of a proximal tubule (Fanconi type) dysfunction but <u>no</u> aminoacidemia:

Cystinosis   Lowe's Syndrome
Fructose Intolerance   Tyrosinosis
Galactosemia   Wilson's Disease

2) Non-inherited, transient and/or acquired causes of generalized aminoaciduria:

Aminoaciduria of Normal Newborns
Body Irradiation
Heavy Metal Toxicity
Hepatic Necrosis (Tyrosine, Leucine, Proline)
Hyperparathyroidism (Hydroxyproline)
Neurosecretory Tumors (Cystathionine)
Nephrotic Syndrome
Outdated Tetracycline Ingestion
Pregnancy
Renal Transplantation
Salicylate Toxicity
Steroid Therapy
Deficiency of Vitamins B, C, or D
Hyperalimentation

3) Inherited disorders of renal amino acid transport (Normal plasma amino acids with aminoaciduria):

Disorder	Amino Acids in Urine
Cystinuria	Arginine, Cystine, Lysine, Ornithine
Diabasic Aminoaciduria	Arginine, Lysine, Ornithine
Hartnup Disease	Neutral Aminoaciduria
Hypercystinuria	Cystine
Iminoglycinuria	Glycine, Hydroxyproline, Proline
Methionine Malabsorption	Methionine (mainly), also Tyrosine, Phenylalanine, Valine
Glucoglycinuria	Glycine
Glycinuria with Hypophosphatemia	Glycine
Glycinuria	Glycine
Familial Protein Intolerance	Lysine, sometimes Arginine

3. Tests of Gastrointestinal Function

    A. Cholecystokinin/Secretin Stimulation Test (Quantitative Assessment of Exocrine Pancreatic Function)

        1) Method: Fast overnight, sedate with diazepam 1-2 mg/kg IM. Using a pediatric size 3 lumen double balloon duodenal tube, intubate the duodenum under fluoroscopy such that the first balloon is near the ligament of Treitz and the second balloon is in the first part of the duodenum.

        2) Samples: Collect duodenal fluid at rest for 20 minutes. Then stimulate pancreatic secretion with cholecystokinin (2 units/kg) followed in 20 minutes by secretin (2 units/ kg). Give both hormones by slow IV injection over 2 minutes.

        3) Measure: Volume, HCO_3 concentration, pH, lipase activity, amylase, trypsin, chymotrypsin, and carboxypeptidase A. Continue collection in 10 minute blocks for 50 minutes.

        4) Normal values:

Test	Observed Range (after stimulation)
Volume (ml/kg/50 mins)	1.8-8.1
Bicarbonate (mEq/kg/50 mins)	0.08-0.37
Trypsin (micrograms/kg/50 mins)	215-2170
Chymotrypsin (micrograms/kg/50 mins)	252-1900
Carboxypeptidase A (IU 10^3/kg/50 mins)	141-2480
Amylase (children over 1 year) (IU/kg/50 mins)	140-2050
Lipase (IU/kg/50 mins)	206-5093
pH	6

NOTE: Amylase output is age-dependent under 1 year of age.

Ref: Hadorn, B, et al.: J Pediatr 73:39, 1968.

    B. D-Xylose Test

        1) Purpose: To estimate the surface area of the duodenojejunal intestinal mucosa by measuring the absorption of an oral dose of D-xylose. Either the elevation in serum concentration or the % urinary excretion of xylose may be used to quantitate D-xylose absorption. Absorption is independent of bile salts, pancreatic exocrine secretions, and intestinal mucosal disaccharidases. The test is unreliable in patients with edema, renal disease, delayed gastric emptying and severe diarrhea.

        2) Method:

            a) Preparation: Older children fast for 8 hours prior to the test; younger infants need fast for only 4-6 hours.

b) Test dose: D-xylose in a dose of 14.5 gm/M^2 as a 5% water solution is given orally or via a gastric tube. Placement in the duodenum minimizes error caused by delayed gastric emptying.

c) Measurement of urinary excretion: Patient voids and all urine for 5 hours is collected. Insure adequate urine flow by supplementary oral or IV fluid. The quantity of xylose is determined colorimetrically.
Normal values: 5 hour urinary excretion of 25% or greater of the administered dose is normal for children over 6 months. Values between 15 and 23% are questionable. Urinary excretion of less than 15% is abnormal. In infants less than 6 months values below 10% are considered abnormal.

d) Measurement of serum concentration (infants): Obtain serum samples for determination of xylose concentration in fasting state and at 30, 60, 90, and 120 minutes following the xylose dose.
Normal values: A normal response is associated with a serum level exceeding 20 mg/dl in any of the post absorptive specimens.
Ref: Santiago-Borrero, P, et al.: Pediatrics 48:55, 1971; Anderson, CM and Burke, A: Pediatric Gastroenterology St. Louis: C.V. Mosby, pp 633-670, 1975; Buts, JP, et al.: J Pediatr 90: 729, 1978.

C. Mono- and Disaccharide Absorption Tests
1) Purpose: To diagnose malabsorption of a specific carbohydrate by measuring the change in blood glucose following an oral dose of the carbohydrate in question.
2) Method:
a) The patient fasts 4-6 hours prior to test.
b) The test carbohydrate (lactose, sucrose, maltose, glucose, galactose) is given orally or by gastric tube in a dose of 1.75 gm/kg as a 10% solution (maximum dose of 100 gms). For maltose, the dose is 1.0 gm/kg.
c) Measure serum glucose prior to the carbohydrate dose and at 15, 30, 60, and 90 minutes following the dose.
d) Note the number and character of the stools, Clinitest determination for reducing substances on all stools passed during the test and for 8 hours after the test is completed.
3) Interpretation:
a) A rise in the blood glucose level of >25 mg/dl over the fasting level within the test period is

considered normal. An increase of 20 to 25 mg/dl is questionable. Increases of <20 mg/dl are abnormal and suggest malabsorption of the test carbohydrate.

    b) Malabsorption is also suggested if during the test or subsequent 8 hour period one notes:

        (1) The onset of diarrhea.
        (2) Stool pH of 6.0 or less.
        (3) >0.25% reducing substances (Clini-test) in the stool.

NOTE: Sucrose is not a reducing substance.

        (4) Crampy abdominal pain or abdominal distention.

D. Quantitative Fecal Fat

    1) Purpose: Quantitative determination of fecal fat excretion to aid in diagnosis or management of fat malabsorption syndromes.

    2) Method:

        a) The patient is given a diet with a fixed percentage of long chain fats for 3 days prior to the collection period. Keep a record of all intake during this time.

NOTE: Adjust amount of fat administered to the child according to age. Attempt to deliver:

>25 gm/day in infants
>50 gm/day in toddlers
>100 gm/day in school-aged children

Exclude medium chain triglyceride oil from diet.

        b) All stools passed within a 72 hour period should be saved.

        c) Total fecal fatty acid content is determined.

    3) Normals:

        a) Absolute values:

6 mo - 1 yr . . . . . . <4.3 gm/day
1 yr - 10 yr . . . . . . <3.1 gm/day
10 yr - adult . . . . . . <5.0 gm/day

        b) Percentage of fat calculated:

Coefficient of absorption (CA) =

$$\text{CA} = \frac{\text{gms fat ingested} - \text{gms fat excreted}}{\text{gms fat ingested}} \times 100$$

Term newborns	CA = 80-85%
6 mo – 1 yr	CA >87%
1 – 2 yr	CA >93%
2 yr – adult	CA >95%

Ref: Shmerling, DH, et al.: Pediatrics 46:690, 1970.

E. Breath Hydrogen Test

Principle: H_2 gas is produced by bacterial fermentation of carbohydrate, then absorbed, and excreted in the breath. Elevation in breath content of H_2 correlates with malabsorption of delivered carbohydrate.

Procedure:

1) Fast infant for 4-6 hrs and older children for 8 hrs.

2) Give 2 gm/kg (max. 50 gm) of carbohydrate.

3) End-expired air is collected by aspirating 3.5 ml of air after each breath to a total of 30 ml via nasal prongs attached to a gas-tight syringe or via gas balloon attached to face mask.

4) H_2 is measured by gas chromatography on baseline sample (before carbohydrate load) and hourly samples for 6 hrs.

5) Elevation in H_2 content >20 ppm above baseline is considered significant.

NOTE: Prior antibiotic use can obliterate normal enteric flora needed for fermentation and cause a false negative result.

Ref: Perman, JA, et al.: J Pediatr 93:17, 1978; Solomon, NW: Current Concepts in Gastroenterology 2:38, 1977.

C A R D I O L O G Y

1. <u>Cardiac Cycle</u>
   See illustration on page 56.

2. <u>Electrocardiography</u>

   A. <u>Placement of Leads</u>
      1) <u>Biopolar leads</u>
         a) Lead I: right arm – left arm
         b) Lead II: right arm – left leg
         c) Lead III: left arm – left leg
      2) Unipolar leads
         a) aVR: right arm
         b) aVL: left arm
         c) aVF: left foot
      3) Precordial leads
         a) V 1: 4th RICS at right sternal border
         b) V 2: 4th LICS at left sternal border
         c) V 3: midway between V 2 and V 4
         d) V 4: 5th LICS at mid-clavicular line
         e) V 5: 5th LICS at anterior axillary line
         f) V 6: 5th LICS at mid-axillary line
         g) V3R: V3 on right chest
         h) V4R: V4 on right chest
         i) V 7: posterior axillary line (use if no Q
                 wave in V6)

   B. <u>Terminology</u>
      See illustration on page 56.

      The P wave represents atrial depolarization.
      The $\overline{QRS}$ Complex represents ventricular depolarization.
      Waves in the QRS Complex are as follows:
      1) $\overline{R}$ Wave – the first positive deflection
      2) $\overline{S}$ Wave – the negative deflection following the R
                       wave
      3) QS Wave – a monophasic negative complex
      4) $\overline{R'}$ Wave – the second positive deflection
      5) $\overline{S'}$ Wave – the second negative deflection
      6) $\overline{T}$ Wave – represents ventricular repolarization
      7) $\overline{U}$ Wave – may follow the T wave

   C. <u>Rate</u>
      ECG machine speed should be set at 25 mm/second.
      Obtain rate by multiplying by 20 the number of com-
      plexes between two vertical lines (3 seconds) at the
      top of the strip. If rate is slow or irregular, a more
      accurate reflection of rate is obtained by multiplying
      by 10 the number of complexes between three vertical
      lines (6 seconds). Record atrial and ventricular rates
      when AV block is present.

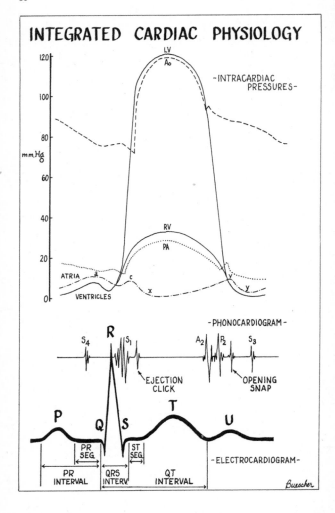

INTEGRATED CARDIAC PHYSIOLOGY

-INTRACARDIAC PRESSURES-

LV
Ao
RV
PA
ATRIA
VENTRICLES
a
c
x
v
y

mm.Hg
120
100
80
60
40
20
0

-PHONOCARDIOGRAM-

S_4 R S_1 A_2 P_2 S_3

EJECTION CLICK

OPENING SNAP

-ELECTROCARDIOGRAM-

P   Q   S   T   U

PR SEG.
ST SEG.
PR INTERVAL
QRS INTERV
QT INTERVAL

Buescher

Alternatively the rate may be estimated from the R-R interval in increments of 0.2 sec:

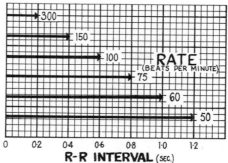

AGE-SPECIFIC HEART RATES

	Heart Rate (beats/min)	
Age	Mean	Range
0–24 hrs.	119.	94–145
1– 7 days	133.	100–175
8–30 days	163.	115–190
1– 3 mos.	154.	124–190
3– 6 mos.	140.	111–179
6–12 mos.	140.	112–177
1– 3 yrs.	126.	98–163
3– 5 yrs.	98.	65–132
5– 8 yrs.	96.	70–115
8–12 yrs.	79.	55–107
12–16 yrs.	75.	55–102

D. **Rhythm**
See pages 61-66 for analysis of disorders of cardiac rhythm.

E. **Intervals**
1) **P-R Interval**

MAXIMUM PR INTERVAL

			Rate			
Age	–70	71–90	91–110	111–130	131–150	151
Under 1 mo			.11	.11	.11	.11
1–9 mos			.14	.13	.12	.11
10–24 mos			.15	.14	.14	.10
3–5 yrs		.16	.16	.16		
6–13 yrs	.18	.18	.16	.16		

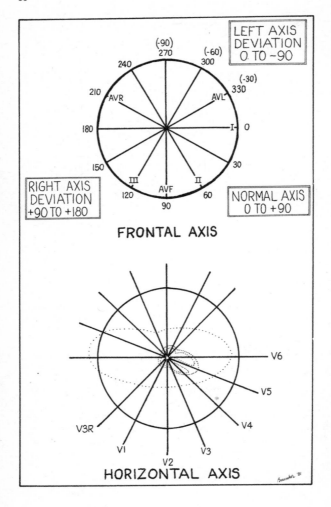

FRONTAL AXIS

HORIZONTAL AXIS

2) QT$_c$ (corrected QT interval)

$$QT_c = \frac{\text{measured QT}}{\sqrt{\text{R-R interval}}};$$

QT$_c$ <u>should</u> <u>not</u> exceed 0.425

F. <u>Axis</u>

1) <u>P Wave</u> <u>Axis</u>. Frontal axis calculated using diagram page 58 is normally 0-90°.

2) <u>QRS</u> <u>Axis</u>: Frontal axis is age specific.

Age	AGE-SPECIFIC QRS AXIS (FRONTAL PLANE) Mean QRS Axis (degrees)	Range
0-24 hrs	135.	60-180
1- 7 days	125.	80-160
8-30 days	110.	60-160
1- 3 mos	80.	40-120
3- 6 mos	65.	20- 80
6-12 mos	65.	0-100
1- 3 yrs	55.	20-100
3- 5 yrs	60.	40- 80
5- 8 yrs	65.	40-100
8-12 yrs	65.	20- 80
12-16 yrs	65.	20- 80

3) <u>T Wave</u> Orientation

NORMAL ORIENTATION OF T WAVE

Age	V1, V2	aVF	I, V5, V6
Birth - 1 day	±	+	±
1 - 4 days	±	+	+
4 days - adolescence	-	+	+
Adolescence - adulthood	+	+	+

+ = T wave positive
- = T wave negative
± = T wave may normally be positive <u>OR</u> negative

G. Atrial Hypertrophy

1) Right atrial hypertrophy (RAH) - suggested by either:

a) Peaked P wave, >2.5 mm in any lead (best seen in L-2, L-3, V3R, and V1)

        b) P/PR segment ratio <1.0 in absence of A-V
            block.
    2) Left atrial hypertrophy (LAH) - suggested by
        any of the following:
        a) P wave duration >0.08 seconds; may have
            "plateau" or "notched" contour (⌒⌒)
        b) Terminal and deep inversion of the P wave
            in V3R or V1 (⌄⌄)
        c) P/PR segment ratio >1.6 in the absence of
            AV block

H. Ventricular Hypertrophy
    1) Normal range for R and S waves:

AMPLITUDE RANGE - RIGHT CHEST LEADS (mm)
(5th - 95th percentiles)

Age	V1		V2	
	R	S	R	S
30 hrs	4.3-21.0	1.1-19.1		
1 mo	3.3-18.7	0.0-15.0		
2-3 mos	4.5-18.0	0.5-17.1		
4-5 mos	4.5-17.4	1.0-16.8		
6-8 mos	3.2-21.2	1.5-25.7		
9 mos-2 yrs	2.5-15.6	2.0-17.2	5.9-25.2	5.0-25.5
2-5 yrs	2.1-13.9	2.1-21.6	4.2-20.8	5.4-29.7
6-13 yrs	1.1-10.7	3.8-22.3	3.7-15.9	8.6-29.8
adult	1.0- 6.0	3.0-13.0		

AMPLITUDE RANGE - LEFT CHEST LEADS (mm)
(5th - 95th percentiles)

Age	V5		V6	
	R	S	R	S
30 hrs	3.1-16.6	2.4-18.5	1.5-11.3	1.0-13.8
1 mo	3.8-24.2	2.8-16.3	1.0-16.2	0.0-9.5
2-3 mos	9.5-26.2	1.2-14.4	5.4-20.8	0.1-9.1
4-5 mos	10.0-28.8	2.6-16.0	4.4-22.4	0.0-8.0
6-8 mos	12.0-29.0	1.5-19.6	6.0-22.0	0.2-4.4
9 mos-2 yrs	7.3-28.4	0.6-10.5	5.7-20.0	0.3-5.2
2-5 yrs	9.4-33.3	0.6-8.9	6.4-22.1	0.0-3.7
6-13 yrs	12.4-33.0	0.0-9.2	7.7-23.3	0.0-4.1
adult	7.0-21.0	0.0-5.0	5.0-18.0	0.0-2.0

    2) Right ventricular hypertrophy (any of below,
        singly or in combination):
        a) R in V1 or V2 above 95th percentile for age
        b) S in V5 or V6 above 95th percentile for age
        c) Upright T in V1 after 4 days
        d) qR in V3R or V1
        e) RSR' in V3R or V1 (This is suggestive of
            diastolic volume overload - eg. ASD)

3) Left ventricular hypertrophy (any of below, singly or in combination):
   a) R in V5 or V6 above 95th percentile for age (suggests volume overload)
   b) Q wave >4 mm in V5 or V6 (suggests volume overload)
   c) R in V1 or V2 below 5th percentile for age (suggests pressure overload)
   d) S in V1 or V2 above 95th percentile for age (suggests pressure overload)

4) <u>NOTE</u>: In the event of abnormal conduction or complex congenital heart disease, these criteria may not be applicable. The electrocardiographic findings in premature infants are not well delineated. Generally, there is a gradual progression from LV to RV predominance as an infant approaches term. Therefore these conventional electrocardiographic criteria for interpretation of ventricular hypertrophy are not reliable in the premature neonate.

Tables and values for electrocardiography section adapted from: Moss, AJ, Adams, FH, and Emmanouilides, GC (eds): <u>Heart Disease in Infants, Children, and Adolescents</u>, 2nd Edition. Baltimore: Williams and Wilkins, 1977, pp. 32-40; Cooksey, JD, Dunn, M, and Massie, E: <u>Clinical Vectorcardiography and Electrocardiography</u>, 2nd Edition. Chicago: Year Book Medical Publishers, Inc., 1977, p. 85; Liebman, J, Plonsey, R, and Gillette, PC (eds): <u>Pediatric Electrocardiography</u>. Baltimore: Williams and Wilkins, 1982, pp. 140-171.

3. <u>Disorders of Conduction and Rhythm</u>
   Abnormalities of rhythm have varying significance depending on the clinical setting. In the child with a structurally normal heart, many arrhythmias have no hemodynamic effects. Arrhythmias may have more serious implications in a child with congenital heart disease. This section catalogues and illustrates some abnormalities seen in children, but does not address issues of clinical significance and therapy. Cardiac resuscitation drugs are charted in the inside front cover, and the formulary includes other useful cardiac medications.

   A. <u>Sinus Arrhythmia</u>
      Variation of the RR interval without morphological changes of the P wave or QRS complex.

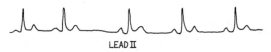

LEAD II

B. <u>Low Atrial Pacemaker</u> ("coronary sinus rhythm").
   Shortened to normal PR interval with negative P in
   L-2, L-3, aVF, and upright in V6. P wave axis is
   180-360°.

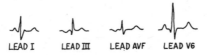

LEAD I   LEAD III   LEAD AVF   LEAD V6

C. <u>Left Atrial Rhythm</u>
   Varying P configurations in limb leads depending on
   site of origin (high, low, mid); however, frequently
   negative in L-2, L-3, aVF, and always negative in V6.
   Dome and dart configuration diagnostic of left atrial
   rhythm with the dome representing the left atrium and
   the dart the right atrium. Best seen in L-2 and V1.
   P wave axis is 90-270°.

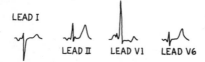

LEAD I

LEAD II   LEAD V1   LEAD V6

D. <u>Premature Atrial Contraction (PAC)</u>
   1)   Premature beat with abnormal P wave, normal
        QRS complexes, and usually not followed by a
        fully compensatory pause.

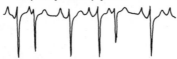

   2)   PAC (with aberrancy) - similar to 1, but with
        wide QRS usually resembling a RBB pattern.
        The initial vector is in the same direction as the
        normal sinus QRS.

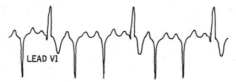

LEAD V1

E. <u>Supraventricular Tachycardia (PAT or SVT)</u>
Normal QRS complexes at a rapid rate with or without
discernible P waves. PAT with RBB, or, less commonly, LBB may be confused with ventricular
tachycardia. Presence of P waves and BBB pattern
are helpful in discerning the two.

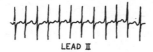

LEAD II

F. <u>Atrial Flutter</u>
Normal QRS complexes, absence of P waves, "flutter
waves" between QRS complexes.

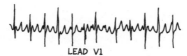

LEAD V1

G. <u>Atrial Fibrillation</u>
Normal QRS complexes, absence of P waves, varying
RR interval.

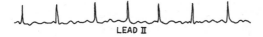

LEAD II

H. <u>First Degree Heart Block</u>
Prolongation of the PR interval beyond normal for age
and rate (see page 57).

I. <u>Second Degree Heart Block</u>
Atrial rate greater than the ventricular rate with conduction of the atrial impluse at regular intervals, i.e.,
every other (2:1 block), every third (3:1 block), three
atrial for every 2 ventricular (3:2 block).

1)   Type I (Wenckebach):   Progressive lengthening
     of the PR interval until an atrial impulse is not
     conducted and the beat is dropped.

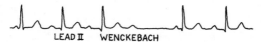

2)   Type II: Dropped beats without lengthening of
     the PR interval.

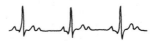

J.   Complete Heart Block
     No conducted atrial impulses, with a slow unrelated
     nodal or ventricular rhythm.

K.   A-V Dissociation
     Failure of conduction of the atrial impulse through the
     A-V node with a faster, independent nodal or ventri-
     cular rhythm.

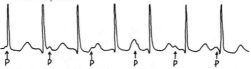

L.   Wolff-Parkinson-White (WPW)
     Prolonged QRS duration and shortened PR interval
     secondary to initial slurring of the upstroke of the
     QRS (delta wave).   Type A has predominantly positive
     QRS complexes in lead V1.   Type B has predominantly
     negative QRS complexes in V1.

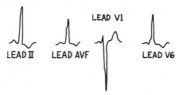

M. Complete Bundle Branch Block
Longest QRS >0.10 second.
1) LBBB: Monophasic R wave in L-1; absence of Q
wave in V6.

LEAD V1

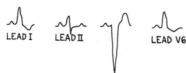

LEAD I   LEAD II   LEAD V6

2) RBBB: Wide S wave in L1, V6; M-shaped QRS in
V-1, RAD.

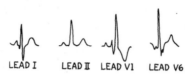

LEAD I   LEAD II   LEAD V1   LEAD V6

N. Left Anterior Hemiblock
Normal QRS duration, left axis deviation; qR in L1, rS
in L3.

O. Left Posterior Hemiblock
Normal QRS duration, right axis deviation without evidence of RVH; rS in L1, qR in L3.

P. Premature Ventricular Contraction (PVC)
QRS complexes are prolonged, ST segments slope away
from QRS, and T waves are inverted. PVC's occur
before the expected atrial beat and are usually followed by a compensatory pause. Bigeminy is alternat-
ing normal and abnormal ventricular complexes.

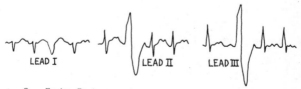

LEAD I   LEAD II   LEAD III

Q. Fusion Beat
Characteristics of both a sinus beat and a PVC. It
has the same early activation of a sinus beat and late
activation of a PVC (see illustration R).

R. Ventricular <u>Tachycardia</u>
Three or more serial PVC's at a rapid rate. P waves, if present, are dissociated. Usually no Q wave in V5-6. QRS complexes tend to be wide and diphasic (R=S) across precordium. Presence of fusion beats prior to onset or at termination of V. tach. is usually diagnostic.

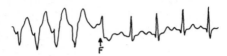

4. <u>Normal Values for Right and Left Heart Pressures</u>
(Ages 2 months to 15½ years)

	Mean	Range
Right Atrial	1	−2 to 6
Right Ventricle		
Systolic	24	15 to 37
End-Diastolic	3	0 to 8
Pulmonary Artery		
Systolic	20	12 to 35
Diastolic	7	3 to 12
Left Atrial	6	2 to 14
Left Ventricle		
Systolic	100	72 to 133
End-Diastolic	7	3 to 14
Aorta		
Systolic	108	84 to 150
Diastolic	64	50 to 83

<u>Ref</u>: Krovetz, LJ and Goldbloom, S: <u>Hopkins Med J</u> <u>130</u>:187-195, 1972.

5. <u>Drug Effects</u>

A. Digoxin
1) Therapeutic effect
   a) PR interval prolonged
   b) QT_c interval is shortened
   c) ST segment changes in direction opposite to QRS complex
   d) Decrease in amplitude of T wave

<u>NOTE</u>: For therapeutic management see page 197.

2) Toxicity (see page 240)
   a) Bradycardia
   b) Various degrees of AV block
   c) Arrhythmias of <u>any</u> type - commonly atrial (e.g. SVT with block) in children
<u>NOTE</u>: Toxicity enhanced by hypoxia, hypokalemia, and acidosis.

B. Quinidine
1) Therapeutic effect
   a) Decrease in amplitude of P wave
   b) Slight prolongation of PR interval
   c) Prolonged QRS duration – correlates with blood level of drug
   d) Prolonged QT_c interval – also correlates with drug level

   NOTE: For therapeutic management see page 180.

2) Toxicity:
   a) Significant prolongation of PR interval
   b) Prolongation of QRS duration by $\geq 50\%$ over initial duration
   c) Sino-atrial or A-V block
   d) Multifocal ventricular premature beats

6. Electrolyte Disturbances

A. Hyperkalemia
1) Earliest manifestation: tall, narrow "tented" T wave.
2) Later, widening of QRS complex occurs; may be mistaken for LBBB.
3) Wide and flattened P waves; may be mistaken for atrial fibrillation.
4) Ectopic rhythms and intraventricular block.
5) Serial EKG changes in an individual can be correlated with serum K^+.

NOTE: Toxic effects are enhanced by sodium or calcium depletion and acidosis. In an individual, signs of severe toxicity may present acutely without earlier manifestations.

B. Hypokalemia
1) Prolonged QT_c interval due to broad, flat T wave.
2) ST segment depressed
3) T wave flattened or inverted
4) Appearance of U wave
5) Ectopic beats: supraventricular and ventricular

NOTE: These effects are enhanced by digitalis intoxication.

C. Hypercalcemia
1) Shortened QT_c interval (due to decreased ST segment)
2) Myocardial irritability – PVC's, ventricular tachycardia
3) Prolonged PR interval, QRS duration, and/or AV block may occur with severe hypercalcemia.

D. Hypocalcemia
Prolonged QT_c interval (due to long ST segment)

E. Hypomagnesemia
Prolonged QT_c interval

7. Echocardiography

A. 2-D Echocardiogram
The two-dimensional echocardiogram can be used to define virtually all structural abnormalities of the heart. These include abnormalities of the great vessels, semilunar valves, A-V valves, atria and atrial septum, ventricles and ventricular septum, the venae cavae, pulmonary veins, and the proximal coronary arteries.

Technique: The 2-D beam is used to image the heart in three separate perpendicular planes as illustrated on the next pages. The short and long axis views are obtained with the transducer on the chest wall and the four chamber view results when the transducer is directed from just below the sternum. (See pages 69-70.)

B. M-Mode Echocardiogram
M-Mode echocardiography is useful especially for accurate measurement of structures, and for calculation of standardized indices. These can be used serially following changes in an individual (e.g. size of the aortic root in a Marfan syndrome patient, or the right systolic time interval in a patient with cor pulmonale), or can be compared to the normal ranges for age.

8. Glossary of Selected Cardiac Surgical Procedures and Shunts

A. Procedures
1) Blalock-Hanlon - closed atrial septectomy.
2) Brock - closed pulmonary valvulotomy or infundibulectomy.
3) Fontan - establishment of continuity between right atrium and pulmonary artery either by atrial appendage - pulmonary artery anastomosis or through use of a conduit or graft between them.
4) Mustard - intra-atrial baffle or patch (usually pericardium) for palliation of simple transposition of great vessels.
5) Park - use of a knife-tipped cardiac catheter to create an atrial septostomy following passage through foramen ovale.

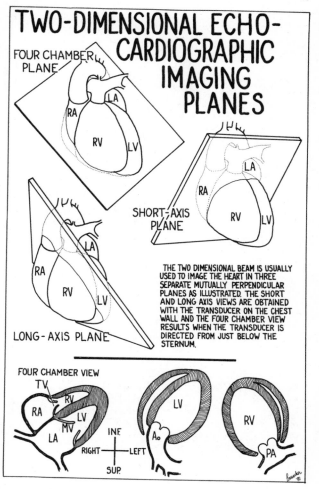

TWO-DIMENSIONAL ECHO-CARDIOGRAPHIC IMAGING PLANES

FOUR CHAMBER PLANE

LA
RA
RV
LV

SHORT-AXIS PLANE

LA
RA
RV
LV

LONG-AXIS PLANE

LA
RA
RV
LV

THE TWO DIMENSIONAL BEAM IS USUALLY USED TO IMAGE THE HEART IN THREE SEPARATE MUTUALLY PERPENDICULAR PLANES AS ILLUSTRATED. THE SHORT AND LONG AXIS VIEWS ARE OBTAINED WITH THE TRANSDUCER ON THE CHEST WALL AND THE FOUR CHAMBER VIEW RESULTS WHEN THE TRANSDUCER IS DIRECTED FROM JUST BELOW THE STERNUM.

FOUR CHAMBER VIEW

TV
RV
RA
LV
MV
LA

INF.
RIGHT — LEFT
SUP.

LV
Ao

RV
PA

70

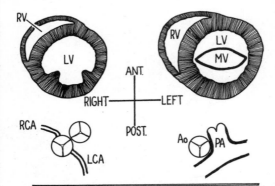

LONG AXIS VIEW

RV
Ao
LV
MV LA

ANT.

INF. — SUP.

POST.

SHORT AXIS VIEW

RV

LV

RV LV MV

ANT.

RIGHT — LEFT

POST.

RCA

LCA

Ao PA

ABBREVIATIONS

ANT: ANTERIOR	INF: INFERIOR
SUP: SUPERIOR	POST: POSTERIOR
RV: RIGHT VENTRICLE	LV: LEFT VENTRICLE
Ao: AORTA	PA: PULMONARY ARTERY
LA: LEFT ATRIUM	RA: RIGHT ATRIUM
MV: MITRAL VALVE	TV: TRICUSPID VALVE
RCA: RIGHT CORONARY ARTERY	
LCA: LEFT CORONARY ARTERY	

6)   Rashkind - use of a balloon-tipped cardiac catheter which is rapidly pulled across the foramen ovale to create a defect in the atrial septum.

7)   Rastelli -
   a) Placement of a valved conduit or graft between right ventricle and pulmonary arteries; used for pulmonary atresia and complex transposition.
   b) Repair of A-V canal by resuspension of mitral and tricuspid valves upon the newly-created atrial septum.

8)   Senning - palliation of simple transposition of the great vessels by means of intra- atrial baffle, using flaps of native atrial septum and atrial wall.

9)   Waldhausen - use of left subclavian artery as an on-lag patch for repair of coarctation of the aorta.

10)   Norwood - complex two-staged palliative procedures for hypoplastic left ventricle. Ref: New Engl J Med 308:23-26, 1983.

B.   Shunts
1) Blalock-Taussig - subclavian to pulmonary artery
2) Glenn - superior vena cava to right pulmonary artery
3) Potts - descending aorta to left pulmonary artery
4) Waterston - ascending aorta to right pulmonary artery

9.   Prophylaxis Against Bacterial Endocarditis in Patients with Structural Cardiac Disease

A.   For Dental Procedures, Tonsillectomy, Adenoidectomy and Bronchoscopy
1) For most patients:
   a) No history of penicillin allergy:
      IM plus oral:

      Aqueous penicillin G 30,000 units/kg (max. dose = 1 million units) plus procaine penicillin 600,000 units IM, followed by oral penicillin V Q6h for 8 doses (Penicillin V dose is 250 mg in children <30 kg and 500 mg in those ≥30 kg.)

      or Oral Only:

      <30 kg: Penicillin V, 1.0 gm PO 30-60 min prior to procedure, then 250 mg PO Q6h for 8 doses.
      ≥30 kg: Penicillin V, 2.0 gm PO 30-60 min prior to procedure, then 500 mg PO Q6h for 8 doses.

b) For patients with penicillin allergy (or those who receive continuous rheumatic fever prophylaxis with oral penicillin):

Erythromycin, 20 mg/kg PO (max. dose = 1.0 gm) 30-60 min prior to procedure, then 10 mg/kg/dose PO (max. dose = 500 mg) Q6h for 8 doses.

2) For patients at higher risk for endocarditis (e.g. those with prosthetic heart valves)
a) No history of penicillin allergy:

Aqueous penicillin G, 30,000 units/kg (max. dose = 1 million units) plus procaine penicillin 600,000 units plus streptomycin 20 mg/kg (max. dose = 1.0 gm), all given IM, followed by oral penicillin V Q6h for 8 doses (Penicillin V dose is 250 mg in children <30 kg and 500 mg in those >30 kg).

b) For patients with penicillin allergy:

Vancomycin, 20 mg/kg (max. dose 1.0 gm) IV over 30-60 min, begun 30-60 min before procedure, then erythromycin 10 mg/kg/dose PO (max. dose = 500 mg) Q6h for 8 doses.

B. For Gastrointestinal or Genitourinary Surgery Instrumentation, and for Surgery of Infected Tissues
1) No history of penicillin allergy:

Aqueous penicillin G, 30,000 units/kg (max. dose = 2 million units) IM or IV, or ampicillin, 50 mg/kg (max. dose = 1.0 gm) IM or IV, PLUS gentamicin, 2 mg/kg (max. dose = 80 mg) IM or IV or streptomycin, 20 mg/kg (max. dose = 1.0 gm) IM given 30-60 min before procedure; repeat Q8h for 2 more doses if gentamicin is used, or Q12h for 2 more doses if streptomycin is used.

2) For patients with penicillin allergy:

Vancomycin 20 mg/kg (max. dose = 1.0 gm) IV over 30-60 min, plus streptomycin 20 mg/kg (max. dose = 1.0 gm) IM, each given 30-60 min before procedure. Repeat doses in 12 hrs.

NOTE: Modify antibiotic doses in patients with significant renal insufficiency (see pages 207-212).

Adapted from: Committee on Rheumatic Fever and Bacterial Endocarditis, American Heart Association; Circulation 56:139A, 1977.

E N D O C R I N O L O G Y

1. Normal Endocrinologic Values

NOTE: Normal values may differ among laboratories.

A. Gonadotropins

	FSH mIU/ml	LH mIU/ml
Adult males	0.6-11.2	3.0-12.0
Adult females	1.6-12.8	1.5-15
Adult females (mid cycle)	variable	variable
Prepubertal children	<3 mIU/ml	<3 mIU/ml

Ref: Johns Hopkins Hospital Pediatric Endocrine Labs, 1983.

B. Steroid Hormones
   1) Plasma
      a) Testosterone

Adult male	=	560 ± 150 ng/dl
Adult female	=	48 ± 14 ng/dl
Male Tanner 2	=	25-85 ng/dl
3	=	52-328 ng/dl
4	=	134-532 ng/dl
5	=	293-564 ng/dl
Prepubertal (<7 yrs)	=	12 ± 5 ng/dl

      b) Estradiol
         Adult male = 1-6 ng/dl
         Adult female = 3-30 ng/dl (varies with cycle)
         Prepubertal = <1 ng/dl
      c) Androstenedione
         Adult male = 115 ± 20 ng/dl
         Adult female = 180 ± 60 ng/dl
         Prepubertal = 20 ± 15 ng/dl
         (<7 yrs)
      d) 170H-Progesterone
         Adult male = 95 ± 30 ng/dl
         Adult female (non-pregnant)
            follicular = 60 ± 20 ng/dl
            luteal = 270 ± 60 ng/dl
         Prepubertal (<7 yrs) = 35 ± 25 ng/dl
         CVAH in good control = 190 ± 120 ng/dl
      e) Cortisol
         8 AM = 11 ± 2.5 mcg/dl (range 8-18 mcg/dl)
         8 PM = 3.5 ± 0.15 mcg/dl
   2) Urine
      a) 17-ketosteroids
         Adult male = 7-17 mg/24h
         Adult female = 4-13 mg/24h
         Prepubertal
            1-2 wks = as high as 2 mg/24h
            1 mo - 5 yrs = <0.5 mg/24h
            6-8 yrs = 1.0-2.0 mg/24h
            >8 yrs = gradually increases to
                     adult levels

b) 17OH-corticosteroids = 3 ± 1 mg/M²/24h
c) Pregnanetriol = <2.5 ng/24h (adult)

Ref: Migeon, CJ, in Collu, R, et al. (eds): Pediatric Endocrinology, Raven Press, New York: 1981, pp. 475, 482, 484; Penny, R: Ped Clin North Am 26:113, 1979; Johns Hopkins Hospital Pediatric Endocrinology Labs, 1983.

C. Tests for Pheochromocytoma

24 hour urine with results expressed as mg/g creatinine

Age	VMA	HVA	Metanephrines
1-12 mo	1.40-15.0	1.20-35.0	0.001-4.6
1- 2 yr	1.25- 8.0	4.0 -23.0	0.27 -5.38
2- 5 yr	1.50- 7.5	0.7 -13.5	0.35 -2.99
5-10 yr	0.50- 6.0	0.5 - 9.0	0.43 -2.7
10-15 yr	0.25- 3.25	0.25-12.0	0.001-1.87
15-18 yr	0.1 - 2.75	0.5 - 2.0	0.001-0.67
Adult	0.25- 3.5	0.25- 2.5	0.05 -1.20

Total free catecholamines: 20-270 mcg/g creatinine

Ref: Gitlow, SE, et al.: J Lab Clin Med 72:612, 1968.

D. Thyroid Function Tests

Test	Normals		Comment
T₄RIA	Cord	7.4-13.0	Direct measurement of total
	1- 3 wk	11.8-22.6	thyroxine by radioimmunoassay,
	1- 2 wk	9.8-16.6	mcg/dl. See values for pre-
	2- 4 wk	7.0-15.0	mature infants below.
	1- 4 mo	7.2-14.4	
	4-12 mo	7.8-16.5	
	1- 5 yr	7.3-15.0	
	Adult	6.5-13.5	
T₃RU	25-35%		Measures thyroid hormone binding, not T₃
T index	1.63-4.73		T₄RIA X T₃RU
Free T₄	0.9-2.0 ng/dl		Metabolically active form
T₃RIA	Cord	15- 75	Measures triiodothyronine by
	1- 3 d	32-216	radioimmunoassay, ng/dl
	2- 4 wk	160-240	
	1-4 mo	117-209	
	4-12 mo	110-280	
	1- 5 yr	105-269	
	Adult	70-204	
TSH-RIA	0-7 mcU/ml		Best sensitivity for primary hypothyroidism

Thyroid anti- bodies	Antithyroglobulin <1:8 Antimicrosomal <2+ at 1:4	High titers suggest Hashimoto's thyroiditis

Ref: LaFranchi, SH: Ped Clin North Am, 26:46, 1979; Johns Hopkins Hospital In Vitro Laboratory, 1983.

Thyroid Function Tests in Premature Infants
estimated gestational age (wks)

Serum T_4 Mean ±1 SD	30-31	32-33	34-35	36-37	Term
Cord	6.5±1.0	7.5±2.1	6.7±1.2	7.5±2.8	8.2±1.8
12-72 hr	11.5±2.1	12.3±3.2	12.4±3.1	15.5±2.6	19.0±2.1
3-10 d	7.7±1.8	8.5±1.9	10.0±2.4	12.7±2.5	15.9±3.0
11-20 d	7.5±1.8	8.3±1.6	10.5±1.8	11.2±2.9	12.2±2.0
21-45 d	7.8±1.5	8.0±1.7	9.3±1.3	11.4±4.2	12.1±1.5
		(30-37 wks)			
45-90 d		9.6±1.7			10.2±1.9

Ref: Cuestas, RA: J Pediatr 92:963-967, 1978.

2. Puberty - Normal, Precocious, and Delayed

   A. Normal Ages of Pubertal Development in American Children
      1) Onset of puberty
         females   8.0 - 14.9 yrs
         males   9.7 - 14.1 yrs
      2) Completion of puberty
         females   12.4 - 16.8 yrs
         males   13.7 - 17.9 yrs

   Ref: Lee, PA: J Adolesc Health Care 1:26-29, 1980.

   B. Tanner Staging of Secondary Sex Characteristics
      1) Breast development
         I. Pre-adolescent with elevation of papilla only.
         II. Breast bud stage with elevation of breast and papilla as small mound and enlargement of areolar diameter.
         III. Further enlargement and elevation of breast and areola, with no separation of their contours.
         IV. Projection of areola and papilla to form a secondary mound above the level of the breast.
         V. Mature stage with projection of papilla only, due to recession of the areola to the general contour of the breast. (Stages IV and V are not distinct in some.)

2) Genital development (male)

   I. Pre-adolescent with testes, scrotum, and penis approximately the same size and proportion as in early childhood.

   II. Enlargement of scrotum and of testes. The skin of the scrotum reddens and changes in texture. There is little or no enlargement of the penis at this stage.

   III. Enlargement of penis, which occurs at first mainly in length. Further growth of testes and scrotum.

   IV. Increased size of penis with growth in breadth and development of glans. Further enlargement of testes and scrotum and increased darkening of scrotal skin.

   V. Genitalia adult in size and shape.

3) Pubic hair (male and female)

   I. Pre-adolescent. The vellus over the pubes is no further developed than that over the abdominal wall, i.e. no pubic hair.

   II. Sparse growth of long, slightly pigmented downy hair, straight or only slightly curled, appearing chiefly at the base of the penis or along the labia.

   III. Considerably darker, coarser and more curled. The hair spreads sparsely over the junction of the pubes.

   IV. Hair now resembles adult in type, but the area covered by it is still considerably smaller than in the adult. No spread to the medial surface of thighs.

   V. Adult in quantity and type with distribution of the horizontal pattern.

   VI. Spread up the linea alba - "male escutcheon."

Ref: Tanner, JM: Growth at Adolescence, 2nd Edition. Oxford: Blackwell Scientific Publications, 1962, p. 32-37.

DIFFERENTIAL DIAGNOSIS OF PREMATURE ONSET OF SECONDARY SEX CHARACTERISTICS

Disorder	Breast tissue	Sexual hair	Linear growth	Bone age	Serum estrogen[1]	Serum[4]/urinary[3] androgens	Gonadotropin response to LHRH[4]	Estrogen effect in vaginal smear
Premature thelarche (isolated breast tissue development)	Usually 2-4 cm diameter	None	Normal growth percentile & velocity	Comparable with chronologic & height age	Normal for prepubertal level	Normal for prepubertal level	Prepubertal response; greater FSH response than LH; magnitude small	Absent or minimal
Premature adrenarche (isolated development of sexual hair growth)	None	Present	Normal or slightly advanced height percentile & velocity	Comparable with height age	Normal for prepubertal	Early or midpubertal level	Prepubertal response	Usually absent or minimal
Precocious puberty (onset <8 yrs, girls; <9.7 yrs, boys)	Buds, with prominent nipples	Early stage possible; later stage, present	Usually accelerated height percentile & velocity	Accelerated bone age compared to height age or chronologic age	Usually early pubertal level	Pubertal level	Pubertal response; LH response >FSH; magnitude >prepubertal	Usually moderate or good

[1] Serum estrogens=estradiol (E_1) and estradiol-17-β(E_2)
[2] Serum androgens=testosterone, androstenedione, 17OH-progesterone
[3] Urinary androgens=17-ketosteroids, pregnanetriol
[4] LHRH=luteinizing hormone releasing hormone
Ref: Pang, S: Pediatr Ann 10:29-34, 1981.

78

Mean Ages of Pubertal Events (±1 SD) in American Adolescents

	Females	Males
Br Tanner 2	11.2±1.6	
G Tanner 2		11.9±1.1
PH Tanner 2	11.9±1.5	12.3±0.8
G Tanner 3		13.2±0.8
Gynecomastia		13.2±0.8
Voice Break		13.5±1.0
Peak Height Velocity	12.5±1.5	13.8±1.1
Peak Weight Gain	12.4±1.4	13.9±0.9
Axillary Hair	13.1±0.8	14.0±1.1
Br Tanner 3	12.4±1.2	
Menarche	13.3±1.3	
PH Tanner 3	12.7±0.5	13.9±0.9
Voice Change		14.1±0.9
Acne	13.2±0.5	14.3±1.3
G Tanner 4		14.3±0.8
Regular Menses	13.9±1.0	
PH Tanner 4	13.4±1.2	14.7±0.9
Br Tanner 4	13.1±0.7	
Facial Hair		14.9±1.1
Br Tanner 5	14.5±1.6	
G Tanner 5		15.1±1.1
PH Tanner 5	14.0±1.1	15.3±0.8

Br = Breast   G = Genitalia   PH = Pubic hair

Ref: Lee, PA: J Adolesc Health Care 1:26-29, 1980.

4) Vaginal smear
Tests for estrogenization of vaginal mucosa, useful in evaluation of precocious puberty as well as in determination of the phase of the menstrual cycle.
a) Preparation:
Instill a few drops of normal saline in the vagina. Spread vaginal secretions on a clean glass slide. Add a few drops of saline to make a wet mount. Methylene blue may be used to stain the nuclei. The unstained preparation can also be read. A permanent slide can be made in a manner similar to that for a pap smear by sending slide in fixative (95% ethanol) to cytopathology lab.
b) Interpretation:
(1) Low estrogen states - round or oval basal cells, with vesicular nuclei comprising 1/3 of total cell area.
(2) High estrogen states - polygonal, cornified cells with small, deeply pigmented, homogeneous nuclei.

Ref: Gupta, PK, Johns Hopkins Cytopathology Laboratory, Personal Communication, 1984.

5) Dexamethasone suppression test
The source of androgen excess (in premature adrenarche and precocious puberty) is frequently not obvious; therefore adrenal gland suppression with oral dexamethasone may be necessary.

Day	1	2	3	4	5	6
Urinary 17-KS	X	X			X	X
Urinary 17-OHCS	X	X				X
Urinary pregnanetriol	X					X
Dexamethasone 1.25 mg per M²/day divided Q6h			X	X	X	X

Interpretation: Increased, but suppressible, urinary 17-KS and pregnanetriol confirm the diagnosis of CAH. Incomplete suppression of 17-KS, but complete suppression of pregnanetriol, suggests that the patient has already entered into puberty. Markedly increased, nonsuppressible 17-KS suggest the presence of an androgen-producing tumor, most likely adrenal in origin.

Ref: Bacon, GE, et al.: Pediatric Endocrinology, 2nd Edition. Chicago: Year Book Medical Publishers, Inc., 1982, p. 209.

6) Gonadotrophin releasing hormone stimulation test
Measures pituitary LH and FSH reserve. Helpful in the differential diagnosis of precocious sexual development.
a) Method
Inject LHRH 2.5 mcg/kg IV bolus (adult dose = 100 mcg) and collect samples at -15, 0, 15, 30, 45, 60, 90, and 120 minutes.
b) Interpretation
A pubertal or adult response shows an LH response within the adult range within 30 minutes. Normal prepubertal children should show no or minimal response.

Ref: Bacon, GE, et al.: Pediatric Endocrinology, 2nd Edition. Chicago: Year Book Medical Publishers, Inc., 1982, p. 205; Kelch, RP, et al; J Clin Endocrinol Metab 40:53-61, 1975; Ayerst Laboratories Synthetic LHRH Product Information, 1983.

7) HCG stimulation test
Measures the responsiveness of the gonad to gonadotropin stimulation and determines the functional capacity of cryptorchid testes.
a) Method
This is a 6 week test. Inject HCG (human chorionic gonadotropin) 3000 U/M² (minimum 1000 U, maximum 5000 U) IM on days 1-5

during week 1 and days 1, 3, and 5 of weeks 2-6. Examine the patient and measure serum testosterone on days 0 and 6 and at the end of the third and sixth weeks.

b) Interpretation
Normal rise in serum testosterone, FSH, LH, and androstenedione to adult levels and descent of cryptorchid testes with an increase in its size. The best time for administration of HCG is controversial.

Ref: Lee, PA, et al.: Johns Hopkins Medical Journal, 146:159, 1980; Garagorri, et al: J Pediatr 101:923-927, 1982.

3. Ambiguous Genitalia

A. Buccal Smear, Y-Fluorescence, and Karyotype
A karyotype is much more accurate and preferred over a buccal smear. When a result is needed quickly, Y fluorescence can be done within 3 days (karyotype usually takes 2 weeks) and is also preferred over the buccal smear.

B. Other Useful Diagnostic Studies
1) Urinary 17-KS and pregnanetriol in 24 hour studies. If elevated, a diagnosis of congenital adrenal hyperplasia (CAH) can be made. However, it may take one to two weeks for the 17-KS in a patient with CAH to rise above the normally high newborn levels. Additional information supporting the diagnosis of CAH would be hyponatremia, hyperkalemia, high 17-OH- progesterone, and high androstenedione.
2) Retrograde genitourography through the urogenital orifice to assess internal structures.
3) Pelvic ultrasonography.

Ref: Bacon, GE, et al.: Pediatric Endocrinology, 2nd Edition. Chicago: Year Book Medical Publishers, Inc., 1982, pp. 182-184.

C. Penile Standards for Newborn Male Infants
The mean term stretched penile size is 3.5 x 1.1 cm. The third and ninety-seventh percentile for the penile length are 2.8 and 4.2 cm and for the diameter 0.9 and 1.3 cm, respectively. A phallic length which is 2.5 or more standard deviations below the mean should be considered abnormal; for an infant of 0-5 months, the lower limit is 1.9 cm.

Ref: Feldman, KW and Smith, DW: J Pediatr 86:395-398, 1975; Lee, PA, et al.: Johns Hopkins Medical Journal 146:156-163, 1980.

4. Growth

A. Delayed Growth
Depending on history, physical exam, and growth data (increments, velocity) lab studies which may be indicated are electrolytes, calcium, phosphorus, alkaline phosphatase, total protein, albumin, CBC with differential, ESR, BUN, creatinine, liver function tests, urinalysis, thyroid function tests, bone age, somatomedin C, growth hormone test, karyotype, sweat test, and other tests of pituitary insufficiency.

B. Tests for Growth Hormone (GH)
GH is often low; therefore, provocative tests are necessary to document deficiency. Diagnosis requires two abnormal definitive tests (not screening tests).

1) Screening tests
   a) Sleep specimen
      Most subjects will have a rise in GH 45-60 minutes after the onset of nocturnal sleep. A single value >10 ng/ml rules out GH deficiency.
   b) Exercise test
      80% or more of normal persons will release significant amounts of GH after vigorous exercise. Fast the patient for at least 4 hours and draw a baseline GH sample. Exercise the patient for 20 minutes (steady jogging). Obtain a second GH sample immediately. Values >10 ng/ml rule out GH deficiency.

Ref: Eisenstein, E, et al.: Pediatrics 62:526, 1978.

2) Stimulation tests
   GH >10 ng/ml effectively rules out GH deficiency. (Note that some labs use 7 ng/ml as the cut-off for normal/abnormal rather than 10.) Values between 5-10 ng/ml are equivocal and may indicate partial deficiency. Results less than 5 ng/ml are definitely abnormal. GH deficiency diagnosis requires two abnormal tests (i.e. AITT or L-dopa and glucagon).
   a) Arginine-insulin tolerance test (AITT)
      Draw baseline GH. Infuse 0.5 g/kg arginine HCl (not to exceed 20 g) IV over 30 minutes. Sample GH at 15, 30, 45, 60, and 90 minutes. At 90 minutes, give 0.1 U/kg insulin (diluted to 1 U/ml) rapidly via IV push. Collect GH and glucose samples at 20, 30, 45, and 60 minutes. As each sample is collected, centrifuge and separate serum. Observe the patient continuously for hypoglycemia. $D_{50}W$ should be by the bedside and IV access established. A valid test requires either clinical or chemical ($\geq$50% drop in glucose) hypoglycemia.

Ref: Bacon, GE, et al.: Pediatric Endocrinology, 2nd Edition. Chicago: Year Book Medical Publishers, Inc. 1982, pp 85-86.

    b) L-dopa stimulation test
       Give L-dopa orally (125 mg, <15 kg; 250 mg, 15-30 kg; 500 mg, >30 kg) to fasting patient. Collect GH samples at 0, 20, 40, 60, 90, and 120 minutes.

Ref: Weldon, VV, et al.: J Pediatr 87:540-544, 1975.

    c) Glucagon stimulation test
       Draw baseline GH. Give 0.1 mg/kg glucagon IM. Sample GH at 15, 30, 45, 60, 90, 120, 150, and 180 minutes. Reactive hypoglycemia is possible.

Ref: Vanderschuren, M, et al.: J Pediatr 85:182-187, 1974.

C. Methods of Adult Height Prediction
See Reference section, pages 332-333, for bone age determination.
When height age = bone age (both less than chronologic age), this usually means constitutional short stature.
When chronologic age = bone age, this usually means familial short stature.
When bone age is much less than height age, consider endocrine abnormality.
1) Bayley-Pinneau Method: uses Greulich and Pyle
2) RWT Method: uses Greulich and Pyle and midparental heights

Ref: Roche, A, et al.: Monogr Paediatr 3:1-114, 1975; Himes, JH, et al.: Monogr Paediatr 13:1-88, 1981.

3) TW-2 Method: Uses Tanner-Whitehouse

Ref: Tanner, JM, et al.: Assessment of Skeletal Maturity and Prediction of Adult Height (TW-2 Method). New York: Academic Press, 1975.

5. Diabetic Ketoacidosis (DKA)

A. Evaluation
1) New or known diabetic? Usual insulin regimen? Last insulin dose? Any infection or other inciting event?
2) Quick history and physical examination.

B. Baseline Studies
1) Fluids
    Normal saline at 20 ml/kg/hr for 1-2 hours. Then 1/2 normal saline + K^+ and/or D_5W as appropriate

(see below) (1/2 normal saline alone is hypotonic), calculated to replace deficit plus maintenance and on-going losses over 24 hours (usually 10% dehydrated). See fluid and electrolyte table, page 224, for estimated deficits.

2) <u>Insulin</u>

Insulin drip is preferred since it allows constant control. There is also less risk of hypoglycemia and too rapid decrease of the serum glucose concentration (hence may lessen risk of cerebral edema).

a) 0.1 unit/kg regular insulin IV bolus
b) Follow with continuous drip 0.1 U/kg/hr regular insulin piggybacked into IV line (50 units insulin/250 ml normal saline). Fresh solutions required every 6 hours.

3) <u>Glucose</u>

Measure dextrosticks or chemstrips hourly. Rate of glucose fall should be between 80-100 mg/dl/hr. Increase insulin to 0.14-0.20 U/kg if glucose falls at <50 mg/dl/hr. If glucose drops too rapidly (>100 mg/dl/hr) continue insulin infusion (0.1 U/kg/hr) and add D_5W to IV. Also, as glucose approaches 250-300 mg/dl, add D_5W to IV.

4) <u>Electrolytes</u>

a) <u>Potassium</u>

Patients with DKA are potassium depleted. Give patients maintenance plus deficit over 24 hours. A general guide is to give 40 meq/L if initial K^+ is < normal. Give no K^+ initially if K^+ is elevated or patient is not making urine.

b) <u>Phosphate</u>

PO_4 is depleted in DKA and will drop further with insulin therapy. PO_4 encourages better oxygenation of tissues. Replace K^+, 1/2 as KCl and 1/2 as K_2PO_4 for the first 8 hours, then all as KCl. However, let caution be your guide as too much PO_4 will cause decreased Ca and tetany.

c) <u>Bicarbonate</u>

This is not administered unless pH is <7.10± HCO_3^- <5. If necessary to give $NaHCO_3$, administer 2 meq/kg IV over 30-60 minutes or add to the first bottle of 1/2 normal saline.

5) <u>Miscellaneous</u>

Follow vital signs, dextrosticks Q1-2h, glucose, pH, pCO_2, electrolytes Q3-4h, EKG periodically to follow K^+.

C. Further Insulin Management

1) When blood glucose approaches 300 mg/dl, blood pH >7.3, and ketosis has cleared, discontinue insulin drip, add 5% glucose, and start "sliding" scale. This is usually in a dosage of 0.25-0.5 units/kg regular insulin to be given subcutaneously Q6-8h.

2) The next day, 1/2-2/3 of the previous day's total insulin dose is given as an intermediate acting form (NPH, Lente) with further regular insulin coverage at 0.25 U/kg according to blood glucose concentration measured before each meal. The usual time required to stabilize the insulin dosage is 3-5 days. Usual daily maintenance dose in children: 0.5 U-1.0 U/kg/24h. Adolescents during growth spurt: 0.8-1.2 U/kg/24h.

Ref: Plotnick, L and Kritzler, R: In: Cole, CH (ed) Therapeutic Shorts, Johns Hopkins Hospital Pediatric Outpatient Dept., 1982; Sperling, MA: Pediatric Clin North Am 26:149-169, 1979.

6. Adrenal and Pituitary Function

A. Pathway of Steroid Hormone Synthesis

Mineralocorticoids	Glucocorticoids	Androgens

Glucocorticoids

CHOLESTEROL
→ 20,22 desmolase
Δ-5-PREGNENOLONE
→ 3,β-ol-dehydrogenase
PROGESTERONE
→ 17-hydroxylase
17-OH-PROGESTERONE
→ 21-hydroxylase
11-DESOXYCORTISOL
→ 11-hydroxylase
CORTISOL

Mineralocorticoids

→ 21-hydroxylase
11-DESOXYCORTICOSTERONE
→ 11-hydroxylase
CORTICOSTERONE
→ 18 "oxidation" defect
ALDOSTERONE

Androgens

→ 17-hydroxylase
17-OH-PREGNENOLONE
↓
DEHYDROEPIANDROSTERONE
→ 3,β-ol-dehydrogenase
ANDROSTENEDIONE
↓
TESTOSTERONE

Ref: Bacon GE, et al.: Pediatric Endocrinology, 2nd Edition. Chicago: Year Book Medical Publishers, Inc., 1982, p. 153.

B. Tests of Adrenal and Pituitary Function (normal values pages 73-74)
   1) Urinary 17-hydroxycorticosteroids (17-OHCS)
      This measures approximately 1/3 of end products of metabolism of cortisol. Collect a 24 hour urine specimen. Refrigerate during collection and process immediately (17-OHCS are destroyed at room temperature).
      Interpretation:
      a) Decreased in inanition states (anorexia nervosa); pituitary disorders involving ACTH; Addison's disease; administration of synthetic, potent corticosteroids (prednisone, dexamethasone, triamcinolone); 21-hydroxylase deficiency; liver disease; hypothyroidism; newborn period (due to decreased glucuronidation).
      b) Increased in Cushing's syndrome; ACTH, cortisone, cortisol therapy; medical or surgical stress; obesity (occasionally), hyperthyroidism; and 11-hydroxylase deficiency.
   2) Urinary 17-ketosteroids (17-KS)
      This measures some end products of androgen metabolism. Collect and refrigerate 24 hour urine specimen.
      Interpretation:
      a) Decreased in Addison's disease, anorexia nervosa, panhypopituitarism.
      b) Increased in adrenal hyperplasia; virilizing adrenal tumors; Cushing's syndrome; exogenous ACTH, cortisone, androgens (except methyltestosterone); stressful illness (burns, radiation illness, etc.); androgen-producing gonadal tumors.
   3) Plasma corticosteroids
      Collect heparinized blood and separate plasma immediately. Measure cortisol (corticosterone and 11-deoxycortisol may sometimes be needed).
      Interpretation:
      Abnormal values occur in the same disorders as for abnormal 17-OHCS; however, usually normal in anorexia nervosa, liver disease, hypo- and hyperthyroidism, and obesity. Elevated levels by protein binding assay occur during pregnancy and during estrogen administration.
   4) Plasma 17-OH Progesterone (17-OHP)
      Collect heparinized blood and separate plasma immediately. Measures precursor which is elevated with certain adrenal enzyme deficiency states (21-and 11-hydroxylase deficiency).

C. Adrenal Capacity Test
   1) IM ACTH test
      Measures maximal capacity of adrenal to produce cortisol.

Procedure:
Days 1 and 2 collect baseline 24 hour urine for 17-OHCS. Days 3, 4, and 5 administer 20 USP U/M² Acthargel every 8 hours. Collect 24 hour urines on days 5 and 6 for 17-OHCS.

a) Normal
   Urinary 17-OHCS = 85±15 mg/M²/24h.
b) Abnormal
   Lack of response in Addison's disease; subnormal in adrenal hyperplasia; hyperresponse at times in Cushing's syndrome.

2) IV ACTH test
   Procedure:
   Give ACTH (Cortrosyn) IV bolus (0.1 mg, <1 year; 0.15 mg, 1-5 years; 0.25 mg, >5 years). Draw serum cortisol at 0, 15, 30, 45, 60, 90, and 120 minutes.

   a) Normal
      Plasma cortisol 32±4 mcg/dl by 2 hours (or >20 mcg/dl or 10 mcg/dl increment). In patients whose adrenals have been suppressed for more than one month, the IV test is usually not prolonged enough to produce adrenal reactivation.
   b) Abnormal
      A lack of response in the presence of Cushing's syndrome is characteristic of adrenal carcinoma. A normal response does not rule out carcinoma. A hyperresponse is indicative of bilateral adrenal hyperplasia. A normal response does not rule out hyperplasia. Lack of response is suggestive but not diagnostic of primary adrenal disease.

   Ref: Migeon, CJ, in Collu, R, et al. (eds): Pediatric Endocrinology. New York: Raven Press, 1981, p. 475; Bacon, GE, et al.: Pediatric Endocrinology, 2nd Edition. Chicago: Year Book Medical Publishers, Inc., 1982, p. 170.

D. Pituitary ACTH Capacity (Metyrapone) Test
   Metyrapone inhibits 11-hydroxylase in the adrenal and blocks cortisol production. With increased ACTH, 11-deoxy precursors of cortisol accumulate and are excreted as 17-OHCS.
   Procedure:
   Collect 24 hour urine for 17-OHCS on days 1 and 2. On day 3 give metyrapone orally 300 mg/M² (max. dose = 750 mg) Q4h x 24h (6 doses) (1800 mg/M²/day) and continue urine collection. Day 4 is the final 24 hour urine.
   1) Normal
      Urinary 17-OHCS increase to >9 mg/M²/24h on day 3 or 4. This test may be modified by giving a single midnight dose of metyrapone IV (35 mg/kg, max. 1 gram). Cortisol and 11-desoxycortisol are measured in an 8 AM sample. Normally a many-fold

rise in 11-desoxycortisol and a precipitous drop in cortisol are seen.

2) Abnormal
Little or no increase in urinary 17-OHCS is seen with pituitary ACTH deficiency, hypothalamic tumors, and pharmacologic doses of steroids.

CAUTION - In patients with reduced adrenal secretory capacity, the drug may cause acute adrenal insufficiency. Precede this test by an adrenal capacity ACTH test in these persons.

Ref: Migeon, CJ, in Collu, R, et al. (eds): _Pediatric Endocrinology_. New York: Raven Press, 1981, p. 475.

E. Insulin-Induced Hypoglycemia
During AITT for growth hormone, plasma cortisol can be measured at 0 and 60 minutes. Normally plasma cortisol increases by 10 mcg/dl and the maximum level is ≥ 20 mcg/dl.

Ref: Bacon, GE, et al.: _Pediatric Endocrinology_, 2nd Edition. Chicago: Year Book Medical Publishers, Inc., 1982, p. 87.

F. Pituitary Dexamethasone Suppression Test
Dexamethasone, a synthetic corticoid, suppresses the secretion of ACTH by the normal pituitary. This decreases endogenous production of cortisol and, hence, also the excretion of 17-OHCS. Dexamethasone is not excreted as 17-OHCS.
Procedure:
Collect 24 hour urine for 17-OHCS on days 1 and 2. Administer dexamethasone 1.25 mg/100 lbs/day po divided Q6h on days 3, 4, and 5 followed by dexamethasone 3.75 mg/100 lbs/day po divided Q6h on days 6, 7, and 8. Collect 24 hour urines on days 1, 2, 4, 5, 7, and 8 for 17-OHCS.
1) Normal:
By day 5, urinary 17-OHCS have fallen to <2 mg/M^2/24h.
2) Abnormal:
Cushing's syndrome of any cause, by day 5, 17-OHCS are >2 mg/24h. Cushing's syndrome secondary to adrenal hyperplasia, by day 8, 17-OHCS are <2 mg/24h unless hyperplasia is secondary to ectopic ACTH production (lung, mediastinal tumor, etc). Cushing's syndrome due to adrenocortical carcinoma, by day 8, 17-OHCS are >2 mg/24h. In certain hypothalamic tumors, no suppression is possible.

Ref: Bacon, GE, et al.: _Pediatric Endocrinology_, 2nd Edition. Chicago: Year Book Medical Publishers, Inc., 1982, p. 170.

G. Water Deprivation Test

Useful for the diagnosis of diabetes insipidus. Requires careful supervision since dehydration and hypernatremia may occur.

1) Procedure:

Begin the test in the morning after a 24 hour period of adequate hydration and stable weight. Fluids are restricted for 7 hours. Have the patient empty his bladder and obtain a baseline weight. Urinary specific gravity and volume and body weight are measured hourly. Serum sodium is measured every 1-2 hours. Urine and serum osmolality are measured every 2 hours. Hematocrit and BUN also may be obtained at these times but are not critical. Subjects must be carefully observed to assure that fluids are not ingested during the test. The test should be terminated if weight loss approaches 5%.

2) Interpretation:

Normal individuals who are water deprived will concentrate their urine between 500 and 1400 mOsm/L and plasma osmolality will range between 288 and 291 mOsm/L. In normal children and those with psychogenic DI, urinary specific gravity rises to at least 1.010 and usually greater. The urinary: plasma osmolality ratio exceeds 2. Urine volume decreases significantly, and there should be no appreciable weight loss. Specific gravity remains below 1.005 in patients with ADH-deficient or nephrogenic DI. Urine osmolality remains below 150 mOsm/L, and there should be no significant reduction of urine volume. A weight loss up to 5% usually occurs. At the end of the test, a serum osmolality >290 mOsm/L, Na >150 mEq/L and a rise of BUN and hematocrit provide evidence that the patient did not receive water.

Ref: Bacon GE, et al.: Pediatric Endocrinology, 2nd Edition. Chicago: Year Book Medical Publishers, Inc., 1982, p. 258.

H. Vasopressin Test

1) Procedure:

The test is preceded by a 24 hour control period during which intake, output, and urinary specific gravity are measured while the patient receives fluids ad lib. (It may also follow the above water deprivation test.) The bladder is emptied and aqueous vasopressin is administered, 0.3 ml/M² SC. (Note that aqueous vasopressin contains 20 U/ml, whereas vasopressin tannate in oil contains 5 U/ml). Intake is monitored, and urinary output and specific gravity are determined every 30 to 60 minutes. A response should occur in 4 to 6 hours.

If there is no effect after 6 hours, the test is repeated using 0.6 ml/M².

2) Interpretation:
Patients with ADH-deficient DI concentrate their urine (to 1.010 and usually greater) and also demonstrate a reduction of urine volume and decreased fluid intake. Patients with nephrogenic DI have no significant change in intake, urine volume, or specific gravity. Constant intake associated with decreased output and increased specific gravity suggests psychogenic DI.

Ref: Bacon, GE, et al.: Pediatric Endocrinology, 2nd Edition. Chicago, Year Book Medical Publishers, Inc., 1982, pp. 258-259.

7. Thyroid Function

A. Thyroid Scan
Useful for assessing thyroidal clearance, for localizing ectopic thyroid tissue, and for structure-function studies of the thyroid such as localization of hyperfunctioning and nonfunctioning thyroid nodules and delineation of the irregular thyroidal iodine kinetics and abnormal distribution of isotope frequently associated with chronic lymphocytic (Hashimoto's) thyroiditis. In the newborn infant, it can differentiate athyreotic or ectopic hypothyroidism from other causes of decreased thyroid function. This information could be important in genetic counseling, as athyreosis or ectopic thyroid tissue usually occurs sporadically, whereas hypofunction due to impaired biosynthesis of thyroid implies an inherited defect. Sensitivity, specificity, convenience, and safety considerations indicate that ^{99M}Technetium-pertechnetate is preferable to the iodide isotopes (e.g., ^{123}I and ^{131}I).

Ref: Heyman, S, et al.: J Pediatr 101:571-574, 1982; Bauman, RA, et al.: J Pediatr 89:268, 1976; Fisher, DA: J Pediatr 82:1-9, 1973.

B. Technetium Uptake
Measures uptake of technetium by thyroid gland. Uptake is measured only for the first 20 minutes. Normal: 0.24-3.4%.

C. Pituitary TSH Reserve Test
No rise in TSH in the face of a high T_4 is confirmatory of hyperthyroidism. No rise in TSH in the face of a low T_4 and low TSH suggests pituitary dysfunction.
1) Method
Blood samples for determination of TSH are drawn at -15, 0, +30, and +60 minutes. Synthetic TRH is

given IV over 15 to 30 seconds starting at time zero. The recommended dose of TRH is 7 mcg/kg, maximum dose 200 mcg. The test should be performed in the morning after an overnight fast, although this is not absolutely necessary. Side effects include nausea, a sensation of facial flushing, the urge to urinate, and occasionally vomiting. These effects last from several seconds to two minutes, but they occur in almost all patients.

2) Interpretation:
The absolute values for TSH responses vary considerably between laboratories and are affected somewhat by the patient's age and sex. Although the pattern for TSH release also must be considered, a maximal rise in serum TSH of between 5 and 25 mcU/ml is considered normal in most labs.

Ref: Bacon, GE, et al.: Pediatric Endocrinology, 2nd Edition. Chicago: Year Book Medical Publishers, Inc., 1982, p. 135.

D. Preparation for Surgery in Hyperthyroid Patients
Patients must be euthyroid at the time of operation. Propylthiuracil can be given at 5 mg/kg/24h divided Q8h (or 150-300 mg/24h for 6-10 yr old or 300-400 mg/24h for >10 yr old) or methimazole at 1/10th the PTU dosages. Lugol's solution, 5 qtts/24h PO should be given for 10 to 14 days before surgery. Propranolol 2.5 mg/kg/24h to start (may be increased to 10 mg/kg/24h max., as needed, to control symptoms) PO divided Q6-8h (unless contraindicated i.e.: asthma, congestive heart failure). Adult dose = 80 mg PO Q8h. The dose on the morning of surgery should not be omitted. It should also be continued for 5 days after surgery.

Ref: Buckingham, BA, et al.: Am J Dis Child 135:112-117, 1981; Feek, CM, et al.: New Engl J Med 302:883-885, 1980; Bacon, GE, et al.: Pediatric Endocrinology, 2nd Edition. Chicago: Year Book Medical Publishers, Inc., 1982, p. 128.

DEVELOPMENTAL EVALUATION

The following screening tests provide the pediatrician with appropriate tools to determine if a child should be referred for more extensive examination for developmental delay.

Development takes place in an orderly and sequential manner and three developmental phenomena should be recognized: delay (significant lag in one or more areas of development), dissociation (a delay in just one or two areas of development), and deviancy (non-sequential development in one or more areas of development). It is essential that testing be done in all areas of development. "Rate of development" is reflected by the developmental quotient (DQ = Developmental age ÷ chronological age x 100) or intelligence quotient (IQ). Two developmental assessments separated by a significant time interval is more predictive than a single assessment.

Language remains the best predictor of future intellectual endowment and should serve as the common denominator comparing its rate of development with other areas which include gross motor, problem solving, adaptive, and social skills.

A child who has a significant delay in all areas of development is probably retarded (delay phenomenon), while a child who is significantly delayed in language but normal in problem solving probably has a language disorder (the dissociation phenomenon). Since the rate of development is sequential and orderly, nonsequential or deviant development places the child at high risk for a developmental disorder, or disability (the deviancy phenomenon).

A developmental history is essential. Parents usually give an accurate developmental history. Thus, the presenting complaint, developmental history, and physical examination along with developmental assessment should result in accurate diagnosis by the pediatrician. For proper therapy to be implemented, a more complete and in-depth evaluation is in order. The following tests are included because of their ease of administration and demonstrated reliability. Milestones are included to assist with developmental history and also emphasize language skills. Note that each of the developmental areas have a minimum of two tests recommended. A list of useful reference data is presented at the conclusion of this chapter.

1. DEVELOPMENTAL MILESTONES/LANGUAGE SKILLS

AGE	GROSS MOTOR	VISUAL MOTOR	LANGUAGE	SOCIAL
1 mo	Raises head slightly from prone, makes crawling movements, lifts chin up	Has tight grasp, follows to midline	Alerts to sound (e.g. by blinking, moving, startling)	Regards face
2 mos	Holds head in midline, lifts chest off table	No longer clenches fist tightly, follows object past midline	Smiles after being stroked or talked to	Recognizes parent
3 mos	Supports on forearms in prone, holds head up steadily	Holds hands open at rest, follows in circular fashion	Coos (produces long vowel sounds in musical fashion)	Reaches for familiar people or objects, anticipates feeding
4-5 mos	Rolls front to back, back to front, sits well when propped, supports on wrists and shifts weight	Moves arms in unison to grasp, touches cube placed on table	Orients to voice 5 mos - turns head toward bell, says "ah-goo," razzing	Enjoys looking around environment
6 mos	Sits well unsupported, puts feet in mouth in supine position	Reaches with either hand, transfers, uses raking grasp	Babbles 8 mos - "dada/mama" indiscriminately	Recognizes strangers
9 mos	Creeps, crawls, cruises, pulls to stand, pivots when sitting	Uses pincer grasp, probes with fore-finger, holds bottle, fingerfeeds	Imitates sounds waves bye-bye 10 mos - "dada/mama" discriminately 11 mos - one word	Starts to explore environment plays pat-a-cake
12 mos	Walks alone	Throws objects, lets go of toys, hand release, uses mature pincer grasp	Follows one-step command with gesture, uses two words 14 mos - uses three words	Imitates actions, comes when called, cooperates with dressing

1. DEVELOPMENTAL MILESTONES/LANGUAGE SKILLS (continued)

AGE	GROSS MOTOR	VISUAL MOTOR	LANGUAGE	SOCIAL
15 mos	Creeps upstairs, walks backwards	Builds tower of 2 blocks in imitation of examiner, scribbles in imitation	Follows one-step command without gesture, uses 4-6 words and immature jargoning (runs several unintelligible words together)	
18 mos	Runs, throws toy from standing without falling	Turns 2-3 pages at a time, fills spoon and feeds himself	Knows 7-20 words, points to one body part when named, uses mature jargoning (includes intelligible words in jargoning)	Copies parent in tasks (e.g. sweeping, dusting), plays in company of other children
21 mos	Squats in play, goes up steps	Builds tower of 5 blocks, drinks well from cup	Points to 3 body parts, uses two-word combinations, points to 5 body parts	Asks to have food and to go to toilet
24 mos	Walks up and down steps without help	Turns pages one at a time, removes shoes, pants, etc., imitates stroke	Uses 50 words, two-word sentences, and three pronouns, names objects in pictures	Parallel play
30 mos	Jumps with both feet off floor, throws ball overhand	Unbuttons, holds pencil in adult fashion, differentiates horizontal and vertical line	Pronouns "I, you, me" discriminately	Tells first and last names when asked, gets himself drink without help

1. DEVELOPMENTAL MILESTONES/LANGUAGE SKILLS (continued)

AGE	GROSS MOTOR	VISUAL MOTOR	LANGUAGE	SOCIAL
3 yrs	Pedals tricycle, can alternate feet when going up steps	Dresses and undresses partially, dries hands if reminded, draws a circle	Uses 3 word sentences, uses plurals, past tense. Knows all pronouns. Minimum 250 words	Group play, shares toys, takes turns, plays well with others, knows full name, age, sex
4 yrs	Hops, skips, alternates feet going downstairs	Buttons clothing fully, catches ball	Knows colors, says song or poem from memory, asks questions	Tells "tall tales", plays cooperatively with a group of children
5 yrs	Skips, alternating feet, jumps over low obstacles	Ties shoes, spreads with knife	Prints first name, asks what a word means	Plays competitive games, abides by rules, likes to help in household tasks

Ref: Capute, AJ and Biehl, RF: Pediatr Clin North Am 20:3-25, 1973; Capute, AJ, et al.: Dev Med Child Neurol. In Press, 1984; Capute, AJ and Accardo, PJ: Clin Pediatr 17:847-853, 1978.

GESELL FIGURES

15 MOS. IMITATES SCRIBBLE

18 MOS. SCRIBBLES SPONTANEOUSLY

2 YRS. IMITATES STROKE

2½ YRS. DIFFERENTIATES HORIZONTAL AND VERTICAL LINE

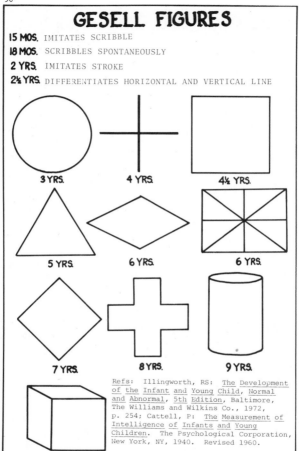

3 YRS.　4 YRS.　4½ YRS.

5 YRS.　6 YRS.　6 YRS.

7 YRS.　8 YRS.　9 YRS.

11 YRS.

Refs: Illingworth, RS: The Development of the Infant and Young Child, Normal and Abnormal, 5th Edition, Baltimore, The Williams and Wilkins Co., 1972, p. 254; Cattell, P: The Measurement of Intelligence of Infants and Young Children. The Psychological Corporation, New York, NY, 1940. Revised 1960.

2. Assessment Tests
    Visual-motor Tests (Problem Solving): Gesell Figures - The
    child copies the forms. Scoring depends upon correct per-
    ception of these images and technique of construction. It is
    more important to observe <u>how</u> the child copies the forms than
    to merely observe the final product. See page 96.

3. Gross Motor

Reflex	Present by (months)	Gone by (months)
A. Primitive Reflexes:		
Palmar grasp	birth	4
Plantar grasp	birth	9
Automatic stepping	birth	2
Moro	birth	3-6
Tonic Neck:		
Asymmetric ("fencer")	birth	4
Symmetric	5	8
B. Placing Reactions		
Lower extremity placing	1 (day)	–
Upper extremity placing	3 (mos)	–
Downward lower extremity	3	–
C. Postural Reflexes		
Head up in prone position	1½	–
Landau (extension of head, trunk, legs in prone)	3	12-24
Derotational righting	4	–
Anterior propping	6	–
Lateral propping	8	–
Posterior propping	10	–

Adapted in part from: Milani-Comparetti, A and Gidoni,
EA: <u>Dev Med Child Neurol</u> 9:631, 1967; Capute, AJ, et
al.: <u>Dev Med Child Neurol</u>. In press, 1984.

D. Cerebral Palsy: non-progressive disorder of movement
    and posture due to a cerebral insult that occurs during
    the development period.
        Physiologic classification: spastic, extrapyramidal
        (non-spastic), mixed types.
        Subclassification: spastic type may be monoplegia,
        hemiplegia, diplegia, quadriplegia.

4. Denver Developmental Screening Test
    A useful screen for social, fine motor skills, in addition to
    gross motor and language areas.

5. Reference Data
    This section presents information regarding classification of
    severity of mental retardation as well as a glossary of
    psychodiagnostic tests most commonly encountered by pediat-
    ric practitioners.

    A. Levels of Mental Retardation Based on Wechsler Scales of
        Intellectual Functioning.

Degree of Mental Retardation	Measured Intelligence Quotient	Expected Mental Age as an Adult (yrs)
"Dull Normal"	80-90	–
"Borderline"	70-79	–
Mild (Educable)	55-69	9-11
Moderate (Trainable)	40-54	5-8
Severe	25-39	3-5
Profound	Below 25	Below 3

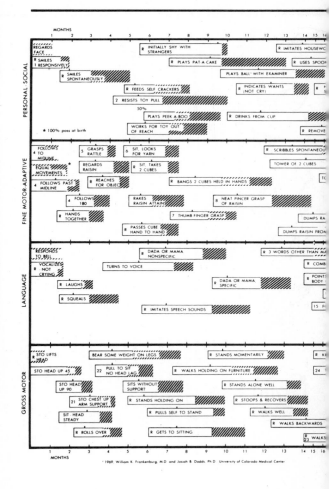

Denver Developmental Screening Test

1969. William K. Frankenburg, M.D. and Josiah B. Dodds, Ph.D. University of Colorado Medical Center

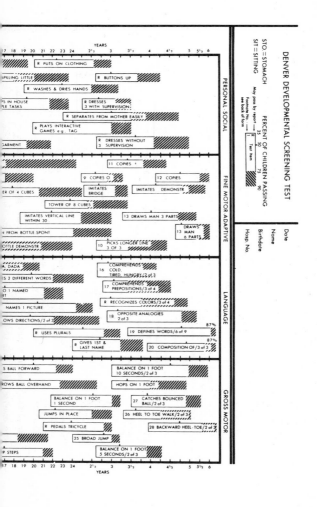

B. PSYCHO-DIAGNOSTIC PROCEDURES

	Age Range	Value
1. Intelligence		
Bayley Scales of Infant Development	2 - 30 mos	Measurement of general developmental levels,
Cattell Infant Intelligence Scale	2 - 30 mos	weighted toward sensory-motor items
Stanford-Binet Intelligence Scale	2 years - adult	Test of general intelligence, without subtest breakdown
McCarthy Scales of Children's Ability	2 1/2 - 8 yrs	Test subdivided into five components which add up to a general cognitive quotient
Wechsler Preschool and Primary Scale of Infant Intelligence (WPPSI)	3 - 6 1/2 yrs	Tests subdivided into five verbal and five performance components, with full-scale IQ
Wechsler Intelligence Scale for Children-Revised (WISC-R)	6 - 16 yrs	indicating overall intellectual level
Vineland Social Maturity Scale	infancy - 25 yrs	Performance of socially adaptive tasks as reported by mother
2. Achievement		
Metropolitan Readiness Test	5 yrs	Test of pre-reading, pre-writing and number skills needed for first grade understanding
Peabody Individual Achievement Test	School age	Individual tests in five areas
Wide-Range Achievement Test (WRAT)	School age	Screen of academic skills, comparing peers
Metropolitan Achievement Tests	School age	of same age or grade level
Gray Oral Reading Test	School age	Individual test of reading achievement

B. PSYCHO-DIAGNOSTIC PROCEDURES (continued)

	Age Range	Value
Key Math Test	School age	Individual test of arithmetic abilities
Woodcock-Johnson Psychoeducational Battery	School age	Individual test of many academic areas
3. Visual Motor		
Bender-Gestalt Test	5 yrs - adult	Visual motor test to identify perceptual disorganization due to organic or emotional cause
Frostig Developmental Test of Visual Perception	4 - 8 yrs	Screen of visual perceptive skills, with breakdown into five areas
Goodenough Draw-A-Person Test	3 - 13 yrs	Measurement of IQ in addition to insight into child's self-concept and emotions
4. Speech and Language		
Zimmerman Preschool Language Scale	1 - 7 yrs	Test of auditory comprehension and verbal ability (expressed as language age)
Illinois Test of Psycho-Linguistic Abilities	2 - 10 yrs	Survey of receptive and expressive language skills
Wepman Auditory Discrimination Test	3 1/2 yrs - adult	Screen for ability to discriminate between phonemes.
5. Projective		
Children's Apperception Test (CAT)	3 - 10 yrs	Survey of potential emotional conflict areas
Thematic Apperception Test (TAT)	preadolescence - adult	

RADIOLOGIC PROCEDURES

1. <u>Psychological Preparation</u>
   A child should be prepared for the examination either by hospital personnel or by his parents. Parents and child should be told about the examination, how the examination is done, and what the child will experience so there will be no surprises.

2. <u>Protection from Radiation</u>
   In order to <u>avoid inadvertent irradiation of a fetus or embryo</u>, elective diagnostic roentgenograms of the abdomen, pelvis, hips, and upper thighs of girls age 12 or older should be made only during the first 10 days of the menstrual cycle. This policy does not apply to girls who have an intra-uterine device or who have been on birth control pills for more than one month. If a girl is or could be pregnant, the physician should either: 1) write on the requisition that the examination is necessary despite the known or possible pregnancy or 2) schedule the examination at a later date.

3. <u>Use of Bisacodyl (Dulcolax)</u>

   A. <u>Contraindications</u>
      Acute surgical abdomen, acute ulcerative colitis.

   B. <u>Tablets</u>
      Tablets must be swallowed whole; they <u>must</u> <u>not</u> <u>be</u> <u>chewed or crushed</u>. Use suppositories unless you are certain that the child can swallow the tablets whole. They should not be taken within 1 hour of antacids or milk. <u>Dose</u>: below 40 kg: 1 tablet h.s.; above 40 kg: 2 tablets h.s.

   C. <u>Suppositories</u>
      May be used at any age; for infants and children under 10 kg use one-half suppository. <u>If the first suppository does not produce a good bowel movement within 45 minutes, administer a second suppository</u>.

4. <u>X-Ray Examinations</u>

   A. <u>Upper Gastrointestinal Series</u>
      A small bowel follow-through is part of most gastrointestinal series, except when there is severe gastric or duodenal obstruction.
      1) Patient <18 months: NPO for 3 hours before the study.
      2) Patient 18 months and older:
         a) Clear liquids only after supper. No carbonated beverages on day of study.

b) Bisacodyl pill(s) or suppositories (see Section 3B) the evening before the examination.

c) Nothing by mouth for 4 hours before the examination.

B. Barium Enema
1) Infants <18 months: Liquid diet starting evening before the study. No carbonated beverages.
2) 18 months and older
   a) Liquid diet for 24 hours before study. No carbonated beverages.
   b) *Bisacodyl pill(s) or suppository (see Section 3B) the evening before the examination.
   c) *Bisacodyl suppository the morning of the study.
   d) *Patients 10 years and older: enemas until clear the morning of the examination.
      *Omit steps b, c, and d when evaluation is for possible Hirschsprung's disease, ulcerative colitis, or acute surgical abdomen.
3) Air contrast barium enema (over 18 months of age)
   a) Clear liquid diet 24 hours before study. No carbonated beverages.
   b) Bisacodyl pill(s) or suppository (see Section 3B) the evening before the examination.
   c) Tap water (luke warm) enemas until clear-- i.e., no stool in the water. This usually takes 2 enemas.
   d) Bisacodyl enema will be given in radiology 1 hour before the examination.

C. Intravenous Urogram (IVP)
(Note: An ultrasound exam of the kidneys frequently can substitute for an IVP.)
All patients should be normally hydrated, but have an empty stomach. Notation must be made on requisition of previous drug reactions and allergies. The examination usually will not be done if the child has a history of allergy to iodine or a previous severe reaction to contrast agent. The hospital requires that one of the child's parents signs the special consent form for administration of intravenous contrast agents.
1) Infants <18 months should be kept NPO before the exam for the same length of time as the usual interval between feedings.
2) 18 months or older:
   a) Bisacodyl pill(s) or suppository (see Section 3B) the night before the examination.
   b) Nothing by mouth 4 hours before examination.

D. Voiding Cystourethrogram (VCUG)
No preparation is required.

E. Gallbladder
    1) The first examination should be with ultrasound.
    2) In those rare cases when a cholecystogram is
        indicated, consult a pediatric radiologist for special
        instructions.

    (Since the pediatric dose of iopanoic acid (Telepaque) is
    not readily available, it seems advisable to list it here.
    Darling recommended 0.5 gm (one tablet) for each 10 kg
    of body weight, not to exceed 3.0 gm (six tablets).
    Never administer more than the recommended dose. If a
    repeat dose is given within 48 hours, use only 1/2 the
    above dose. Contraindications: renal or hepatic failure.

    Ref: Darling, DB: Radiography of Infants and
    Children, 1st Edition, Charles C Thomas, Publisher,
    Springfield, Illinois, p. 147, 1962.

F. Head and Body Computed Tomography (CT)
    1) Small children may need to be sedated to prevent
        motion.
    2) Oral and/or intravenous contrast agents may be
        necessary, depending upon specific examination and
        information required. (Only intravenous contrast
        for Head CT scans). No intravenous contrast is
        given if there is an allergy to iodine or history of
        severe reaction to a contrast agent. The hospital
        requires that a special consent form for adminis-
        tration of intravenous contrast agents be signed by
        one parent.
    3) Infants should be kept NPO 3 to 4 hours if possi-
        ble. The meal before the exam should be held for
        all children.
    4) These are useless exams if child cannot be trans-
        ported to the scanner or hold still.

5. Ultrasound Examination

    A. Advantages
        1) No ionizing radiation.
        2) Minimal advance patient preparation.
        3) Bedside exams can be done with real-time scanners.
        4) No need for oral or intravenous contrast agents.
        5) Children have relatively little retroperitoneal fat,
            which is an asset for ultrasonography.

    B. Disadvantages
        Sound waves do not penetrate bone, gas, or barium.
        (Sonograms should be obtained before any barium con-
        trast studies.)

C. Indications
1) Abdominal or pelvic masses. Should usually be initial diagnostic examination.
    a) Determine location, organ of origin, and internal characteristics of mass (solid or cystic). This permits a directed approach when further radiographic evaluation is needed.
    b) Abscesses and other fluid collections may be localized and aspirated with ultrasonic guidance.
2) Unexplained hepatomegaly or splenomegaly.
3) Jaundice and/or right upper quadrant pain.
4) Routine screening of the kidneys of patients with disorders that have an increased incidence of renal anomalies, neoplasms and/or cystic disease (e.g., hemihypertrophy, tuberous sclerosis).
5) May frequently substitute for (or compliment) intravenous urography. Especially for patients with poor or non-functioning kidneys, or who have had severe reactions to contrast material, or who are allergic to iodine.
6) Cranial ultrasonography in infants.
    a) Intracranial bleeding.
    b) Enlargement of ventricles; position of shunt tube.
    c) Congenital malformations.
    d) Central nervous system infections.

D. Preparation
1) Pelvis and lower abdomen:
    Full bladder necessary. Patients should be well hydrated with oral or intravenous fluids and should not void (if possible) for 1-3 hours before exam.
2) Liver, gallbladder, and biliary tree:
    a) Infants: NPO 3-4 hours (if possible) before exam.
    b) Children: NPO 6-12 hours before exam.

E. Sedation
1) Usually unnecessary for routine ultrasonography.
2) May be required for invasive procedures (aspiration of abscess, etc.).

6. Nuclear Medicine Examinations
The hallmark of nuclear medicine examinations is their non-invasiveness. Strengths include functional, physiological, and biochemical information which may compliment other anatomical studies. The general rules about radiation protection stated above apply for all nuclear studies. Except in emergencies, menstruating girls should receive radio-isotopes only during the first 10 days after the start of their menstrual period (first day of bleeding) unless they have an intrauterine device or have regularly taken birth control pills for at least one month before the examination.

Most procedures do not require patient preparation. Consultation with the nuclear medicine physician is encouraged before a study is performed or ordered. Selected studies are discussed below:

A. Bone Imaging
    This study is usually positive for osteomyelitis before radiographic changes become evident. A flow study should be ordered for suspected infection. Bone scans are sensitive for metastatic disease. Bone scanning is performed with Technetium (Tc99m) methylene diphosphonate (MDP) while bone marrow imaging uses Tc99m sulfur colloid.

B. Gallium - 67 Imaging
    Gallium-67 is very useful for detecting occult abscesses and tumors in children. This is mediated via binding to transferrin, lactoferrin and intracellular lysosomes. Because Gallium-67 is excreted in part through the colon, a standard barium enema preparation regimen (see Section 4B) should be given with a tap water enema just before sending the patient to nuclear medicine. It is not necessary to keep children NPO. Images are usually obtained at 24, 48, and 72 or 96 hours after injection.

C. Cerebral Imaging
    1) Early encephalitis, especially herpes simplex, may be discovered by brain scan well before abnormalities can be detected by CT.
    2) Brain death. Cerebral flow imaging may be helpful in assessing the presence or absence of cerebral perfusion.

D. Nuclear GI Studies
    1) Acutely traumatized child: Liver-spleen scans to detect hematomas or lacerations.
    2) Gastroesophageal reflux.
    3) Hepatobiliary function.
    4) Biliary atresia.
    5) Meckel's scans: Do before barium studies, since barium interferes with the study.

E. GU Studies
    1) DTPA for renal function and GFR determinations.
    2) DMSA provides evaluation of relative cortical function and added information about renal structure.
    3) Glucoheptinate is an alternate renal radiotracer.

F. Nuclear Cardiology
    Thallium (perfusion) and gated blood pool studies (MUGA) for ventricular function are the studies performed in young patients. The latter may be useful in following oncology patients receiving cardiotoxic drugs or

the evaluation of congenital heart disease. Lung scanning may also evaluate lung perfusion and shunt patency in congenital heart disease patients.

G. Sedation
Patient motion commonly degrades the quality of pediatric nuclear imaging studies. Gentle handling and sometimes physical restraints, usually are all that are needed for successful examinations. Sedation is occasionally required in some patients. The final judgement about sedation rests with the child's physician.

Ref: Kirchner, PT (ed.): In: Nuclear Medicine Review Syllabus, 1980, Society of Nuclear Medicine, New York.

7. Recommendations for Specific X-ray Procedures

A. Skull Films in Pediatric Head Trauma
The following criteria have been found to give a high yield of radiologic findings following head trauma:
1) History:
   a) Unconsciousness more than five minutes
   b) Retrograde amnesia more than five minutes
   c) Vomiting
   d) Gunshot wound or accident at work
   e) Nonvisual focal symptoms
2) General physical examination
   a) Palpable bony malalignment
   b) Discharge from ear
   c) Discharge from nose
   d) Ear drum discoloration
   e) Bilateral black eyes
3) Neurologic examination
   a) Stupor, semiconsciousness, or coma
   b) Irregular breathing or apnea
   c) Babinski reflex
   d) Other reflex abnormality
   e) Anisocoria
   f) Other cranial nerve abnormality

Ref: Rosman, NP et al.: Ped Clin North Am 26:707, 1979.

B. Comparison Radiographs of Limbs
Comparison views of the normal limb are valuable for:
1) Suspected osteomyelitis or pyarthrosis.
2) Suspected knee or ankle effusion.
3) Possible elbow fracture. A relative large number of ossification centers appear at various times, which may be confusing.
4) Occasionally helpful to identify or rule out subtle fractures in other sites.

Ref: Merten, DF et al.: Pediatrics 65:646. 1980.

C. Cranial Computed Tomography (CT)

    May be recommended in children in the following clinical situations:

    1) Increased intracranial pressure (headache, vomiting, papilledema).
    2) Rapidly enlarging head size (using standardized head growth charts).
    3) Progressive focal neurologic signs (hemiparesis, localized weakness).
    4) Coma of unknown cause.
    5) Suspected intracranial hemorrhage in the neonate.
    6) Postoperative and postradiation therapy follow-up.
    7) Tuberous sclerosis (including study of family members for genetic counseling).
    8) Serious head trauma.

    Ref: Ferry, PC: J Pediatr 96:961, 1980.

D. Body Computed Tomography (CT)

    Body computed tomography may be useful in these situations:

    1) More detailed evaluation after initial ultrasound and/or radiographic evaluation.
    2) Evaluate masses in the chest, lungs, and mediastinum. Can differentiate pleural, lung, and mediastinal lesions.
    3) Evaluate masses in the abdomen, pelvis, and limbs.
    4) Hepatomegaly. Detect metastases. Recognize certain metabolic diseases.
    5) Retroperitoneal evaluation (e.g., adenopathy).
    6) Determine extent of tumor involvement or response to therapy. May localize metastatic disease.
    7) Evaluate extent of bone marrow involvement for localized bone tumors.
    8) Trauma -- specifically pelvic and hip fractures.

FORMULARY

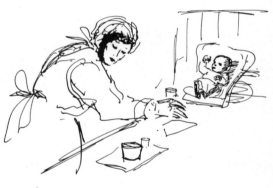

aaron sopher

DRUG INDEX

Prostaphlin	Oxacillin	166
Prostigmine	Neostigmine	164
Prostin VR	Alprostadil	120
Proventil	Albuterol	120
PTU	Propylthiouracil	179
Purinethol	Mercaptopurine	196
Pyopen	Carbenicillin	129
Pyribenzamine	Tripelennamine	191
Pyridium	Phenazopyridine	170
Pyrinal	Pyrethrins	180
Questran	Cholestyramine	133
Reglan	Metaclopramide	158
RID	Pyrethrins	180
Rifadin, Rimactane	Rifampin	181
Ritalin	Methylphenidate	161
Robinul	Glycopyrrolate	148
Rocaltrol	Calcitriol	127
Rubidomycin	Daunorubicin	195
Seconal	Secobarbital	182
Selsun	Selenium sulfide	182
Septra	Trimethoprim-sulfamethoxazole	190
Serpasil, Serpate	Reserpine	181
Shohl's solution	Citrate mixture	133
Slo-phyllin	Theophylline	202
Solu-Cortef	Hydrocortisone	150
Solu-medrol	Methylprednisolone	161, 205
Somophyllin	Aminophylline	202
SSKI	Potassium iodide	173
Staphcillin	Methicillin	160
Sucostrin	Succinylcholine	184
Sudafed	Pseudoephedrine	179
Sulamyd	Sulfacetamide	184, 214
Sus-phrine	Epinephrine	214
Symmetrel	Amantadine	122
Synthroid	L-Thyroxine	155
Tagamet	Cimetidine	133
Tapazole	Methimazole	160
Tegopen	Cloxacillin	134
Tegretol	Carbamazepine	129
Tempra	Acetaminophen	118
Tensilon	Edrophonium	143
Theo-Dur	Theophylline	202
Theophyl	Theophylline	202
Thorazine	Chlorpromazine	133
Ticar	Ticarcillin	187
Tigan	Trimethobenzamide	190
Tinactin	Tolnaftate	189
Tofranil	Imipramine	151
Tolectin	Tolmetin	188
Trimox	Amoxicillin	124
Trobicin	Spectinomycin	183
Tylenol	Acetaminophen	118
Unipen	Nafcillin	163
Urecholine	Bethanechol	126

DRUG DOSES

Drug	Supplied	Dose and Route	Remarks
Acetaminophen (Tylenol, Tempra, Datril, Liquiprim)	Tabs: 80, 325, 500, 650 mg Syrup: 160 mg/5 ml Supp: 120, 125, 130, 300, 325, 500, 600, 650 mg Drops: 80 mg/0.8 ml Elixir: 160 mg/5 ml Liquid: 500 mg/15 ml	0-3mo: 40 mg 4-11mo: 80 mg 12-24mo: 120 mg 2-3yr: 160 mg 4-5yr: 240 mg 6-8yr: 320 mg 9-10yr: 400 mg 11-12yr: 480 mg Alternate: 5-10 mg/kg/dose give 4-5 x daily Adult: 300-650 mg Q4h Max. dose: 1000 mg QID	Overdose may cause hepato- toxicity, often delayed. T1/2 = 1-3 hrs. Contrain- dicated in patients with known G6PD deficiency.
Acetazolamide (Diamox)	Tabs: 125, 250 mg Vials (sodium): 500 mg/5 ml Caps (Sustained Release): 500 mg	Diuretic: Child: 5 mg/kg/dose QD-QOD (PO or IV) Adult: 250-375 mg/dose QD- QOD (PO or IV) Glaucoma: Child: 5-10 mg/kg/dose IM or IV Q6h; 10-15 mg/kg/ day PO Q6-8h. Adult: 250 mg/dose PO Q6h; for rapid decrease in pres- sure give 500 mg/dose IV. Seizures: 8-30 mg/kg/day PO to max. dose of 1 gm/day Q6-8h.	Renal excretion. T1/2 is 4-10h. Paresthesias, poly- uria, drowsiness, gastrointes- tinal irritation (vomiting, diarrhea), transient hypo- kalemia, reduced urate excretion, and acidosis may occur with long-term therapy; alkalinize urine. IM injec- tion may be painful and should be avoided.

Drug	Preparations	Dosage	Comments
Acetylcysteine (Mucomyst)	Vials: (10% or 20%) 4 ml, 10 ml, 30 ml	Nebulizer: 3-5 ml of 20% solution (diluted with equal vol. of H₂0 or sterile saline), or 6-10 ml of 10% solution. Administer TID-QID. Direct instillation: 1-2 ml of 10% or 20% solution Q1-4h. For acetaminophen poisoning: Treat within 24 hrs of ingestion. Administer 20% acetylcysteine solution (diluted 1:4 in carbonated beverage). Loading dose: 140 mg/kg PO or NG, followed by 70 mg/kg Q4h x total of 18 doses	May induce bronchospasm, stomatitis, rhinorrhea, and nausea.
ACTH (Corticotropin, Acthar)	1 unit = 1 mg Aqueous (Injection): 25, 40 U/vial Gel: 40, 80 U/ml Gel: 1 & 5 ml vials	Aqueous: 1.6 U/kg/day IV, IM, or SC Q6-8h. Gel: 0.8 U/kg/day Q12-24h. Infantile spasms: Many regimens exist. Gel: 25-80 U/day (usually 40 U/day) IM or SQ Q24-72h. Gradually taper after 4 wks.	Contraindicated in acute psychoses, CHF, Cushing's disease, Tb, peptic ulcer, ocular herpes, fungal infections, recent surgery, sensitivity to pork. IV administration for diagnostic purposes only.
Acyclovir	Vial - 500 mg/5 ml	Children <12 yrs: 250 mg/M² IV over 1 hr Q8h. Adults: 5 mg/kg IV over 1 hr Q8h.	FDA approved for initial and recurrent mucosal cutaneous herpes simplex in immunocompromised patients and in severe initial episodes of herpes genitalis; often causes renal impairment; adequate hydration essential to prevent renal tubular crystallization. Encephalopathic reactions have been reported.

Albumin, human serum (normal serum albumin)	Injection (vials): 5% (5 gm/dl; 0.18 mEq Na/ml); 25% (25 gm/dl; 0.15 mEq Na/ml) 5%: 20, 50, 100 ml bottles 25%: 50, 250, 500 ml bottles	Administration: IV: Hypoproteinemia: 0.5-1 gm/kg/dose. Repeat Q1-2 days as calculated to replace ongoing losses. Hypovolemia: 0.5-1 gm/kg/dose, repeated PRN. Max. dose: 6 gm/kg/day	Contraindicated in severe anemia or CHF. Use with caution in hypervolemia. Allergic reactions are unusual but may occur.
Albuterol (Proventil, Ventolin)	Tabs: 2, 4 mg Aerosol inhaler: 90 µg/dose	Children >12 yrs and adults: Initial: 2-4 mg/dose PO TID or QID Advance: up to 8 mg PO QID Inhalations: 1-2 puffs Q4-6h	May cause tachycardia, tremor, nervousness, GI symptoms, and headaches.
Alprostadil (PGE_1, Prostin VR)	Amps: 500 µg/ml	Neonates: Initial: 0.1 µg/kg/min. Advance to 0.4 ug/kg/min. Maintenance: when increase in pO_2 is noted, decrease immediately to lowest effective dose (e.g. 0.01 ug/kg/min). Administer in large vein or umbilical artery catheter at ductal opening.	For palliation only. Continuous vital sign monitoring essential. May cause apnea, fever, seizures, flushing, bradycardia, hypotension, and diarrhea. Decreases platelet aggregation.
Allopurinol (Zyloprim)	Tabs: 100, 300 mg	<6 yr: 150 mg/day given TID 6-10yr: 300 mg/day >10yr: 100-200 mg/day min. dose Alternative: 10 mg/kg/day ÷ TID. Max. dose: 800 mg/day	Maintain alkaline urine flow. Decrease dosage with renal insufficiency. Rash, neuritis, hepatotoxicity and GI disturbances may occur. Follow serum uric acid levels.

Aluminum Hydroxide (Amphojel AlternaGel) (and many other brands)	Caps: 475, 500 mg Gel susp.: 320 mg/ 5 ml (360 ml bottle) Tablets: 300, 600 mg Gel liquid: 600 mg/ 5 ml (150, 360 ml bottle)	Titrate to desired clinical response. Route: PO, very little absorbed. Dose: Peptic Ulcer: Child: 5-15 ml PO Q3-6h or 1 and 3h PC and HS Adult: 15-45 ml PO Q3-6h or 1 and 3h PC and HS Prophylaxis of GI Bleeding: Infant: 2-5 ml/dose Q1-2h per NG tube Child: 5-15 ml/dose Q1-2h per NG tube Adult: 30-60 ml/dose Q1h per NG tube Hyperphosphatemia: 50-150 mg/kg/day Q4-6h	May cause constipation, phosphorus depletion. Inhibits gastric emptying. Interferes with absorption of several drugs. 10 ml neutralizes 13 mEq acid. 5 ml contains <0.3 mEq Na.
Aluminum Hydroxide with magnesium hydroxide (Maalox and many other brands with varying concentration)	Tabs: 400, 800 mg Susp: 180, 360 ml bottles	Same as for Al(OH)$_3$	Limit to 80 ml suspension daily. 5 ml ≅ 400 mg tab. Magnesium containing antacids are laxative. May cause hypokalemia. Use in caution with renal failure.

| Amantadine (Symmetrel) | Cap: 100 mg
Susp: 50 mg/5 ml | Children
1-9 yrs: 4-8 mg/kg/day BID or TID. Do not exceed 150 mg/day
9-12 yrs: 100 mg BID
Adults: 200 mg/day QD or BID
Prophylaxis - continue until 90 days past exposure; for continuing exposure give Influenza A vaccine and continue for 2-3 wks. If vaccine not available continue for 90 days.
Symptomatic - continue for 24-48 hrs after disappearance of symptoms. | May cause depression, CHF, and orthostatic hypotension, and urinary retention. Adjust dose in renal failure. |
| Amikacin Sulfate (Amikin) | Injection: 50 mg/ml (2 ml vial); 250 mg/ml (2, 4 ml vials) | Newborn:
Loading dose: 10 mg/kg
Maintenance: 15 mg/kg/day Q12h
Children and Adults: 15 mg/kg/day Q8h.
Max. dose: 1.5 gm/day
Infusion rate:
Infant: 1-2h
Children and Adults: 30-60 min | Ototoxicity, nephrotoxicity, rash, fever, eosinophilia, and headache may occur. Monitor levels. Therapeutic levels: peaks between 25-30 ug/ml; troughs 5-8 ug/ml. Adjust dose with renal impairment. |

Aminophylline	Injection (IV): 25 mg/ml (79% theophylline) Liquid (oral): 105 mg/5 ml (Somophyllin) (85% theophylline) Tablets: 100, 200 mg (79% theophylline)	Loading: 6 mg/kg IV over 20 min. Maintenance (continuous drip): Neonates: 0.2 mg/kg/hr Infants (<1 yr): 0.2-0.9 mg/kg/hr Children 1-9 yr: 1.0 mg/kg/hr 9-16 yr and young adult smokers: 0.8 mg/kg/hr Adults, non-smokers: 0.5 mg/kg/hr. Individual variation of serum half life is great. In many instances these doses will need to be adjusted.	Suggest monitoring serum levels especially in infants and young children. Therapeutic level: for asthma, 10-20 µg/ml; for neonatal apnea, 6-13 µg/ml. Side effects: restlessness, GI upset, arrhythmias. See Theophylline preparations, page 202.
Ammonium Chloride	Tabs: 300, 500 mg; 1 gm Caps: 300, 500 mg Solns./Syrup: 500 mg/5 ml Injection: 0.4 mEq/ml (2.14%); 4.0 mEq/ml (21.4%); 5.0 mEq/ml (26.75%)	Urinary acidification: Child: 75 mg/kg/dose Q6h PO or IV. Adol. & Adult: 1.5 gm/dose IV Q6h. Max. dose: 6 gm/day IV or 8-12 gm/day PO (QID) Injection: Dilute to concentration not >0.4 mEq/ml. Infusion not to exceed 50 mg/kg/hr or 1 mEq/kg/hr	May produce acidosis; do not use in hepatic or renal insufficiency; use with caution in infants. May cause GI irritation.

Drug	How Supplied	Dosage	Comments
Amobarbital (Amytal)	Tabs: 15, 30, 50, 100 mg. Caps: 65, 200 mg. Injection: 250, 500 mg vials. Elixir: 44 mg/5 ml in 34% alcohol	Not recommended in child <6 yr of age. Sedation: Child: 2-6 mg/kg/day Q6-8h. Adult: 30-50 mg/dose BID-TID. Max. dose for sedation 120 mg/dose BID or QID. Anticonvulsant: 3-5 mg/kg/dose (IM, IV). Inject slowly IV.	Contraindicated in liver dysfunction, porphyria, allergy to barbiturates, or respiratory distress.
Amoxicillin (Amoxil, Larotid, Trimox, Wymox, Utimox, Amcill)	Chewable tabs: 125 mg. Caps: 250, 500 mg. Drops: 50 mg/ml (15 ml). Susp: 125, 250 mg/5 ml (80, 100, 150 ml)	Child: 25-100 mg/kg/day Q8h PO. Adult: 250-500 mg/dose Q8h PO. Gonorrhea (acute uncomplicated): 3 gm as single PO dose with 1 gm probenecid	Renal elimination. Achieves serum levels about twice those achieved with equal dose of ampicillin. Less GI effects, but otherwise similar to ampicillin.
Amphotericin B (Fungizone)	Injection: 50 mg vials. Cream: 3%. Lotion: 3%	Topical: apply BID-QID. IV: (mix with D_5W to concentration 0.1 mg/ml, pH >4.2) Infuse over 6-12 hr. Test dose: 0.1 mg/kg/day IV up to max. 1 mg/dose. Initial dose: 0.25 mg/kg/day. Increase to 1 mg/kg/day as tolerated by increments (0.125-0.25 mg/kg/day QD or QOD. Max. dose: 1.5 mg/kg/day. Alternate day dose: 1.5 mg/kg/day QOD.	Fever, chills, nausea, vomiting are common side effects. May premedicate with acetaminophen and diphenhydramine 30 min before and 4 hrs after infusion. Hydrocortisone 10-20 mg added to bottle also helps prevent immediate adverse reactions. Monitor renal, hepatic, electrolyte, and hematologic status closely. Hypercalciuria, RTA, renal failure, acute hepatic failure, and phlebitis may occur.

Ampicillin (Omnipen, Polycillin, Principen)	Caps: 250, 500 mg Injection: 125, 250, 500 mg; 1, 2, 4 gm Drops: 100 mg/ml Susp: 125, 250 mg and 500 mg/5 ml	Neonates: <7 days: 50-100 mg/kg/day ÷ Q12h IM or IV >7 days: 100-200 mg/kg/day ÷ Q8h IM or IV Mild-moderate infections: <40 kg: 50-100 mg/kg/day ÷ Q6h PO, IM, or IV >40 kg: 2-4 gm/day ÷ Q6h PO, IM, or IV Severe infections: <40 kg: 200-400 mg/kg/day ÷ Q4-6h IM or IV >40 kg: 8-12 gm/day ÷ Q4-6h IM or IV. Max. dose: 12 gm/day. Uncomplicated gonorrhea: 3.5 gm PO with 1 gm probenicid PO.	Same side effects as penicillin, with cross-reactivity. Rash commonly seen at 5-10 days. May cause interstitial nephritis.
Aspirin (ASA)	Tabs: 65, 75, 200, 300, 325, 500, 600, 650 mg Tabs (chewable): 65, 81 mg Caps: 325 mg Supp: 60, 65, 130, 150, 195, 200, 300, 325, 600 mg and 1.2 gm	Antipyretic: 10-15 mg/kg/dose Q4h up to total 60-80 mg/kg/day (max. dose: 3.6 gm/day) Q4h Antirheumatic: 100 mg/kg/day PO Q4h	Use with caution in platelet and bleeding disorders. Follow serum levels when used as antirheumatic. Therapeutic levels: 15-30 mg/dl. May cause GI upset, allergic reactions, hepatotoxicity. Overdosage may cause salicylism.

Atropine Sulfate	Tabs: 0.3, 0.4, 0.6 mg Injection: 0.1, 0.3, 0.4, 0.5, 0.6, 0.8, 1.0, 1.2, 2 mg/ml Vials: 0.3, 0.4, 0.5, 0.6, 1.0 mg/ml	General dose recommendation: Child: 0.01 mg/kg/dose PO, SC, IV (max: 0.4 mg/dose); may repeat Q4-6h Adult: 0.5 mg/dose Cardiopulmonary resuscitation: 0.01-0.03 mg/kg/dose IV Q2-5 min. x 2-3 PRN. Min. dose: 0.1 mg. Max. dose: 0.4 mg for children and 0.5 mg/dose for adults.	Dry mouth, blurred vision, fever, tachycardia, constipation, urinary retention, CNS signs (dizziness, hallucinations, restlessness). Contraindicated in glaucoma. Caution with use in asthma.
Beclomethasone (Vanceril, Beclovent)	Aerosol (17 gm dispenser): each 200 metered doses. 1 dose = 42 µg	Inhalant: 6-12 yr: 1-2 inhalations Q6-8h; max: 10 inhalations/day >12 yr: 2 inhalations Q6-8h; max: 20 inhalations/day (1 inhalation = 42 µg)	Rinse mouth and gargle with water after inhalation; may cause thrush. No systemic affects with doses <1 mg/day. Wean cautiously off steroids once inhalant is used. Not recommended for children <6 yrs.
Bethanechol (Urecholine and other brand names)	Tabs: 5, 10, 25, 50 mg Injection: 5 mg/ml	Oral: 0.6 mg/kg/day ÷ Q6-8h PO SC: Use 1/3-1/4 of oral dose For gastroesophageal reflux: 2.9 mg/M²/dose Q8h PO (Ref: J Pediatr 96:321, 1980) Adults: 10-50 mg PO Q6-12h	Contraindicated in asthma, GI, or GU obstruction, peptic ulcer. May cause hypotension, nausea, bronchospasm, salivation, flushing. Atropine is specific antidote.
Bisacodyl (Dulcolax and various other names)	Tabs: 5 mg Supp: 10 mg	Oral: 0.3 mg/kg/dose, 6h before desired effect. Adult: 10-15 mg Rectal: <2 yr: 5 mg >2 yr: 10 mg; usually effective within 15-60 min.	Do not chew tablets; do not give within 1 hr of antacids or milk.

Bretylium (Bretylol)	Amp: 50 mg/ml	Not approved for children <12 yr. 5-10 mg/kg/dose IV over 10-30 min. 5-10 mg/kg/ dose Q1-2h IM OR IV if arrhythmia persists on maintenance dose. Maintenance dose: 5-10 mg/kg/ dose infuse over 10 min Q6h or constant infusion of 1-2 mg/ min.	For treatment of life-threatening ventricular arrhythmias. Often causes hypotension. May cause transient hypertension or PVC. Adjust dose in renal failure.
Calcitriol (1,25-dihydroxy-cholecalciferol, Rocaltrol)	Caps: 0.25, 0.50 μg	Children: Dose not established; suggested doses range 0.01-0.05 μg/kg/day, some with hepatic osteodystrophy may require more. Titrate increments Q2-4 wks based on clinical response. Adults: Initial: 0.25 μg/day Increment: 0.25 μg/day Q2-4 wks	Most potent vitamin D metabolite available. Monitor serum calcium and phosphorus. Avoid concomitant use of Mg++ containing antacids. Discontinue if hypercalcemia occurs.
Calcium chloride (27% calcium)	Solution: 100 mg/ml (10%) (1.36 mEq Ca++/ ml); 13.6 mEq Ca++/gm salt; 73 mg salt/mEq Ca+)	Infant/Child: 200-300 mg/kg/day PO as 2% soln ÷ Q6h Adult: 4-8 gm/day PO QID For Cardiac Arrest: Infant/Child: 20 mg/kg/dose (0.2 ml/Kg/dose) IV Q 10 min. Adult: 250-500 mg/dose (2.5-5 ml/dose) IV Q 10 min. Do not exceed 1 ml/min with IV infusion.	May cause GI irritation, phlebitis. Use intravenously with extreme caution. Acidifying effect; give only 2-3 days, then change to another Ca+ salt.
Calcium Glubionate (Neocalglucon) (6% calcium)	Syrup: 1.8 gm/5 ml (5.6 mEq Ca++/5 ml; 115 mg Ca++/5 ml)	Maintenance: Infant/Child: 600-2000 mg/kg/ day PO QID (max. dose: 9 gm/day) Neonatal hypocalcemia: 1200 mg/ kg/day PO Q4-6h Adult: 6-18 gm/day QID	Administer before meals for best absorption. Absorption inhibited by high phosphate load. High osmotic load of syrup (20% sucrose) may cause diarrhea.

Calcium Gluconate (9.4% calcium)	Tabs: 500, 650, 1000 mg Solution (10%): 100 mg/ml (0.45 mEq Ca^{++}/ml; 224 mg salt/mEq Ca^{++})	Maintenance: IV: 200-500 mg/kg/day or 100 mg/kg/dose slowly PO: Infants: 400-800 mg/kg/day Q6h Child: 200-500 mg/kg/day Q6h Adult: 5-15 gm/day IV or PO Q6h. Not for IM injection. For Cardiac Arrest: Infants and Children: 100 mg/kg/dose IV Q10 min. Adults: 10 ml/dose IV Q10 min.	If given IV, watch for bradycardia, hypotension, extravasation. May produce arrhythmias in digitalized patients. Precipitates with bicarbonate. Tissue necrosis may result from infiltrates. Do not use scalp veins.
Calcium Lactate (13% calcium)	Tabs: 325, 650 mg (6.5 mEq Ca^{++}/gm salt; 154 mg salt/mEq Ca^{++})	Infant/Child: 400-500 mg/kg/day PO Q4-8h Adult: 1.5-3 gm PO TID	Give with meals. Tablets do not dissolve in milk.
Captopril (Capoten)	Tabs: 25, 50, 100 mg	Children (>12 yrs) and Adults Initial: 25 mg PO TID and then increase weekly if necessary by 25 mg/dose to max. of 450 mg/day.	Adjust with renal failure. May cause rash, proteinuria, neutropenia, hypotension, or diminution of taste perception. Known to decrease aldosterone production.

| Carbamazepine (Tegretol) | Tabs: 200 mg | 6-12 yr old:
Initial: 10 mg/kg/day PO QD or BID or 100 mg/dose BID
Increment: 100 mg/day at intervals of 1 day (÷ TID or QID) until best response
Maintenance: 20-30 mg/kg/day PO TID or QID
Max. dose: 1000 mg/day
>12 yrs - adult:
Initial: 200 mg BID
Increment: 200 mg/day at intervals of 1 day using TID or QID schedule until best response.
Maintenance: 600-1200 mg/day TID or QID
Max. 12-15 yr: 1000 mg/day adult: 1200 mg/day | Obtain pretreatment CBC. Monitor for hematologic, hepatic toxicity. Therapeutic blood levels: 4-12 ug/ml. Many potential side effects, including; neuritis, drowsiness, dizziness, tinnitus, diplopia, urinary retention, nausea. |
| Carbenicillin disodium (Geopen, Pyopen) | Injection: 1, 2, 5, 10 gm vials
Tabs: 382 mg | Neonates:
Initial: 100 mg/kg/dose
Maintenance:
<2 kg: 225 mg/kg/day Q8h x 7 days, then 400 mg/kg/day Q6h
>2 kg: 300 mg/kg/day x 3 days, then 400 mg/kg/day Q6h
Oral (for UTI only):
Children: 100 mg/kg/day PO Q4h
Adults: 300-500 mg/kg/day PO Q2-4h
Parenteral (IM or IV) for Children/Adult: UTI - 50-200 mg/kg/day Q4-6h
Severe infection - 400-500 mg/kg/day Q4-6h;
Max. dose: 40 gm/day | May cause anaphylaxis, platelet destruction. Unpredictable interaction with gentamicin. Give through separate IV tubing. May lead to urinary K⁺ loss. Adjust dose with renal failure. Use with caution in patients with penicillin allergies. (1 gm carbenicillin = 4.7 mEq Na). |

Cefaclor (Ceclor)	Caps: 250, 500 mg Susp: 125, 250 mg/ 5 ml in 75 and 150 ml bottles	Child: 20-40 mg/kg/day Q8h PO. Max. dose: 1 gm/day. Adult: 250-500 mg/dose Q8h PO. Max. dose: 4 gm/day	Not recommended for < 1 mo. Use with caution in penicillin-allergic patient or in presence of renal impairment.
Cefamandole (Mandol)	Injection: 0.5, 1.0, 2.0 gm vials	Children: Mild-moderate infection: 50-100 mg/kg/day Q4-8h IM or IV. Severe infection: 150 mg/kg/day ÷ Q4-8h IM or IV. Adult: 2-6 gm/day Q4-8h IM or IV. Max. dose: 12 gm/day	Not recommended in patients < 1 mo. Use with caution in penicillin-allergic patients or in renal impairment. 1 gm cefamandole = 3.3 mEq Na. Associated with hemostatic abnormalities.
Cefazolin (Ancef, Kefzol)	Amp: 250, 500, 1000 mg	Children: 25-100 mg/kg/day ÷ Q6-8h IV or IM. Adult: 750 mg-6 gm/day Q6-8h. Max. dose: 12 gm/day	See cephalexin. Use with caution in renal impairment or in penicillin-allergic patients. May cause phlebitis, hematologic abnormalities. Not recommended in patients < 1 mo.
Cefotaxime (Claforan)	Injection: 0.5, 1.0, 2.0 gm vials	Infant: 0-1 wk: 100 mg/kg/day IV Q12h; 1-4 wk: 150 mg/kg/day IV Q8h; >4 wk: 50-180 mg/kg/day IV, IM Q4-6h. Children (<50 kg): 50-180 mg/ kg/day Q4-6h IV or IM. Use higher doses in serious infections. Adult (>50 kg): 2-12 gm/day IV or IM Q4-12h	Use with caution in penicillin-allergic patients or in presence of renal impairment.

Drug	Forms	Dosage	Comments
Cefoxitin (Mefoxin)	Injection: 1, 2 gm vials	Children (>3 mos): 80-160 mg/kg/day Q4-6h IV Adult: 1-2 gm/dose Q6-8h Max. dose: 12 gm/day	Use with caution in penicillin-allergic patients or in presence of renal impairment.
Cefuroxime (Zinacef)	Injection: 750 mg and 1.5 gm vials	Children (>3 mos): 50-100 mg/kg/day IV Q6-8h Meningitis: 200-240 mg/kg/day Q6-8h Adults: 750 mg-1.5 gm IV Q8h	Use with caution in penicillin-allergic patients or in presence of renal impairment.
Cephalexin (Keflex)	Tabs: 1000 mg Caps: 250, 500 mg Susp: 125, 250 mg/5 ml Drops: 100 mg/ml	Children: 25-100 mg/kg/day ÷ Q6h PO Adult: 250-1000 mg/dose Q4-6h Max. dose: 4 gm/day	Some cross-reactivity with penicillins. GI disturbance frequent. Use with caution in renal insufficiency.
Cephalothin (Keflin)	Vials: 1, 2, 4 gm	Children: 80-160 mg/kg/day ÷ Q4-6h IV or deep IM. Max. dose: 12 gm/day Adults: 4-12 gm/day Q4h	See cephalexin. May cause phlebitis.
Charcoal, activated	Powder: ≅3-4 gm/tbsp	0.3-0.5 gm/ml (e.g. 30 gm in 60-90 ml water). Stir constantly. Children: 0.5-1 gm/kg/dose Adults: 30-50 gm/dose	Stains clothing. Will absorb Syrup of Ipecac if given concomitantly.
Chloral Hydrate (Noctec, Aqua-choral)	Caps: 250, 500 mg Syrup: 250, 500 mg/5 ml Supp: 325, 500, 650	Children: Sedative: 25 mg/kg/dose Q8h PO or rectally Hypnotic: 50-75 mg/kg/dose PO or rectally Adult: Sedative: 250 mg/dose TID Hypnotic: 500 mg to 2 gm/dose PO or rectally	Irritating to mucous membranes; may cause laryngospasm if aspirated. Avoid large doses in severe cardiac disease. GI irritation. Contraindicated in hepatic or renal impairment.

132

Drug	Formulations	Dose	Recommendations
Chloramphenicol (Chloromycetin)	Caps: 250 mg Susp: 150 mg/5 ml Vials: 1 gm (100 mg/ml) Otic sol'n: 0.5% Ophthal sol'n: 0.16, 0.25, 0.5% Ophthal ointment: 1% Topical cream: 1%	Loading dose (severe infections): 20 mg/kg IV or PO Maintenance: *Neonates $\leq$7 days (premature and full term) - 25 mg/kg/day $\div$ Q6h IV 7-28 days Premature: 25 mg/kg/day $\div$ Q6h IV Full term: 50 mg/kg/day $\div$ Q6h Infants, children, adults: 50-100 mg/kg/day $\div$ Q6h IV or PO. *NOTE: Initiate maintenance therapy for neonates <7 days of age at 24 hrs after loading dose. Max. adult dose: 2 gm/day	Dose recommendations are guidelines for therapy; monitoring of blood levels is essential in neonates and infants. Drug is poorly absorbed IM. Follow hematologic status for dose-related or idiosyncratic marrow suppression. Check levels in face of hepatic or renal dysfunction. Therapeutic levels: 15-25 µg/ml.
Chlorothiazide (Diuril)	Tabs: 250, 500 mg Susp: 250 mg/5 ml Vials: 500 mg (20 ml)	<6 mos: 20-30 mg/kg/day PO Q12h >6 mos: 20 mg/kg/day PO Q12h Adults: 250-500 mg/dose QD or intermittently. Max. dose: 2 gm/day	Use with caution in liver and severe renal disease. May cause hyperbilirubinemia, hypokalemia, alkalosis, hyperglycemia, hyperuricemia.

Drug	Preparations	Dosage	Remarks
Chlorpromazine (Thorazine, Promapar, Chloramend)	Tabs: 10, 25, 50, 100, 200 mg. Spansules: 30, 75, 150, 200, 300 mg. Syrup: 10 mg/5 ml. Supp: 25, 100 mg. Oral Conc: 30, 100 mg/ml. Injection: 25 mg/ml (1 and 2 ml vials).	IM or IV: 0.5 mg/kg/dose or or 2 mg/kg/day Q6-8h. PO: 0.5 mg/kg/dose Q4-6h. Rectal: 1 mg/kg/dose Q6-8h. Max. dose: <5 yrs: 40 mg/day. 5-12 yrs: 75 mg/day.	Adverse effects include drowsiness, jaundice, lowered seizure threshold, extrapyramidal symptoms, hypotension, arrhythmias, agranulocytosis. May potentiate effects of narcotics, sedatives, other drugs. Monitor BP closely.
Cholestyramine (Questran, Cumid)	Powder: 9 gm packets. Tins: 378 gm (4 gms of active ingredient Anhydrous Cholestyramine in 9 gms Questran Powder)	Children: 240 mg/kg/day cholestyramine ÷ TID. Give PO as slurry in water, juice, etc. Adult: 4 gm TID	May cause constipation, diarrhea, vomiting, vitamin deficiencies (A, D, E, K), alter absorption of other drugs. Give other oral medications 1 hr before or 4-6 hrs after cholestyramine doses. Hyperchloremic acidosis may occur with prolonged use.
Cimetidine (Tagamet)	Tabs: 200, 300 mg. Vials: 150 mg/ml (2, 8 vials). Syrup: 300 mg/5 ml	Children: 20-40 mg/kg/day PO, IV ÷ Q6h. Max. dose: 2400 mg/day. Adults: 300 mg/dose QID	Use with caution in all patients. Diarrhea, rash, myalgia, neutropenia, gynecomastia, dizziness may occur.
Citrate Mixtures, Oral	Each ml contains: (mEq) Na K Citrate Polycitra 1 1 2 Polycitra K 0 2 2 Bicitra (Shohl's) 1 0 1	Children: 5-15 ml/dose PO Q6-8h; or 2-3 mEq/kg TID-QID. Adult: 15-30 ml PO Q6-8h. Dilute dose in water.	Adjust dose to maintain desired urine pH. 1 mEq of citrate is equivalent to 1 mEq HCO_3. Use with caution in patients already receiving potassium supplements.

Clindamycin (Cleocin)	Caps: 75, 150 mg Oral liquid: 75 mg/ 5 ml Injection: 150 mg/ml	Children: 8-25 mg/kg/day ÷ Q6-8h PO. 15-40 mg/kg/day ÷ Q6-8h IM or IV. Adults: 150-450 mg Q6h PO 600-2700 mg/day Q6-12h IM or IV. Max. dose: 4.8 gm/ day	Not indicated in meningitis. Use with caution in infants and neonates, in hepatic or renal insufficiency. Colitis may occur up to several wks after cessation of therapy, but is generally uncommon in pediatric patients.
Clonazepam (Clonopin)	Tabs: 0.5, 1.0 and 2.0 mg	Children: Up to 10 yr or 30 kg: Initial: 0.01-0.03 mg/kg/day ÷ Q8h Increments: not >0.25-0.5 mg Q3 days, up to maximum maintenance dose of 0.1-0.2 mg/kg/day ÷ Q8h Adult: Initial: 1.5 mg/day TID Increment: 0.5-1 mg Q3 day Max. dose: 20 mg/day	CNS depression, drowsiness and ataxia common. May cause behavioral changes, and other CNS symptoms; increased bronchial secretions, GI, CV, GU, and hematopoietic toxicity may occur. Use with caution in renal impairment.
Clotrimazole (Lotrimin, Mycelex)	Cream: 1% Solution: 1% Vaginal tabs: 100 mg Vaginal cream: 1%	Topical: apply to skin BID Vaginal Candidiasis: 1 tab in vagina daily x 7 days	May cause erythema, blistering, or urticaria where applied.
Cloxacillin (Tegopen, Cloxapen)	Caps: 250, 500 mg Oral Sol'n: 125 mg/ 5 ml	<20kg: 50-100 mg/kg/day ÷ Q6h PO >20kg: 1-2 gm/day ÷ Q6h PO. Max. dose: 4 gm/day	Same side effects as other penicillins. Give on an empty stomach.

Drug	Formulation	Dosage	Comments
Codeine	Tabs (sulfate): 15, 30, 60 mg; Amp (phosphate): 30, 60 mg/ml	Analgesic: Children: 0.5-1.0 mg/kg/dose Q4-6h IV or PO; Adults: 30-60 mg/dose Q4-6h IV or PO; Antitussive: Children: 1-1.5 mg/kg/day Q4h to max. of 30 mg/day; Adults: 10-20 mg/dose Q4-6h PRN	CNS and respiratory depression. Constipation, cramping. May be habit forming. For analgesia, use with acetaminophen orally.
Cortisone Acetate	Tabs: 5, 10, 25 mg; Vials: 25, 50 mg/ml	Physiologic replacement: 30-32 mg/M²/day ÷ Q8h PO 15-16 mg/M²/day IM single daily dose OR 45 mg/M²/dose IM Q3 days; Stress: 2-4 x physiologic replacement dose	See pages 205-206. IM slowly absorbed over several days.
Cromolyn (Intal)	Caps: 20 mg (must be administered via "spin haler"); Ampule: 20 mg for nebulization	Inhalant: 20 mg Q6h (for adults and children >5 yrs)	Not for acute asthmatic attack. Allow 2-4 wks for adequate trial. May cause rash, cough, bronchospasm, nasal congestion. Not recommended in children <5 yrs or in patients with renal or hepatic dysfunction.
Crotamiton (Eurax)	Cream (10%): 60 gm; Lotion (10%): 60 ml	Massage into skin of whole body from chin down, with particular attention to folds and creases; reapply 24 hrs later. Cleansing bath should be taken 48 hrs after last application.	Change clothing and bed linens. Clean immediately after treatment. Do not apply to raw or weeping skin. Avoid eyes and mouth.

Drug	Preparation	Dosage	Comments
Cyproheptadine (Periactin)	Tabs: 4 mg Syrup: 2 mg/ 5 ml	0.25–0.5 mg/kg/day PO ÷ Q6-8h. Max. total dose: 0.5 mg/kg/day Adult: 4-20 mg/day TID	Contraindicated in neonates. Use with caution in asthma. Anticholinergic (atropine-like) effects.
Dantrolene (Dantrium)	Cap: 25, 50, 100 mg IV: 0.32 mg/ml in 70 ml vials	Chronic spasticity: Children (>5 yrs): Initial: 0.5 mg/kg PO BID, then give 0.5 mg/kg PO TID or QID and increase by 0.5 mg/kg up to 3 mg/kg QID - do not exceed 100 mg PO QID Adults: Initial: 25 mg PO QD, then give 25 mg PO 2-4 x day and increase by 25 mg increments up to 100 mg PO QID if necessary. See package insert for use with malignant hyperthermia.	Contraindicated in active hepatic disease. Monitor transaminases for hepatotoxicity. May cause change in sensorium, weakness, and diarrhea. A decrease in spasticity sufficient to allow daily function not otherwise attainable should be therapeutic goal. Discontinue if benefits are not evident in 45 days.
Deferoxamine (Desferal)	Injection: 500 mg	Iron poisoning: Test dose: 2 gm IM. If urine positive (pink) then begin: 20 mg/kg Q4-6h IM or 10-15 mg/kg/hr by continuous or intermittent IV infusion. Do not exceed 15 mg/kg/hr. Lavage stomach with deferoxamine solution containing 2 gm/L in water buffered with NaHCO₃ to maintain gastric pH >5.0. After lavage, give per NG tube a solution containing 10 gm deferoxamine/50 ml H₂O, buffered with NaHCO₃ (gastric pH >5.0).	May cause hypotension, flushing, urticaria. Contraindicated in patients with severe renal disease or anuria. Use intravenous route with caution - risk of hypotension increased; vital signs must be closely monitored.

Drug	Preparation	Dosage	Comments
Desmopressin Acetate (DDAVP)	Nasal solution: 0.1 mg/ml (in 2.5 ml vial with applicator)	> 3 mos - 12 yrs: 0.05-0.3 ml/day as 1-2 doses intranasally. Adults: 0.1-0.4 ml/day in 2-3 doses. Titrate dose to achieve control of excessive thirst and urination. Max. adult dose: 0.4 ml/day	For intranasal use only. Adjust fluid intake to decrease risk of water intoxication. Use with caution in hypertension and coronary artery disease. Duration of effect is 8-12 hrs.
Desoxycorticosterone (DOCA, Percorten)	Injection: 5 mg/ml (in oil) Pellets: 125 mg	1-5 mg/day IM (in oil) as single dose, or implant 1 pellet Q8-12 mos for each 0.5 mg of daily IM dose	(See pages 205-206.) 1 mg DOCA = 0.1 mg 9α-fluoro-cortisol. IM preferred route. Use pellets only after IM dose is well established.
Dexamethasone (Decadron and other brand names)	Tabs: 0.25, 0.5, 0.75, 1.5, 4 mg Vials: 4, 10, 24 mg/ml Oral liquid: 0.5 mg/5 ml Inhalation: 0.143% (0.084 mg/metered dose)	Increased intracranial pressure: Initial loading dose: 0.5-1.5 mg/kg IV or IM. Maintenance: 0.25-0.5 mg/kg/dose ÷ Q6h IV, IM x 5 d, then taper. Airway edema: 0.25-0.5 mg/kg/dose Q6h PRN for croup or beginning 24 hrs before elective extubation, then x 4-6 doses. Shock: 3-6 mg/kg/dose Q4-6h (max. of 48-72 hrs).	(See pages 205-206.) IM route preferred unless patient is in shock or acutely ill (use IV). Toxicity - same as for prednisone.

		Dose for Attention Deficit	
Dextro-amphetamine (Dexedrine and many other brand names)	Tabs: 5, 10 mg Elixir: 5 mg/5 ml Sustained-release caps: 5, 10, 15 mg	**Disorder:** 3-5 yrs: 2.5 mg/day initially; increase daily dose by 2.5 mg increments at weekly intervals (range 2.5-40 mg/day) >6 yrs: double above dose (range 2.5-40 mg/day) **Dose for Narcolepsy:** 6-12 yrs: 5 mg/day; increase by 5 mg/day at weekly intervals (range 5-60 mg) >12 yrs: double above dose (range 5-60 mg)	Use with caution in presence of hypertension or cardiovascular disease. Not recommended for <3 yr. Interrupt administration occasionally to determine need for continued therapy. Many side effects including insomnia, restlessness, and anorexia. Tolerance develops.
Diazepam (Valium)	Tabs: 2, 5, 10 mg Amp: 5 mg/ml (for injection)	**Sedative/muscle relaxant:** <u>Children:</u> IM or IV: 0.04-0.2 mg/kg/dose Q2-4h (max. dose: 0.6 mg/kg within an 8 hr period) PO: 0.12-0.8 mg/kg/day TID-QID <u>Adults:</u> IM or IV: 2-10 mg/dose Q3-4h PRN PO: 2-10 mg/dose Q6-8h PRN **Status epilepticus:** <u>1 mo-5 yr:</u>0.2-0.5 mg/kg/dose IV Q15-30 min. (max. total dose: 5 mg). May repeat in 2-4h PRN. <u>>5 yrs:</u> 1 mg/dose IV Q15-30 min. (max. total dose: 10 mg) May repeat in 2-4h PRN Adults: 5-10 mg/dose IV Q10-15 min (max. total dose: 30 mg) May repeat in 2-4h PRN	Hypotension and respiratory depression may occur. Use with caution in glaucoma, shock, and depression. Give undiluted - do not mix with IV fluids. Not recommended for use in neonates. In status epilepticus, diazepam must be followed by long acting anticonvulsants.

Diazoxide (Hyperstat, Proglycem)	Amp: 15 mg/ml (injection) Caps: 50, 100 mg Susp: 50 mg/ml	Hypertensive crisis: Children: 3-5 mg/kg IV as bolus injection given as fast as possible. May repeat in 30 min, and Q3-10h PRN. Adults: 1-3 mg/kg up to 150 mg; repeat 5-15 min PRN, then Q4-24h Hypoglycemia (due to insulin producing tumors): Newborns and infants: 8-15 mg/kg/day ÷ Q8-12h PO or IV Children and adults: 3-8 mg/kg/day ÷ Q8-12h PO or IV (start at lowest dose)	May cause hyponatremia, salt and water retention, GI disturbances, ketoacidosis, hyperuricemia, hypertrichosis and arrhythmias. Monitor BP closely for hypotension. Hyperglycemia occurs in majority of patients. Hypoglycemia should initially be treated with IV glucose; diazoxide should be introduced only if refractory to glucose infusion.
Dicloxacillin sodium (Dynapen, and many other brand names)	Caps: 125, 250, 500 mg Oral Susp: 62.5 mg/5 ml	Children (<40 kg): 25-75 mg/kg/day Q6h Adults (>40 kg): 250 mg-1 gm Q6h	Similar toxicity and side effects as with cloxacillin. Give 1-2 hrs before meals. Limited experience in neonates and very young infants.
Dihydro-tachysterol USP	Caps: 0.125 mg Sol'n (in oil): 0.25 mg/ml Tabs: 0.125, 0.2, 0.4 mg	Hypoparathyroidism: Neonates: 0.05-0.1 mg/day Infants/Young Children: 0.1-0.5 mg/day Older Children/Adults: 0.5-1.0 mg/day Hypophosphatemic Vit. D-resistant rickets: 0.25-1.0 mg/day Nutritional rickets: 5 mg x 1 dose Renal osteodystrophy: 0.6-6 mg/day until healing occurs, then 0.25-0.6 mg/day	Monitor serum Ca++ and PO4. Action faster than that of Vit. D. Titrate dosage with patient response. Oral Ca++ supplementation may be required. 1 mg equiv. to 120,000 units Vit. D2. Activated by 25-hydroxylation in liver; does not require 1-hydroxylation in kidney.

Dimenhydrinate (Dramamine and other brand names)	Tabs: 50 mg Sol'n: 15.0 mg/5 ml Amp: 50 mg/ml (injection) Supp: 100 mg	Children (<12 yr): 5 mg/kg/day ÷ Q6h PO, IM, or rectal. Max. IM dose: (children) 300 mg/day Adult: 50-100 mg Q4h PO; 100 mg QD-BID PR; 50 mg PRN IM	May mask vestibular symptoms. Caution when taken with ototoxic agents. Causes drowsiness.
Dimercaprol (B.A.L., British anti-Lewisite)	Injection (in oil): 100 mg/ml (3 ml amp)	Give all injections deep IM Dose: Lead poisoning: For symptomatic patients with blood lead 70-100 µg/100 ml: 333 mg/M² /day x 2-3 day. For encephalopathic patients or with blood level >100 µg/100 ml: 500 mg/M² /day Q4h x 3-5 day.	May cause hypertension, tachycardia, GI disturbance, headache, fever (30% of children). (Symptoms are usually relieved by anti-histamines.) Contra-indicated in hepatic or renal insufficiency. Urine must be alkaline. May result in renal toxicity. Use cautiously in patient with G6PD deficiency. Do not use concomitantly with iron. See section on lead poisoning page 242.
Diphenhydramine (Benadryl and other brand names)	Caps: 25, 50 mg Tabs: 50 mg Elixir: 12.5 mg/5 ml Injection: 10, 50 mg/ml	Children: 5 mg/kg/day PO or deep IM ÷ Q6h Adult: 10-50 mg/dose Q6-8h For anaphylaxis or phenothia-zine overdose: 1-2 mg/kg IV slowly. Max. total dose: 300 mg/day	Side effects common to anti-histamines. CNS side effects more common than GI distur-bances. Contraindicated in infants and neonates.

Drug	Preparations	Dosage	Comments
Dobutamine (Dobutrex)	Injection: 250 mg/ 20 ml vials	Continuous IV infusion: 2.5-15 $\mu g/kg/min$. To prepare for infusion: $6 \times$ wt(kg) $\times$ desired dose ($\mu g/kg/min$) = IV infusion rate (ml/hr) mg of drug to be added to 100 ml of IV fluid Max. recommended dose: 40 $\mu g/kg/min$	Monitor blood pressure and vital signs. T1/2 = 2 min. Contraindicated in IHSS. Side effects of tachycardia hypertension, arrhythmias (PVC's) may occasionally occur (especially at higher infusion rates). Adjust rate and duration of therapy according to patient response. Correct hypovolemic states before use. Increases AV conduction, may precipitate ventricular ectopic activity.
Docusate (Colace and many other brand names)	Caps: 50, 100, 120, 240 mg Syrup: 20 mg/5 ml Tab: 50, 100 mg Drops: 10 mg/1 ml	PO: (take with liquids) <u><3 yr:</u> 10-40 mg/day QD-QID 3-6 yr: 20-60 mg/day QD-QID 6-12 yr: 40-120 mg/day QD-QID >12 yr: 50-240 mg/day QD-QID Rectal: <u>Older children and adults:</u> add 50-100 mg to enema solution	PO requires 1-3 days for notable effect. Incidence of side effects is exceedingly low.
Dopamine (Intropin)	Injection: 40 mg/ml 80 mg/ml (5 ml/vial)	Continuous IV infusion: Effects are dose dependent. Titrate to achieve desired effect. Low dose (2-5 $\mu g/kg/min$): Increases renal blood flow. Less effect on heart rate and cardiac output. (CONTINUED)	Monitor vital signs and blood pressure continuously. Correct hypovolemic states. Tachyarrhythmias, ectopic beats, hypertension, vasoconstriction, vomiting may occur. Extravasation may cause tissue necrosis. Use cautiously with phenytoin.

Dopamine (Introprin)	(CONTINUED)	Intermediate doses (5-15 μg/kg/min): Increases renal blood flow, heart rate, cardiac contractility, and cardiac output. High doses (>20 μg/kg/min): Alpha adrenergic effects are prominant. Decreases renal perfusion. To prepare for infusion: $$\frac{6 \times wt(kg) \times \text{desired dose } (\mu g/kg/min)}{IV \text{ infusion rate (ml/hr)}} =$$ mg of drug to be added to 100 ml of IV fluid Max. dose recommended: 20-50 μg/kg/min.	
Doxycycline (Vibramycin and other brand names)	Caps: 50, 100, 300 mg Tabs: 100 mg Oral sol'n: (as Calcium salt) 50 mg base/5 ml; (as Monohydrate) 25 mg base/5 ml Injection: 100, 200 mg/vial	Initial: <45 kg - 4.4 mg/kg/day ÷ Q12h PO or IV x 1 day; >45 kg - 200 mg/day ÷ Q12h PO or IV x 1 day Maintenance: <45 kg - 2.2 mg/kg/day as single dose or ÷ Q12h PO or IV >45 kg - 100 mg/day as single dose or ÷ Q12h PO or IV Max. adult dose: 300 mg/day	Use with caution in hepatic and renal disease. May cause increased intracranial pressure. Use in children <8 yrs may result in tooth enamel hypoplasia and discoloration. May cause GI symptoms, photosensitivity, hemolytic anemia, hypersensitivity reactions. Infuse over 1-4 hrs IV; avoid extravasation. See tetracycline.

Edrophonium (Tensilon)	Injection: 10 mg/ml (1 ml)	Test for myasthenia gravis (IV): Neonate: 1.0 mg single dose Infant, child, and adult: 0.2 mg/kg/dose. Give 20% of the test dose slowly; if no response in 1 min give 1 mg increments Max. total dose: 5-10 mg	Keep atropine available in syringe and have resuscitation equipment ready. May precipitate cholinergic crisis, arrhythmias, bronchospasm. Hypersensitivity to test dose (fasciculations or intestinal cramping) is indication to delay further administration of the drug.
EDTA Calcium disodium	Amp: 200 mg/ml (5 ml)	Lead poisoning: 1-1.5 gm/M²/day, ÷ Q4-12h and given x 3-5 days depending on severity. Do not exceed 7 days duration of administration. Can add procaine (final conc. 0.5%) when giving IM. IM route preferred.	May cause renal tubular necrosis. Do not use if anuric. Follow urinalysis and renal function. Monitor EKG continuously when giving IV. Rapid IV infusion may cause sudden increase in intracranial pressure in patients with cerebral edema. May cause zinc deficiency by chelation effect.
Ephedrine	Tabs: 25 mg Syrup: 20 mg/5 ml or 11 mg/5 ml Caps: 25, 50 mg Amp: 25, 50 mg/ml Nasal drops: 0.5%	Children: 0.5-1.0 mg/kg/dose Q4-8h (max. dose: 3 mg/kg/day) Adults: IM, SC, or PO: 25-50 mg Q3-4h. IV: 5-25 mg slow push; repeat in 5-10 min PRN	May potentiate actions of theophylline or precipitate arrhythmias. Insomnia, nervousness, headache, sweating are other side effects.

Epinephrine (Adrenalin)	1:1000 (Aqueous): Amp: 1 mg/ml (1 ml) Vials: 1 mg/ml (30 ml) 1:200 (Sus-phrine): Vials: 5 mg/ml (5 ml) 1:10,000 (Aqueous): Prefilled syringes 10 ml Aerosol (15 ml): each contains 300 metered doses equivalent to 0.16 mg/dose or 0.2 mg/dose of epine-phrine.	1:1000 (Aqueous): 0.01 ml/kg/dose SC (max. single dose 0.3 ml); repeat Q15 min x 3-4 or Q4h PRN 1:200 (Sus-phrine): 0.005 ml/kg/dose SC (max. single dose 0.15 ml); repeat Q8-12h PRN 1:10,000 (Aqueous) 0.1 ml/kg/dose IV Q5-10 min (max. 10 ml for adult) Inhalation: 1-2 puffs during attack. Repeat Q4h PRN	May produce arrhythmias, tachycardia, hypertension, headaches, nervousness, nausea, vomiting. Necrosis may occur at site of repeated local injection.
Epinephrine, Racemic (Vaponefrin, Micronefrin Asthmanefrin)	Sol'n: 2.25%	Croup: 0.05 ml/kg/dose diluted to 3 ml with saline. Given via nebulizer PRN, but not more frequently than Q2h. Max. dose: 0.5 ml	"Rebound" common. Tachyar-rhythmias, headache, nausea, palpitations reported.
Ergocalciferol (Drisdol, Calciferol) Vit. D$_2$	Caps: 0.62 mg (25,000 IU); 1.25 mg (50,000 IU) Sol'n: 0.25 mg/ml (10,000 IU) Injection: 12.5 mg (500,000 IU)/ml Drops: 8,000 IU/ml (0.2 mg) (200 IU/gtt) 1 mg = 40,000 IU	Maintenance: 400 IU/day Renal osteodystrophy: 25,000-250,000 IU/day until healing occurs, then 10,000-25,000 IU/day Rickets: Vit. D dependent: 5,000-15,000 IU/day Vit. D resistant: 25,000-1,000,000 IU/day Nutritional: 10,000 IU/day x 30 days	Monitor serum Ca++, PO$_4$, and alk. phos. Titrate dosage to patient response. Maintain serum Ca++ 8.5-10.0 mg/dl, and urinary Ca++ <3 mg/kg/day. Watch for symptoms of hypercalcemia. Vit. D$_2$ is activated by 25-hydroxylation in liver and 1-hydroxylation in kidney.

Erythromycin Salts (Erythrocin, Pediamycin, Ilosone, E-Mycin and others)	Erythromycin: Tabs: 250, 500 mg Erythromycin Ethyl Succinate: Susp: 200, 400 mg/ 5 ml Drops: 100 mg/2.5 ml Tabs: 200, 400 mg Erythromycin Lactobionate: Vials: 500, 1000 mg Erythromycin Estolate (Ilosone): Tabs: 500 mg Chewable tabs: 125, 250 mg Drops: 100 mg/ml Caps: 125, 250 mg Susp: 125, 250 mg/5ml Erythromycin Stearate Tabs: 125, 250, 500 mg	Oral: Children: 30-50 mg/kg/day ÷ Q6-8h Adults: 1-4 gm/day ÷ Q6h Parenteral: 10-20 mg/kg/day ÷ Q6h IV Rheumatic fever prophylaxis: 500 mg/day ÷ Q12h PO Max. adult dose: 4 gm/day	Avoid IM route (pain, necrosis). GI side effects common (nausea, vomiting, abdominal cramps). Use with caution in liver disease. Estolate causes cholestatic jaundice, although hepatotoxicity uncommon (<2% of reported cases). May produce elevated digoxin and carbamazepine levels.
Erythromycin Ethylsuccinate and Acetyl Sulfisoxazole (Pediazole)	Susp: 200 mg erythro and 600 mg sulfa/5 ml	Otitis media: 50 mg/kg/day (as erythro) and 150 mg/kg/day (as sulfa) ÷ Q6h PO Max. dose: 6 gm sulfisoxazole/day	See adverse effects of erythromycin and sulfisoxazole. Not recommended in infants <2 mos.

Drug	Supplied	Dosage	Comments
Ethambutol (Myambutol)	Tabs: 100, 400 mg	Children >12 yrs and adults: 15-25 mg/kg/day as single PO dose. Not recommended for children <12 yrs. Should be used concurrently with another antituberculosis drug.	May cause optic neuritis, especially with larger doses. Obtain baseline ophthalmologic studies before beginning therapy and then monthly. Follow visual acuity, visual fields, and (green) color vision. Discontinue if any visual deterioration occurs. Monitor uric acid, liver function, heme status and renal function. May cause GI disturbances. Adjust with renal failure.
Ethosuximide (Zarontin)	Caps: 250 mg Syrup: 250 mg/5 ml	Initial: 3-6 yr: 250 mg/day PO BID or QD >6 yr: 500 mg/day PO BID or QD Increase as necessary: 250 mg every 4-7 days Maintenance: 20-30 mg/kg/day Max. dose: 1.5 gm/day Therapeutic levels: 40-100 µg/ml	Monitor levels. Use with caution in hepatic and renal disease. Ataxia, anorexia, GI distress are adverse effects; rashes and blood dyscrasias are rare idiosyncratic reactions. May increase frequency of grand mal seizures in patients with mixed type seizures.
Fluoride	Drops: 0.125 mg, 0.25 mg/drop Solution: 0.2 mg/ml Chewable tabs: 0.25, 0.5, 1.0 mg	Dose (mg/day): Concen. of Fluoride in Drinking Water (ppm) Age / <0.3 / 0.3-0.7 / >0.7 2 wk-2 yr: 0.25 / 0 / 0 2-3 yr: 0.5 / 0.25 / 0 3-16 yr: 1.00 / 0.50 / 0	Acute overdose: GI distress and salivation. Chronic excess use: mottled teeth and bone changes.

9α-Fluoro-cortisol (Florinef)	Tabs: 0.1 mg	0.05-0.1 mg/day PO Usual dose: 0.1 mg/day	Preferably administered in conjunction with cortisone or hydrocortisone. If elevated BP develops, decrease dose to 0.05 mg/day. 0.1 mg 9α-fluorocortisol = 1 mg DOCA. See pages 205-206.
Flurazepam (Dalmane)	Caps: 15, 30 mg	15-30 mg PO QHS Max. dose: 30 mg	Dizziness, GI symptoms, hematologic abnormalities, hepatic dysfunction. Rarely causes paradoxical hyperactivity. Not recommended for children <15 yrs.
Furosemide (Lasix and others)	Tabs: 20, 40, 80 mg Amp: 10 mg/ml Oral liquid: 10 mg/ml	Oral: Infants and Children: 2 mg/kg/dose Q6-8h PRN; may increase by 1-2 mg/kg/dose Adult: 20-80 mg/day QD or BID; may increase 20 or 40 mg up to total of 600 mg/day Parenteral: Infants and Children: 1 mg/kg/dose Q12h IM or IV PRN; may increase by 1 mg/kg/dose Adult: 20-80 mg/dose IM or IV Max. single dose (PO, IM, IV): 6 mg/kg	Ototoxicity may occur in presence of renal disease. Use with caution in hepatic disease. May cause hypokalemia, alkalosis, dehydration, and increased calcium excretion. Prolonged use in premature infants may result in nephrocalcinosis.

Gamma Benzene Hexachloride (Kwell, Lindane)	Shampoo: 1% Lotion: 1% Cream: 1%	Shampoo: Use < 30 ml per application Lotion: apply to skin, leave on 12-24 hr, then wash off. Change clothing and bed sheets after starting treatment. Treat family members. NOTE: Second application not usually necessary - may repeat application in 7-10 days if lice persist.	Systemically absorbed. Risk of toxic effects is greater in young children; use other agents in infants, young children, and during pregnancy. Avoid contact with face or mucous membranes. CNS toxicity reported with repeated use.

Gentamicin (Garamycin and others)	Vials: 10, 40 mg/ml
	Ophth ointment: 3 mg/gm
	Drops: 3 mg/ml
	Topical ointment: 0.1%
	Intrathecal amp: 2 mg/ml
		Parenteral (IM or IV):
		Neonates
		  <7 days - 5 mg/kg/day ÷ Q12h;
		  >7 days, infants - 7.5 mg/ kg/day ÷ Q8h
		Children: 5-7.5 mg/kg/day Q8h
		Adults: 3-5 mg/kg/day ÷ Q8h
		Intrathecal/intraventricular:
		  >3 mos - 1-2 mg daily;
		  Adult - 4-8 mg daily
		Ophth drops: 1-2 gtts Q4h
		Ophth oint: apply Q6-8h
			Monitor levels (peak and trough). Therapeutic levels: 6-10 µg/ml (peak); <2 µg/ml (trough). Monitor renal status; watch for ototoxicity. Higher than recommended doses may be necessary when based on serum levels. Intrathecal or intraventricular administration is adjunctive to parenteral administration. Arachnoiditis, phlebitis are seen uncommonly.

Glycopyrrolate (Robinul)	Tabs: 1, 2 mg
	Vials: 0.2 mg/ml
		Respiratory antisecretory:
		  Children: 0.004-0.010 mg/kg/ dose IV Q4-8h
		  Adults: 0.1-0.2 mg/dose IV Q4-8h. Max. dose: 0.2 mg/dose or 0.8 mg/day
		Reverse neuromuscular block: 0.2 mg per each mg neostigmine IV
		Oral: Adult: 1-2 mg BID-TID
		  Children: Dose not established
			Atropine-like side effects. Use with caution in hepatic and renal disease, ulcerative colitis, asthma.

Griseofulvin Microcrystalline (Grifulvin V, Grisactin, Fulvicin)	Microsize tabs: 125, 250, 500 mg Caps: 125, 250, 500 mg Susp: 125 mg/5 ml Ultramicrosize tabs: 330 mg = 500 mg microsize	Children >2 yrs: 5-10 mg/kg/day PO ÷ Q6-24h. Give with meals. May need to treat wide-spread infections with 20 mg/kg/day initially). Adult: 500 mg/day QD. Decrease dose accordingly if using ultramicrosize. Max. adult dose: 1 gm/day	Monitor hematologic, renal, and hepatic function. Possible cross-reactivity in penicillin-allergic individuals. Contraindicated in porphyria, hepatic disease. Usual treatment period 4-6 wks (for tinea unguum, 4-6 mos). Photosensitivity reactions may occur.
Heparin sodium	Injection: 10, 100, 1,000, 5,000, 10,000, 20,000, 40,000 units/ml Repository injection: 20,000 U/ml 120 U = approx. 1 mg	Infants and Children: Initial: 50 U/kg IV bolus Maintenance: 10-25 U/kg/hr as continuous infusion, or 100 U/kg/dose IV Q4h Adults: Initial: 10,000 U IV bolus Maintenance: 5,000-10,000 units Q4h IV intermittently or as constant infusion.	Adjust dose to give clotting time of 20-30 min or PTT of 1½-2½ x control value before dose. Antidote: Protamine sulfate (1 mg per 100 U heparin in previous 4 hr)
Hepatitis B immune globulin (HBIG, Hyperhep)	Vials: 1, 5 ml	IM: 0.06 ml/kg IM to max. of 3-5 ml given within 7 days of exposure. Repeat 30 days after exposure.	Contraindicated in patients with allergy to human Ig, coagulopathies, IgA deficiency, thrombocytopenia. Recommended for post-exposure prophylaxis following parenteral exposure, direct mucous membrane contact, or oral ingestion of HB$_s$ AG positive materials.

Hydralazine (Apresoline)	Tabs: 10, 25, 50, 100 mg; Amps: 20 mg/ml	Hypertensive crisis: Children: 0.1-0.2 mg/kg/dose IM or IV Q4-6h PRN; Adults: 20-40 mg IM or IV Q3-6h PRN; Chronic hypertension: Children: 0.75-3 mg/kg/day PO Q6-12h; Adults: 10-50 mg/dose PO QID	Use with caution in severe renal and cardiac disease. May cause lupus- and arthritis-like syndromes. CV, neurologic, GI, hematologic, dermatologic reactions may be seen. Follow blood pressure closely.
Hydrochlorothiazide, USP (Esidrix, Hydrodiuril)	Tabs: 25, 50, 100 mg	Infants and Children: 2-3 mg/kg/day PO Q12h; Adult: 25-100 mg/day QD or BID; Max. adult dose: 200 mg/day	See chlorothiazide.
Hydrocortisone (Solu-cortef)	Tabs: 5, 10, 20 mg; Oral susp: 2 mg/ml; Na Phosphate: Vials: 50 mg/ml; Na succinate (Solu-Cortef): Vials: 100, 250, 500, 1000 mg/ml; Acetate: Vials: 25, 50 mg/ml	Physiologic replacement: 12.5 mg/M^2/day IM; 25 mg/M^2/day PO ÷ Q8h; Shock: (Na succinate): initial dose 50 mg/kg IV; subsequently - 50-75 mg/kg/day ÷ Q6h IV; Status asthmaticus: Loading: 4-8 mg/kg/dose, then 10 mg/kg/day ÷ Q6h IV	See pages 205-206.
Hydroxyzine (Atarax, Vistaril)	Tabs (HCl): 10, 25, 50, 100 mg; Caps (pamoate): 25, 50, 100 mg; Syrup (HCl): 10 mg/5 ml; Susp (pamoate): 25 mg/5 ml; Vials (HCl): 25, 50 mg/ml	Oral: Children: 2 mg/kg/day ÷ Q6h; Adult: 25-100 mg/dose QID; Parenteral: Children: 0.5-1.0 mg/kg/dose Q4-6h IM PRN; Adult: 25-100 mg/dose IM PRN; Max. adult dose: 600 mg/day	May potentiate barbiturates, meperidine and other depressants. May cause dry mouth, drowsiness, tremor, convulsions.

Ibuprofen (Motrin)	Tabs: 300, 400, 600 mg	Adults: 400 mg/dose Q4-6h Max. adult dose: 2.4 gm/day Not FDA approved for children	GI distress (lessened with milk), rashes, ocular problems. Inhibits platelet aggregation. Use cautiously in patients with aspirin hypersensitivity.

Imipramine (Tofranil)	Tabs: 10, 25, 50 mg
	Caps: 75, 100, 125, 150 mg
	Vials: 12.5 mg/ml
		Antidepressant: Not recommended for children <12 yr
		Adult:
		  Initial: 75-150 mg/day BID;
		  Maintenance: 50-300 mg/day QD at bedtime
		  Max. adult dose: 300 mg/day
		Enuresis: Not recommended in children <6 yr
		  Initial: 10-25 mg Q HS
		  Increment: 10-25 mg/dose at 1-2 wk intervals until max. dosage for age or desired effect is achieved. Continue x 2-3 mos, then taper.
		  Max. dose:
		    6-8 yr: 50 mg/day
		    8-10 yr: 60 mg/day
		    10-12 yr: 70 mg/day
		    12-14 yr: 75 mg/day
			Caution in presence of MAO inhibitors, arrhythmias, glaucoma. May effect sensorium. Use cautiously in patients with cardiovascular diseases, urinary retention, or seizure disorder.

Indomethacin (Indocin)	Caps: 25, 50 mg Injection: investigational drug	Anti-inflammatory: >14 yrs old: 1-3 mg/kg/day (max. dose: 100 mg/day) TID or QID Adults: 50-150 mg/day BID-QID Closure of ductus arteriosus: 0.2-0.3 mg/kg/dose. Repeat at intervals of 24h up to total of 3 doses. Not FDA approved.	In neonates: monitor renal and hepatic function before and during use. May ↓ platelet aggregation. GI disturbances, headache, blood dyscrasias may occur.
Insulin		See insulin preparations. Pages 203-204.	See Endocrine section: DKA, and subsequent insulin management. Pages 82-84.
Ipecac, Syrup of	Syrup: 7% 15 and 30 ml available over the counter	<1 yr: 5-10 ml PO (followed by 200 ml water) >1 yr: 15 ml PO (followed by 200 ml water). Repeat in 20 min. x 1 only if no result Adults: 15-30 ml PO (followed by 200-300 ml water). Repeat x 1 only if no result.	If no results, remove ipecac from stomach by lavage. Cardiac toxicity (arrhythmias); GI irritation. Do not give to unconscious patients. Emesis will occur only if stomach is distended with fluid.
Iron Dextran (Imferon and others) (2% Fe)	Amp: 2, 5, 10 ml (IM or IV) (contains 50 mg elemental Fe/ml)	Total dose in mg Fe: a) surface area (M^2) x 55 x (13.5-Hb in gm%) = mg Fe needed IM or IV OR b) Wt (kg) x 2.5 x (13.5 - pt's Hb in gm%) = mg Fe needed IM or IV Note: Add 10-50% to above for iron stores replenishment. Max. IV dose: 2 ml/day Max. daily dose: <5 kg: 0.5 ml <10 kg: 1.0 ml <50 kg: 2.0 ml >50 kg: 5.0 ml	Oral therapy with iron salts is preferred. Numerous side and adverse effects, including anaphylaxis, fever, myalgias, arthralgias. Use "Z-track" technique for IM administration. Inject test dose (0.5 ml) on first day. Give IV at rate of <1 ml/min. undiluted, up to 2 ml/day.

Iron Salts	Ferrous sulfate (20% Fe):
	  Drops (Fer-in-sol):
	    75 mg (15 mg Fe)/
	    0.6 ml
	  Syrup (Fer-in-sol):
	    90 mg/5 ml (18 mg
	    Fe/5 ml)
	  Elixir (Feosol):
	    220 mg (44 mg Fe)/
	    (5 ml)
	  Caps & Tabs: 200 mg
	    (40 mg Fe), 300 mg
	    (60 mg Fe)
	Ferrous gluconate
	(Fergon): (11.5% Fe):
	  Elixir: 300 mg
	    (35 mg Fe)/5 ml
	  Tabs: 320 mg (37 mg
	    Fe)
	  Caps (sustained-
	    release): 435 mg
	    (50 mg Fe)
	  Caps: 325 mg (38 mg
	    Fe)
		<u>Treatment of iron deficiency</u>
		<u>anemia:</u> 6 mg elemental
		  Fe/kg/day ÷ TID PO
		<u>Prophylaxis:</u> (single dose or
		  ÷ BID-TID, PO)
		  Preterm infant - 2 mg elemental
		    Fe/kg/day
		  Full-term infant - 1 mg
		    elemental Fe/kg/day
		  Max. prophylactic dose: 15 mg/
		    day as elemental Fe
			Do not use in hemolytic dis-
			orders. Less GI irritation
			when given with meals.
			Vitamin C 200 mg per 30 mg
			iron enhances absorption.

Isoetharine (Bronkosol and others)	Aerosol (10, 20 ml dispensers): 20 metered doses/ml Each dose 340 µg isoetharine Solution: 1% (10 mg/ ml)	Aerosol: 1-2 puffs Q3-4h PRN Nebulization: 0.25-0.5 ml 1% solution diluted to 2 ml in NS (1:8-1:4 dilution) Q4h PRN. May be used more frequently with careful monitoring.	Toxicity: nausea, tachy- cardia, hypertension, anxiety, headache.

154

Drug	Preparations	Dosage	Comments
Isoniazid (INH)	Tabs: 50, 100, 300 mg Amp: 100 mg/ml	**Therapeutic:** Infants and children: 10-20 mg/kg/day as single dose or ÷ Q12h PO or IM. (max. dose: 300-500 mg/day); Adults: 5 mg/kg/day QD (max. dose: 300 mg/day) **Prophylaxis:** Infants and children: 10 mg/kg/day as single daily dose or ÷ Q12h PO (max. dose: 300 mg/day) Adults: 300 mg/day QD	CNS, hepatic side effects may occur with higher doses. Hepatotoxicity is rare in children, but discontinue drug if hepatic dysfunction occurs. Supplemental pyridoxine (1-2 mg/kg/day) is recommended.
Isoproterenol (Isuprel)	Isoproterenol HCL: Tabs: 10, 15 mg Solutions (vials): 1:400 (2.5 mg/ml) 1:200 (5 mg/ml) 1:100 (10 mg/ml) Aerosol (15 ml dispensers): 80 μg, 120 μg/dose Injection: 200 ug/ml (1:5000)	Sublingual: 5-10 mg/dose Q6-8h PRN (max: 30 mg/day). Aerosol: 1-2 puffs up to 5 times/day Nebulized solution: Children: 0.01 ml/kg/dose (max.: 0.05 ml/dose) diluted with NS to 2 ml. Give Q4h PRN; Adult: 0.25-0.5 ml diluted with NS to 2 ml Q4h PRN. IV: 0.1-1.5 ug/kg/min. Begin with 0.1 ug/kg/min. and increase every 5-10 min. by 0.1 ug/kg/min. until desired effect or heart rate >180 bpm or arrhythmia occurs. Usual max. dose: 1.5 μg/kg/min. To prepare for infusion: $\frac{6 \times wt(kg) \times desired\ dose\ (ug/kg/min)}{IV\ infusion\ (ml/hr)}$ = milligrams of drug to be added to 100 ml of IV fluid	Use with care in CHF. May precipitate arrhythmias in combination with epinephrine. Avoid "abuse" of inhaler. Patients with continuous IV infusion should be followed by continuous monitoring for arrhythmias and hypertension.

Kanamycin (Kantrex)	Caps: 500 mg Vials: 37.5 mg/ml, 250 mg/ml, 333 mg/ml	For IM (or IV) administration: <table><tr><td>Neonates</td><td><7 days</td><td>>7 days</td></tr><tr><td>BW ≤2000 gm</td><td>15 mg/ kg/day Q12h</td><td>20 mg/ kg/day Q12h</td></tr><tr><td>BW >2000 gm</td><td>20 mg/ kg/day Q12h</td><td>30 mg/ kg/day Q8h</td></tr></table>Infants and children 30 mg/kg/day ÷ Q8-12h Max. dose: 1.5 gm/day	Renal, ototoxicity. Administer over 30 min. if IV. Reduce dosage frequency with renal impairment. Therapeutic levels: peak: 25-30 µg/ml; trough: < 6 µg/ml
Lactulose (Cephulac)	Syrup: 3.3 gm/5 ml	Infant: 2.5-10 ml/day ÷ TID-QID PO Older children, adolescents: 40-90 ml/day TID-QID PO Adults: 30-45 ml/dose TID or QID	Use with caution in diabetes mellitus. GI discomfort, diarrhea may occur. If initial dose causes diarrhea, reduce immediately. Discontinue drug if diarrhea persists.
Levothyroxine (Synthroid)	Tabs: 25, 50, 100, 150, 200, 300, 400 µg Injection solution: 0.1 mg/ml Vials: 500 µg/vial	Neonates: PO: 25-50 µg/dayQD; IV: 20-40 µg/dayQD 4 wk - 1 yr: PO: 50 µg/day QD (5-6 µg/kg/day); IV: 40 µg/dayQD (CONTINUED)	Use with caution in patients on anticoagulants. Titrate dosage with clinical status and serum T_4. (100 µg thyroxine = 65 mg thyroid USP).

	(CONTINUED)		

Levothyroxine (Synthroid)		Children/Adolescents:
		PO:
		   Maintenance: 3-5 μg/kg/day
		   Initially give 1/4 of daily
		   maintenance dose. Increase
		   by increments of 1/4 main-
		   tenance dose at weekly
		   intervals;
		IV: 75% of oral dose. All
		   given as single daily dose
		Adults:
		PO:
		   Initially 25-50 μg/day
		   Increase by 25-50 μg/day
		   at intervals of 1 month.
		   Maintenance: 100-200 μg/day
		   (1.4-3 μg/kg/day);
		IV: 75% of oral dose	

Lidocaine (Xylocaine)	Vials: 0.5, 1, 1.5, 2, 4, 5% (1% solution = 10 mg/ml) Cream: 3% Ointment: 2.5, 5% Susp (viscous): 2% Jelly: 2% Prefilled syringes: 10 mg/ml (1%) 100 mg/5 ml (2%)	Anesthetic: apply or infiltrate locally PRN (max. total dose: 4-5 mg/kg) Anti-arrhythmic: Single bolus 1 mg/kg/dose slowly IV; may repeat Q5-10 min PRN (max. dose: 3-4.5 mg/kg/hr) Continuous infusion (IV): 20-50 μg/kg/min To prepare infusion: 6 x wt(kg) x desired dose <u> (μg/kg/min)</u> = IV infusion rate (ml/hr) ml of drug to be added to 100 ml of IV fluid	Topical use facilitates sen- sitization. Use sparingly orally to minimize aspira- tion. Side effects: hypo- tension, seizures, asystole, respiratory arrest. Decrease dose in presence of hepatic or renal failure. Contra- indicated in Stokes-Adams attacks, SA, AV, or intraven- tricular block. Prolonged (24 hr) infusion may result in toxic accumulation of lidocaine in plasma, neces- sitating reduction of infusion rate.

Lypressin (Diapid)	Nasal spray: 50 U/ml (2.0 U/spray) (8 ml/dispenser)	Diabetes insipidus: 1-2 sprays into each nostril QID and HS. If patient requires more than 2-3 sprays per dose, increase frequency of doses rather than larger amounts/dose	Titrate dose with thirst, urinary frequency. Coronary vasoconstriction may occur with large doses.
Magnesium Citrate	Solution: 300 ml bottles	4 ml/kg/dose PO Max. dose: 200 ml	Use with caution in renal insufficiency.
Magnesium Hydroxide (Milk of Magnesia)	Suspension (USP Magma): 8% Tabs: 300, 325 mg (equivalent to 3.75 ml suspension)	Children: 0.5 ml/kg/dose or 40 mg/kg/dose PO PRN Adults: 15-30 ml/dose	See Mg citrate.
Magnesium Sulfate	Injection: 100 mg/ml (0.8 mEq/ml) (10%) 500 mg/ml (4 mEq/ml) (50%) Oral solution: 50% (Epsom salts)	Cathartic: Child: 0.25 gm/kg/dose PO; Adult: 10-30 gm dose PO Hypomagnesemia: IV or IM: 25-50 mg/kg/dose Q4-6h x 3-4 doses. Repeat PRN; PO: 100-200 mg/kg/day QID. Maintenance: 0.25-0.50 mEq/ kg/day or 30-60 mg/kg/day IV to max. dose: 1000 mg/day	When given IV, monitor BP, respirations, and serum level. Calcium gluconate (IV) should be available as antidote. Use with caution in renal insufficiency.
Mannitol	Injection: 50, 100, 150, 200, 250 mg/ml (5, 10, 15, 20, 25%)	Anuria, Oliguria: (Test dose) 0.2 gm/kg/dose over 3-5 min. If there is no diuresis within 2 hrs, give no more mannitol. Edema: 1-2 gm/kg infused over 2-6 hr as 15-20% solution Cerebral edema: Acute Intra- cranial hypertension: 0.25 gm/ kg IV push, repeat Q5 min. PRN. (CONTINUED)	May cause circulatory over- load and electrolyte distur- bances. Keep serum osmolality at 310-320 mOsm/kg. Caution: may crystallize with concen- tration >20%.

Mannitol	(CONTINUED)	(Give furosemide 1 mg/kg concurrently or 5 min. before mannitol.) Dose of mannitol may be increased gradually to 1 gm/kg/dose if necessary for satisfactory response. Preoperative for Neurosurgery: 1.5-2 gm/kg IV over 30-60 min.	
Medium Chain Triglycerides (MCT oil)	Oil supplied in quarts	As calculated for necessary caloric supplement. Begin with 0.5 ml QO feed; advance to Q feed. Then increase in increments of 0.25-0.5 ml/feeding at intervals of 2-3 days as needed.	MCT derived from coconut oil. Provides 8.2 kcal/gm or 7.7 kcal/ml. Diarrhea may result if advanced rapidly or given in excessive amounts. Contraindicated in patients with cirrhosis.
Mebendazole (Vermox)	Tabs (chewable): 100 mg	Pinworms: 100 mg x 1, repeat in 2 wks Hookworms, Roundworms (Ascaris), Whipworm (Trichuris): 100 mg BID x 3 days	May cause diarrhea and abdominal cramping in cases of massive infection. Use with caution in children <2 yr.
Meperidine HCL (Demerol)	Tabs: 50, 100 mg Elixir: 50 mg/ml Vials: 25, 50, 75, and 100 mg/ml	PO, IM, IV: Children: 1-1.5 mg/kg/dose Q3-4h PRN or 6 mg/kg/day Q4-6h PRN Adults: 50-100 mg/dose Q3-4h PRN. 75 mg Demerol is equivalent to 10 mg morphine. Max. dose: 100 mg	Contraindicated in cardiac arrhythmias, asthma, increased intracranial pressure; potentiated by MAO inhibitors, phenothiazines, isoniazid and other CNS-acting agents.
Metoclopramide (Reglan)	Tabs: 10 mg Injection: 10 mg/ml Syrup: 1 mg/ml	Children: 1-6 yr: 0.1 mg/kg/dose 6-14 yr: 2.5-5 mg/dose Adult: 10 mg/dose	Max. dose: 0.5 mg/kg/day to avoid extrapyramidal effects.

Metaproterenol (Metaprel, Alupent)	Syrup: 10 mg/5 ml Tabs: 10, 20 mg Inhaler: each metered dose = 0.65 mg (15 ml containers) Inhalant solution: 5% (10 ml bottle)	Inhalation: Aerosol: 1-3 puffs Q3-4h to max. of 12 puffs/day Nebulized solution: Give undiluted solution by hand nebulizer (usual single dose = 10 inhalations, range 5-15) or dilute 0.2-0.3 ml in 2.5 ml NS for administration by IPPB or nebulizer. May repeat Q4h Oral: <6 yr: (Dose not well-established in this age group) 1.3-2.6 mg/kg/day TID or QID 6-9 yr: 10 mg/dose TID-QID >9 yr - Adult: 20 mg/dose TID-QID	Metaproterenol not approved in children <12 yrs. Adverse reactions as with other β-adrenergic agents. Excessive use may result in cardiac arrhythmias.
Methadone	Tabs: 5, 10 mg Vials: 10 mg/ml	Children: 0.7 mg/kg/day ÷ Q4-6h PO or SC PRN pain Adults: 2.5-10 mg/dose Q4-8h PRN pain Detoxification or maintenance: see package insert	Respiratory depression, hypotension. Generally not indicated in children <6 yrs old.
Methenamine Mandelate (Mandelamine)	Tabs: 250, 500, 1000 mg Susp: 250 mg/5 ml, 500 mg/5 ml Powder: 500 mg, 1 gm packets	<6 yrs: 50 mg/kg/day to max. of 250 mg/dose QID 6-12 yrs: 500 mg/dose QID >12 yrs - Adult: 1 gm/dose QID	Contraindicated in renal insufficiency. May cause dysuria and GI irritation. Maintain urine pH <5.5.

Methicillin (Staphcillin)	Vials: 1, 4, 6 gms	Newborn: <7 days: 50-100 mg/kg/day ÷ Q12h >7 days: 100-200 mg/kg/day ÷ Q6-8h Children: 100-400 mg/kg/day ÷ Q4-6h Adult: 4-12 gm/day Q4-6h Max. adult dose: 12 gm/day.	Allergic cross-reactivity with and same toxicity as penicillin. May cause hematuria and nephritis. (Contains 2.5 mEq Na/gm)
Methimazole (Tapazole)	Tabs: 5, 10 mg	Children: Initial: 0.4-0.7 mg/kg/day (TID) Maintenance: 1/2 initial dose (TID) Max: 30 mg/day Adults: Initial: 15-60 mg/day TID Maintenance: 10-30 mg/day BID or TID	Readily crosses placental membranes; blood dyscrasias, dermatitis, hepatitis, arthralgia, CNS reactions, hypothyroidism may occur. T1/2 = 6h
Methoxamine hydrochloride (Vasoxyl)	20 mg/ml	0.1 mg/kg IV	May cause sustained excessive BP elevation, headache, nausea.
Methsuximide (Celontin)	Caps: 150, 300 mg	Initial: 300 mg/day x 1 wk For Increase: 300 mg/day/wk x 3 wk to max. of 1.2 gms/day	GI symptoms, blood dyscrasias, CNS symptoms, and behavioral changes may occur. Use with caution in presence of renal or liver disease. Follow LFT and urinalysis.

Methyldopa (Aldomet)	Tabs: 125, 250, 500 mg Amp: 50 mg/ml	10 mg/kg/day PO ÷ Q8-12h; increase PRN at 2 day intervals. Max. dose: 65 mg/kg or 3 gm/day, whichever is less. Hypertensive crisis: 20-40 mg/kg/day IV Q6h	Contraindicated in pheochromocytoma and active hepatic disease. False positive Coombs, fever, hemolytic disease, leukopenia, sedation, GI disturbance.
Methylene blue	Amp: 10 mg/ml (1%)	Methemoglobinemia: 1-2 mg/kg/dose IV over 5 min.	
Methylphenidate (Ritalin)	Tabs: 5, 10, 20 mg Slow release 20 mg (8 hr duration)	Hyperactivity: Children >6 yrs old: 5 mg before breakfast, 5 mg before lunch; may increase dose by 5-10 mg/day increments at weekly intervals to max. of 60 mg/day. Same total daily dose for SR tablets.	In high dose may suppress height and growth. May increase BP and heart rate, suppress appetite, and interfere with sleep. Contraindicated in glaucoma. May interact with pressors. Close supervision advised.
Methylpred-nisolone (Medrol, Solu-Medrol, Depomedrol)	Tabs: 2, 4, 8, 16, 24, 32 mg; 34 mg extended release caps Injection (IV or IM): Na succinate (Solu-Medrol): 40, 125, 500, 1000 mg vials Injection (IM Repository): 20, 40, 80 mg/ml	Anti-inflammatory/Immunosuppressive: 0.4-1.6 mg/kg/day Q6-12h. Shock: 30 mg/kg/dose Q6h for max. of 48-72 hr Status Asthmaticus: Loading: 1-2 mg/kg/dose x 1, Maintenance: 0.5-1 mg/kg/dose Q6h up to 5 days before changing to oral route	See pages 205-206. Dose of methylprednisolone = 1/6 of cortisone dose. Repository used mainly for local therapy. Can be used IM for systemic effects as infrequently as Q week.

Metronidazole (Flagyl)	Tabs: 250 mg Vag. supp: 500 mg Injection: 500 mg (not currently approved for children <12 yr)	**Amebiasis:** Children: 35-50 mg/kg/day PO TID x 10 days. Adults: 750 mg PO TID x 5-10 days **Giardiasis:** Children: 5 mg/kg/dose PO TID x 10 days **Gardnerella vaginalis vaginitis:** 500 mg PO BID x 7 days **Trichomonas vaginitis:** Children: 5 mg/kg/dose PO TID x 7 days Adults: 250 mg/dose PO TID x 7 days or 2 gm PO x 1, IV - loading dose 15 mg/kg. Follow by 7.5 mg/kg Q6h	Nausea, diarrhea, urticaria, leukopenia, vertigo. Candidiasis may worsen. Patients should not ingest alcohol for 24 hr after dose (disulfuram type reaction). Potentiates anticoagulants.
Miconazole (Monistat)	Cream: 2% Lotion: 2% Vaginal cream: 2% Injection: 10 mg/ml	**Topical:** Apply BID x 2-4 wks **Vaginal:** 1 applicator - measured dose QHS x 7 days. IV: >1 yr.: 20-40 mg/kg/day Q8h, max. of 15 mg/kg/dose Adults: 200-1200 mg/dose Q8h.	Side effects of IV therapy: phlebitis, pruritus, rash, nausea, vomiting, fever, drowsiness, diarrhea, anorexia and flushes. Decrease in Hct and plt. have been reported.
Minocycline (Minocin)	Caps: 50, 100 mg Syrup: 50 mg/5 ml Vials: 100 mg	Children: (8-12 yrs): Initial: 4 mg/kg/dose x 1 Maintenance: 2 mg/kg/day Q12h Adolescents/Adults: Initial: 200 mg/dose x 1 Maintenance: 100 mg/day Q12h	High incidence of vestibular dysfunction. Hepatic metabolism and renal excretion. T1/2 = 18 hrs

Drug	Formulation	Dosage	Comments
Mithramycin (Mithracin)	Vials: 2500 μg (refrigerate)	<u>IV</u>: has been used in hypercalcemia associated with malignancies. 25 μg/kg/dose in 1 L D₅W or NS over 4-8 hrs, QD x 1-4 days. Repeat at weekly intervals if necessary or maintain 1-3 doses weekly.	Bone marrow depression, hemorrhagic diathesis with coagulopathy, cellulitis on extravasation, nausea, vomiting, hypocalcemia, hepatotoxicity, renal toxicity.
Morphine sulfate	Elixir: 2, 4 mg/ml Tabs: 10, 15, 30 mg Injection: 8, 10, 15 mg/ml	Analgesia and tetralogy (cyanotic) spells: 0.1-0.2 mg/kg/dose SC. Repeat Q2-4h PRN Max. dose: 15 mg/dose.	PO = 1/6 as effective as IM, IV. For respiratory depression see Naloxone. Addicting.
Moxalactam (Moxam)	IV Injection: 1-2 gm	Infants: <u>0-1 wk</u> - 50 mg/kg Q12h; 1-4 wk - 50 mg/kg Q8h Children and Infants >1 mo.: <u>200 mg/kg/day ÷ Q6h or Q8h</u> Adults: 2-6 gm/day ÷ Q6h or Q8h	Coagulation abnormalities responsive to vitamin K; platelet dysfunction, antabuse type reactions with ETOH. Cross reacts with penicillin.
Nafcillin	Caps: 250 mg Tabs: 500 mg Vials: 250 mg/ml Oral solution: 250 mg/5 ml	Newborn: <u><7 days</u>: 40 mg/kg/day ÷ Q12h; >7 days: 60 mg/kg/day ÷ Q6-8h Older infants and children: 50-100 mg/kg/day PO Q6h or 100-200 mg/kg/day IM Q12h or IV Q4h. (15-30 min. infusion) Adults: 4-12 gm/day IM Q6h or IV Q4h	Allergic cross-sensitivity with penicillin. Oral route not recommended due to poor absorption.

Naloxone (Narcan)	Amp: 0.4 mg/ml (400 µg/ml) Neonatal narcan: 0.02 mg/ml	5-10 µg/kg/dose IM or IV. Repeat as necessary Q3-5 min. Adult dose: 0.4 - 2.0 mg/dose Q2-3 min. x 1-3. May give 10 fold higher dose if needed for diagnosis or therapy.	Does not cause respiratory depression. Short duration of action may necessitate multiple doses. For very large ingestions 100-200 µg/kg have been necessary.
Neomycin Sulfate	Tabs: 500 mg Vials: 500 mg Oral susp: 125 mg/5 ml	Prematures and Newborns: 50 mg/kg/day PO ÷ Q6h Infants and Children: 50-100 mg/kg/day PO ÷ Q6h Adult: 50 mg/kg/day PO ÷ Q6h Hepatic Encephalopathy: Acute: 2.5-7 gm/M²/day PO ÷ Q6h x 5-7 days; Chronic: 2.5 gm/M²/day PO QID. Bowel Prep: 90 mg/kg/day Q4h x 3 days	Follow for renal or ototoxicity. Contraindicated in ulcerative bowel disease or intestinal obstruction.
Neostigmine (Prostigmine)	Tabs: 15 mg (bromide) Amp: 0.25, 0.5 mg/ml, 1 mg/ml Vials: 1 mg/ml	Myasthenia Gravis: Test dose: Children: 0.04 mg/kg/dose IM x 1; 0.02 mg/kg/dose IV x 1 Adults: 0.02 mg/kg/dose IM x 1 Treatment: Children: IM, IV, SC: 0.01-0.04 mg/kg/dose Q2-3h PRN. PO: 2 mg/kg/day Q3-4h Adults: IM, IV, SC: 0.5 mg/dose Q3-4h PRN. Max: 10 mg/day; PO: 15 mg/dose Q3-4h (CONTINUED)	Titrate for each patient, but avoid excessive cholinergic effects. Caution in asthmatics. Contraindicated in intestinal and urinary obstruction. May cause cholinergic crisis. Keep atropine available.

Neostigmine (Prostigmine)	(CONTINUED)	Reversal of Nondepolarizing Neuromuscular Blocking Agents: Children: 0.07-0.08 mg/kg/dose IV with atropine Adults: 0.5-2 mg/dose IV with atropine. Max. dose: 2.5 mg/dose	
Netilmicin (Netromicin)	Injection: 100, 25, 10 mg/ml	Neonates <6 wk: 4-6.5 mg/kg/day ÷ Q12h Children 6 wk-12 yr: 5.5 - 8 mg/kg/day ÷ Q8h Adults: >12 yr.: 4 - 6.5 mg/kg/day ÷ Q8h	Ototoxicity, neurotoxicity similar to other amino-glycosides. Also elevates LFTS. Hematologic changes, neuromuscular blockade.
Niclosamide (Yomesan)	Tab: 0.5 gm	For tapeworm: 11-34 kg - 2 tab >34 kg - 3 tab Adult - 4 tab (Given as single dose - chewed thoroughly)	Nausea and abdominal pain. Available from Center for Disease Control.
Nitrofurantoin (Furadantin, Macrodantin)	Tabs 50, 100 mg Susp: 25 mg/5 ml Caps: (Macrocrystal) 25, 50, 100 mg Injection: 180 mg vial	Children: 5-7 mg/kg/day Q6h. Reduce to 2.5-5 mg/kg/day after 10-14 days for chronic therapy. Adults: Prophylaxis: 50-100 mg QHS. Treatment: 50-100 mg/dose Q6h Give with food or milk. Max. adult dose: 400 mg/day	Large range of hypersensitivity reactions. Contra-indicated in severe renal disease, G6PD deficiency, and in infants <1 month of age. Dosage may require reduction in prolonged usage (>2 wks).

Nitroprusside (Nipride)	Vial: 50 mg	Dilute with D_5W and wrap in aluminum foil. Constant infusion: 15 mg/kg x wt(kg) in 250 ml D_5W. Then rate in μg/kg/min = rate in ml/hour. Begin at 1.0 μg/kg/min. Titrate dose to BP. Range 0.5-10 μg/kg/min.	Must be monitored with arterial line. Produces profound hypotension, metabolic acidosis and CNS symptoms when overdosed. Monitor thiocyanate levels with long term use (>48 hr). Levels should not exceed 12 mg/dl.
Nystatin	Tabs: 100,000, 500,000 U. Susp: 100,000 U/ml Topical powder, oint., cream: 100,000 U/gm Vag supp: 100,000 U	Premature and Newborn Infants: 400,000 U/day PO ÷ Q6-8h. Older Infants and Children: 1-2 mil U/day ÷ Q6-8h Vaginal: 1 supp QHS x 10 d Topical: Apply BID-QID until 2-3d after infection has cleared.	May produce diarrhea and GI symptoms.
Oxacillin	Capsules: 250, 500 mg Oral Soln: 250 mg/5 ml	PO: Give on empty stomach. Children: 50-100 mg/kg/day Q6h Adults: 500-1000 mg/dose Q4-6h Limited experience in newborns.	Same as methicillin.
Pancreatic enzymes, (Pancrease, Viokase, Cotazyme)	Enteric coated microspheres (Pancrease): capsules Non-enteric coated (Viokase, Cotazyme) Tablets Powder (Viokase, Cotazyme)	Enteric Coated: 1-2 capsules with meals, and 1 capsule with snacks. Microspheres may be mixed with each feeding for infants. Non-enteric coated: 3-12 tablets or 1-4 tsp. with each meal. Titrate according to patient's needs.	May cause occult GI bleeding, hyperuricemia, and hyperuricosuria with high doses.

Pancuronium Bromide (Pavulon)	Injection: 1, 2 mg/ml	Neonates: (test dose) Initial: 0.02 mg/kg/dose Maintenance: 0.03-0.09 mg/kg/dose Q1/2-4h PRN >1 mo. - Adult: Initial: 0.04-0.10 mg/kg/dose Maintenance: 0.02-0.10 mg/kg/dose Q30-60 min. Defasciculating dose: 0.006-0.01 mg/kg/dose Individualize dosage according to patient's response.	Must be prepared to intubate within 2 min. of induction. Drug effect accentuated by hypothermia, acidosis, neonatal age, decreased renal function, halothane, succinylcholine, hypokalemia and aminoglycoside antibiotics. May cause tachycardia.
Paraldehyde	Amp: 1 gm/ml Oral Solution: 1 gm/ml	Sedative: 0.15 ml (150 mg)/dose PO, IM or PR in equal amount of veg. oil Anticonvulsant: Deep IM: 0.15 ml (150 mg)/kg/dose Q4-6h; PR: 0.3 ml (300 mg)/kg/dose in oil Q4-6h; IV: May infuse continuously at 0.1 to 0.15 ml paraldehyde/kg/h (Dilute to 5% solution in normal saline, max. infusion rate 1 ml/min).	Do not use discolored solution. Avoid plastic equipment. Contraindicated in hepatic or pulmonary disease. Overdose may cause cardiorespiratory depression. IM may give sterile abscesses.
Paregoric (Camphorated Opium Tincture)	Tincture: 2 mg/5 ml (0.4 mg morphine/ml)	Analgesia: Children: 0.25-0.5 ml/kg/dose PO QD-QID Adults: 5-10 ml PO QD-QID Neonatal Opiate Withdrawal: Initial: 0.2-0.3 ml/dose Q3-4h Increment: 0.05 ml/dose until symptoms abate. Max. dose: 1-2 ml/kg/day or 0.7 ml/kg/dose	Same side effects as morphine (constipation, lethargy). Taper neonatal dose after symptoms are controlled for several days by 10% Q2-3 days.

Pemoline (Cylert)	Tabs: 18.75, 37.5, 75 mg Chewable: 37.5 mg	Initial: 37.5 mg/day Increments: 18.75 mg/wk Max. dose: 112.5 mg Not recommended for children <6 yrs old.	Overdosage: tachycardia, hallucinations, agitation. Reactions: insomnia, anorexia, hypersensitivity; follow liver functions; use with caution in renal disease. Effect may not be seen until 3-4 wks of therapy.
Penicillamine (Cuprimine)	Caps: 125, 250 mg	Lead poisoning: Dose not to exceed 500 mg/M²/day IM Q4h x 3-5 days.	Requires close liver, urine, and hematologic monitoring. May cause blood dyscrasias, nephrotic syndrome, liver and skin disorders, cataracts and optic neuritis. Eye exam Q6 mo.

Penicillin G Preparations
<u>Potassium</u>
	Injection: 200,000, 500,000 U/vial; 1, 5, 10, 20 million U/vial
	Oral liquid: 200,000, 400,000 U/5 ml
	Tabs: 100,000, 200,000, 400,000, 500,000, 800,000 Units
		Newborn:
		IV or IM:
		  <7 days: 50,000-150,000 U/kg/day ÷ Q12h;
		  >7 days: 75,000-250,000 U/kg/day ÷ Q6-8h
		Children:
		  IV, IM: 25,000- 500,000 U/kg/day ÷ Q4-6h
		PO:
		  Children: 40,000-80,000 U/kg/day Q6h
		  Adults: 300,000-1.2 mil U/day Q6h
		
		(CONTINUED)
			1 mg = approx. 1600 U
			Salt Content:
			K Salt: 1 million U (625 mg) contains 1.68 mEq K⁺
			Na Salt: 1 million U (625 mg) contains 1.68 mEq Na⁺
			
			NOTE: Pen. G. must be taken 1/2 hr before or 2 hrs after meals.
			Side effects: Anaphylaxis, skin rashes, serum sickness.

<u>Sodium</u>	Injection: 1, 5 million U/vial		

Penicillin Preparations (CONTINUED)			
Benzathine (Bicillin L-A)	Injection: 300,000 and 600,000 U/ml	Newborns: 50,000 U/kg x 1 Infants/Young Children: 300,000-600,000 U x 1 Older Children (>30 kg): 900,000 U x 1 Adults: 1.2 mil. U x 1 Rheumatic fever prophylaxis: 600,000 U Q2 wks or 1.2 mil. U Q month	
Procaine	Injection 300,000, 500,000, 600,000 U/ml	Newborn: 50,000 U/kg/day QD. Avoid use in this age group because of sterile abscesses and procaine toxicity. Children: 100,000-600,000 U/day QD or BID Adults: 600,000-1 mil U/day QD or BID	
Bicillin C-R	Tubex: 300,000 U Procaine + 300,000 U Benzathine/ml	Acute streptococcal infections 1.2 mil. U x 1	
Bicillin C-R 900/300	Tubex: 900,000 U Benzathine + 300,000 U Procaine/2 ml		
Penicillin V Potassium (Pen Vee K, V-Cillin K)	Tabs: 125 mg (200,000 U), 250 mg (400,000 U), 500 mg (800,000 U) Oral Solution: 125, 250 mg/5 ml	Children: 25,000-50,000 U/kg/ day PO ÷ Q6h Rheumatic Fever Prophylaxis: 250 mg (400,000 U)/day PO ÷ Q12h	

Pentamidine Isethionate (Lomidine)	100 mg/ml (sterile water only)	4 mg/kg/dose Q day IM x 10 days for T. gambiense; x 12-14 days for Pneumocystis carinii. (Max. total dose: 56 mg/kg)	Transient hypotension, tachycardia, nausea, vomiting, hypoglycemia, mild hepatotoxicity, mild anemia (megaloblastic) and granulocytopenia, renal toxicity. Available from CDC Parasitic Dis. Branch, Atlanta, GA 30333.
Pentobarbital (Nembutal)	Tabs (prolonged): 100 mg Caps: 30, 50, 100 mg Elixir: 20 mg/5 ml Supp: 30, 60, 120, 200 mg Amp: 50 mg/ml	Sedation: Children: 2-6 mg/kg/dose Adults: 30 mg TID-QID PO Cerebral Edema: Initial: 3-5 mg/kg IV x 1 Maintenance: 2-3.5 mg/kg/dose Q1h as needed	No advantage over phenobarbital for control of seizures. Adjunct in treatment of increased intracranial pressure. May cause drug-related isoelectric EEG.
Phenazopyridine (Pyridium)	Tabs: 100, 200 mg	Children 6-12 yr: 100 mg TID until symptoms are controlled Adults: 200 mg TID until symptoms are controlled	Caution in presence of G6PD deficiency, GI problems or renal insufficiency. May cause methemoglobinemia, hemolytic anemia. Colors urine orange.
Phenobarbital (Luminal)	Drops: 16 mg/ml Tabs: 8, 15, 30, 60 100 mg Elixir: 20 mg/5 ml Spans: 60, 100 mg Vials: 65 mg/ml, 130 mg/ml, 165 mg/ml	Sedation: 2-3 mg/kg/dose PO, IM, or PR Q8h PRN. Slower acting barbiturates are preferred. Status epilepticus: IV: 5-10 mg/kg/dose. Repeat in intervals of 20-30 min. if necessary. Max. total dose: 30-40 mg/kg. Do not exceed 600 mg/day. IM: 10 mg/kg Chronic anticonvulsant: Children: 4-6 mg/kg/day PO ÷ Q12h - follow levels and correlate to clinical response Adult: 150-250 mg/day bid (1-3 mg/kg/day).	IV administration may cause respiratory arrest or hypotension. Contraindicated in hepatic or renal disease and porphyria. T1/2 approximately 96 hours in children. Paradoxical reaction in children (not dose related) may cause hyperactivity, irritability, insomnia.

| Phenylephrine (Neo-Synephrine) | Vials: 10 mg/ml (1% solution)
Nasal drops: 0.125, 0.25, 0.5, 1%
Nasal solution: 0.25, 0.5, 1.0%
Ophthalmic solution: 10%
Elixir: 5 mg/5 ml | **Hypotension:**
Children:
  IM or SC: 0.1 mg/kg/dose Q1-2h PRN
  IV bolus: 5-20 µg/kg/dose Q10-15 min. PRN
  IV drip: 0.1-0.5 µg/kg/min.
Adults:
  IM or SC: 5-10 mg/dose Q1-2h PRN
  IV bolus: 0.25-1 mg/dose Q10-15 min. PRN
  IV drip: 1-4 µg/min (10 mg/100 ml saline - adjust dosage rate to desired effect)
Paroxysmal supraventricular Tachycardia:
  Children: 5-10 µg/kg/dose IV push.
  Adults: 0.25-0.5 mg/dose IV push
Decongestant:
Oral: 1 mg/kg/day Q4h to max. adult dose of 10 mg/dose or 60 mg/day
Topical:
  Infants: 0.125% sol'n Q3-4h up to 3 days
  Children: 0.25% sol'n Q3-4h up to 3 days
  Adults: 0.25-1% sol'n Q3-4h up to 3 days | Use cautiously in presence of hypertension, arrhythmias, hyperthyroidism, or hyperglycemia. May cause tremor, insomnia, palpitations. |

Phenytoin (Dilantin)	Caps: 30, 100 mg Tabs: 50 mg (Infatab) Susp: 30 mg/5 ml (Ped.), 125 mg/5 ml Amps: 50 mg/ml	**Status epilepticus:** IV (loading dose) 15 mg/kg in NS at rate <u>not</u> >50 mg/ min. Max. dose: 1000 mg/day **Maintenance for seizure disorders:** Infants/Children: 4-7 mg/kg/ day IV or PO ÷ QD or BID Adults: 300-400 mg/day IV or PO ÷ QD or BID Therapeutic levels = 10-20 μg/ml **Anti-arrhythmic:** Children: IV: 2-4 mg/kg over 5 min.; PO: 2-5 mg/kg/day Adults: IV: 100 mg Q 5 min. up to total dose: 500 mg, repeat in 2h PRN; PO: 250 mg/dose QID x 1 day, then 250 mg/dose BID x 2 days, then 300-400 mg/day ÷ QD to QID	T1/2 is variable (7-42 hrs) and dose dependent. Useful in ventricular tachycardia and digitalis-induced arrhythmias (esp. PAT with block). Not FDA approved for ventricular arrhythmias. Side effects include gingival hyperplasia, hirsutism, dermatitis, blood dyscrasias, ataxia, lymphadenopathy, liver damage, and nystagmus.
Phosphorus Supplements	(Neutraphos): Per capsule: 250 mg P (14 mEq, 8.1 mM), 7 mEq Na, 7 mEq K (Neutraphos-K): Per capsule: 250 mg P (14 mEq, 8.1 mM), 14 mEq K (Na-P Injection): 94 mg P/ml (3 mM), 4 mEq Na/ml (K-P Injection): 94 mg P/ml (3 mM), 4.4 mEq K/ml	1-2 gm P/day ÷ QID	All can cause GI discomfort and diarrhea. Begin at doses of 0.5-1.0 gm/day and increase slowly. Use of Na salts may aggravate GI symptoms. Injectable forms may also be given PO.

Drug	Form	Dosage	Notes
Physostigmine Salicylate (Antilirium)	Vial: 1 mg/ml	For antihistamine overdose or anticholinergic poisoning: Children: 0.01-0.03 mg/kg/dose, repeat x 1 after 15-30 min. Adults: 0.5-2 mg/dose infusion rate not to exceed 0.01 mg/kg/min. or 1 mg/min. (whichever is slower).	Atropine is the antidote for physostigmine and should always be available. Contraindicated in asthma and GI, GU obstruction. Use of physostigmine should be reserved for severe, symptomatic anticholinergic poisoning.
Piperacillin (Pipracil)	IV Infusion: 2, 4 gm vial	Children >12 yr and adults: 200-300 mg/kg/day ÷ Q4h or Q6h.	Similar to penicillin.
Piperazine (Antepar)	Tabs: 250, 500 mg; Syrup: 500 mg/5 ml; Wafer: 500 mg	Enterobius vermicularis (pinworm): 65 mg/kg/day to max. of 2.5 g/day QD x 7 days. May repeat in 1 week if necessary. Ascaris lumbricoides (roundworm): 75 mg/kg/day QD x 2 days to max. of 3.5 gm/day.	Contraindicated in epilepsy. Large doses may cause vomiting, urticaria, muscle weakness, blurred vision.
Potassium Iodide (SSKI)	Tab: 300 mg; Syrup: 325 mg/5 ml; Saturated sol'n (SSKI): 1 gm/ml	For thyrotoxicosis: Children: 200-300 mg/day BID-TID; Adults: 300-900 mg/day TID	Contraindicated in pregnancy. GI disturbance, metallic taste, rash, inflammation of salivary glands, headache, lacrimation, rhinitis are symptoms of iodism.

Potassium Supplements	Potassium Chloride: (1 gm = 13.3 mEq K) Injection: 2 mEq/ml Powder: 20 mEq/packet Sol'n: 5% (10 mEq/15 ml) 10% (20 mEq/15 ml) 20% (40 mEq/15 ml) Potassium Gluconate: (1 gm = 4.3 mEq K) Elixir: 1.56 gm/5 ml (6.66 mEq K /5 ml) Tab: 5mEq Potassium Triplex: Acetate-Bicarbonate- Citrate. Oral Sol'n: 500 mg of each salt/5 ml. (15 mEq K^+/ 5 ml)	Dose based on clinical require- ments. Starting dose should be determined by considering main- tenance K^+ losses and desired supplementation. Usual starting dose in diuretic therapy: 1-2 mEq/kg/day. Max. rate of infusion 0.5-1 mEq/kg/hour.	May cause GI disturbances and ulcerations. Monitor serum K^+. Hyperkalemia may present with cardiac arrhythmias, cardiac arrest.
Prednisolone	Tabs: 1, 2.5, 5 mg Vials: 20 mg/ml, 25 mg/ml	Same as prednisone. See prednisone.	Also see page 205.
Prednisone	Tabs: 1, 2.5, 5, 10, 20, 50 mg Liquid: 5 mg/5 ml	Physiologic replacement: 20% of cortisone dose (see page 205) or 4-5 mg/M^2/day BID Nephrotic Syndrome: Initial: 2 mg/kg/day (max. of 80 mg/day) TID-QID until urine is protein-free x 5 days or for max. of 28 days. If proteinuria persists, dose may be changed to 4 mg/ kg/dose QOD for an additional 28 days. (CONTINUED)	See page 205. Methylprednisolone preferable in hepatic disease. Long- term, low maintenance doses may be beneficial in relaps- ing nephrotic syndrome.

| Prednisone | (CONTINUED) | Maintenance: 2 mg/kg/dose QOD x 28 days. Then taper over 4-6 weeks.
Asthma:
Acute exacerbation: 20-40 mg/ day x 3-5 days.
Severe refractory asthma: 5-10 mg/dose QD or 10-30 mg QOD. Attempt to taper and/or wean to aerosol corticosteroid.
Anti-inflammatory or Immuno-suppressive: 0.5-2 mg/kg/day or 25-60 mg/M^2/day Q6-12h | |
| Primidone (Mysoline) | Tabs: 50, 250 mg
Susp: 250 mg/5 ml | <8 yrs:
Initial: 125 mg/day QD
Increment: 125 mg/day at weekly interval.
Maintenance: 10-25 mg/kg/day TID-QID
>8 yrs-adult:
Initial: 250 mg/day QD
Increment: 250 mg/day at weekly intervals.
Maintenance: 750-1500 mg/day TID-QID.
Therapeutic level: 7-15 µg/ dl of primidone or 10-40 µg/ ml of phenobarbital | Toxicity - same as phenobar-bital. Measure phenobar-bital and Primidone levels. (Primidone is metabolized to phenobarbital). |

Drug	Preparations	Dosage	Comments
Probenecid (Benemid)	Tabs: 0.5 gm	Use with Penicillin. <u>Children (2-14 yr):</u> 25 mg/kg starting dose, 40 mg/kg/day ÷ QID <u>Adult Dose (>50 kg body wt):</u> 2 gms probenecid ÷ QID. For gonorrhea Rx -- 1 gm probenecid 30 min before PCN or ampicillin.	Alkalinize urine in gouty patients, use with caution if history of peptic ulcer. Headache, GI symptoms, hypersensitivity, anemia. Contraindicated in children <2 yrs and in patients with renal insufficiency.
Procainamide (Pronestyl)	Tabs: 250, 375, 500 mg Tabs (SR): 250, 500 mg Caps: 250, 375, 500 mg Injection: 100, 500 mg/ml	<u>Children:</u> IM: 20-30 mg/kg/day Q4-6h to max. dose of 4 gm/day. (IM is the preferred parenteral route. Peak effect in 1 hr). IV: Loading: 3-6 mg/kg/dose over 5 min. Maintenance: 20-80 µg/kg/ min. by continuous infusion. Max. dose: 100 mg/dose or 2 gm/day PO: 15-50 mg/kg/day Q3-6h Max. dose: 4 gm/day <u>Adults:</u> IM: Loading: 1 gm/dose x 1. Maintenance: 250 mg/dose Q3h. IV: Loading: 100-200 mg/dose, repeat Q5 min. PRN to a total of 1 gm Maintenance: 1-3 mg/min by continuous infusion PO: 250-500 mg/dose Q3-6h (usual dose 50 mg/kg/day or 2-4 gm/day)	Contraindicated in myasthenia gravis, complete heart block. May cause lupus-like syndrome, Coombs positivity, thrombocytopenia. Monitor IV use closely with BP's, EKG. QRS widening >0.02 seconds suggest toxicity. May cause arrhythmias, GI complaints, confusion.

Drug	Forms	Dosage	Toxicity/Comments
Prochlorperazine (Compazine)	Tabs: 5, 10, 25 mg Syrup: 5 mg/5 ml Oral concentrate: 10 mg/ml Supp: 2.5, 5, 25 mg Spans: 10, 15, 30, 75 mg Amp: 5 mg/ml	Children >10 kg or >2 yr: 0.4 mg/kg/day PO or PR ÷ Q6-8h; 0.2 mg/kg/day IM ÷ Q6-8h Adults: PO: 5-10 mg/dose TID-QID PR: 25 mg BID IM: 5-20 mg/dose Q4-6h. Max. IM dose: 40 mg/day	Toxicity as for other phenothiazines. Extrapyramidal reactions, drowsiness may occur. Do not use IV route in children. Do not use in children <10 kg or <2 yr. old
Promethazine (Phenergan, Provigan)	Tabs: 12.5, 25, 50 mg Amp: 25, 50 mg/ml Syrup: 6.25 mg/5 ml, 25 mg/5 ml Supp: 12.5, 25, 50 mg	Antihistaminic: Children: 0.1 mg/kg/dose Q6h and 0.5 mg/kg/dose Q HS PO, PRN Adults: 12.5 mg TID and 25 mg QHS Nausea and Vomiting: Children: 0.25- 0.5 mg/kg/dose IM, PO, or PR Q4-6h PRN Adults: 12.5-25 mg Q4-6h PRN Sedative and Preoperative: Children: 0.5-1 mg/kg/dose IM Q6h PRN Adults: 25-50 mg/dose Motion Sickness: Children: 0.5 mg/kg/dose PO Q12h PRN	Toxicity similar to other phenothiazines (see chlorpromazine).
Propantheline Bromide (Pro-banthine)	Tab: 7.5, 15 mg	7.5-15 mg PO BID	Contraindicated in glaucoma, obstruction of urinary or GI tract and inflammatory bowel disease. May cause sedation, dizziness, mydriasis and cycloplegia.

| Propranolol (Inderal) | Tabs: 10, 20, 40, 80 mg. Injection: 1 mg/ml Formulation for oral form (no commercial product available!): Final concentration 1 mg/ml. Ten 10 mg tabs crushed and mixed with 200 mg Na Benzoate. Add simple syrup QS to 100 cc. Adjust pH = 5.0 with citric acid. Stable x 2 mo in refrigerator | **Arrhythmias:**
 Children: 0.01-0.10 mg/kg/ dose, slow IV push; may repeat Q6-8h PRN (max. single dose: 1 mg); 0.5- 1.0 mg/kg/ day PO ÷ Q6-8h (max. daily dose: 60 mg)
 Adults: 1 mg/dose IV repeated Q5 min up to total 5 mg
 Tetralogy Spells: 0.15-0.25 mg/kg/dose IV slowly -- may repeat in 15 min x 1 (max. single dose: 10 mg) then maintenance: 1-2 mg/kg/dose Q6h PO
 Thyrotoxicosis:
 Neonatal: 2 mg/kg/day PO Q6h
 Adolescents and Adults:
 IV: 1-3 mg/dose x 1 over 10 min
 PO: 10-40 mg Q6h
 Hypertension: Starting dose 0.5-1.0 mg/kg/day ÷ Q6-12h (max. dose: 2 mg/kg/ day)
 Adults:
 Initial: 10 mg/dose PO QID; Increment: 10-20 mg/dose at intervals of 3-7 days Max. dose: 320-480 mg/day PO
 Migraine Prophylaxis:
 <35 kg: 10-20 mg PO TID
 >35kg: 20-40 mg PO TID
 Adults: Initially, 80 mg/day PO TID. Usual effective dose range: 160-240 mg/day. | Contraindicated in asthma and heart block. Use with caution in presence of obstructive lung disease, heart failure, renal or hepatic disease. May cause hypoglycemia, hypotension, nausea, vomiting, depression, weakness. |

Drug	Forms	Dosage	Comments
Propyl-thiouracil (PTU)	Tabs: 50 mg	Children: Initial: 5-7 mg/kg/day PO Q8h or 6-10 yrs: 50-150 mg/day PO Q8h; >10 yrs: 150-300 mg/day PO Q8h Maintenance: Adjust to patient response. Usually 1/3 - 1/2 the initial dose beginning when the patient is euthyroid. Adults: Initial: 300 mg/day PO Q8h. Maintenance: 100-150 mg/day PO Q8h	May cause blood dyscrasias, fever, liver disease, dermatitis, urticaria, malaise, arthralgias. Monitor thyroid function. 100 mg PTU = 10 mg methimazole.
Protamine Sulfate	Amp: 10 mg/ml	Heparin Antidote: 1 mg for every 100 U of heparin in previous 3-4 hr by IV drip. Max. dose: 50 mg/dose. IV rate should not exceed 5 mg/min.	May cause coagulation problems in absence of heparin (120 U of heparin = 1 mg).
Pseudoephedrine (Sudafed, Novafed)	Tabs: 30, 60 mg Syrup: 30 mg/5 ml Capsules (sustained release): 60, 120 mg	Children: 4 mg/kg/day PO ÷ Q6h Adults: 30-60 mg Q6-8h Sustained release: >12 yrs - adults: 1 cap PO Q12h	Use with caution in hypertension. May cause nervousness, restlessness.
Pyrantel Pamoate (Antiminth)	Susp: 250 mg/5 ml	Ascariasis (roundworm), hookworm, enterobiasis (pinworm): In children and adults: 11 mg/kg as single dose (max. dose: 1 gm). May repeat x 1 in 2 wks.	Nausea, vomiting, anorexia, transient SGOT elevations. Use with caution with pre-existing liver dysfunction.

Pyrethrins (A-200 Pyrinate) (Pyrinal) (Rid)	Liquid gel	Apply to hair or body area affected x 10 min. and wash thoroughly, may repeat in 7-10 days.	Avoid eye contact or PO intake. Avoid repeat applications in <24 hrs.
Pyrvinium Pamoate (Povan)	Tabs: 50 mg	Enterobiasis: 5 mg/kg/dose PO as single dose. Repeat in 2 wks. Max. dose: 350 mg	May cause GI symptoms, colors stools red. May stain teeth. Swallow tabs whole.
Quinacrine (Atabrine)	Tabs: 100 mg	Giardiasis: 8 mg/kg/day PO ÷ Q8h. Give single dose 1st day, 2 doses 2nd day and 8 mg/kg/day in 3 doses after meals on 3rd day x 5 days. Max. dose: 300 mg/day. Tapeworms: 15 mg/kg/day PO ÷ into 2 doses 1 hr apart. Saline purge night before 1st dose and 2 hrs after last dose. Max. dose: 800 mg.	May cause GI disturbances, dermatosis, bone marrow depression, psychosis. May cause temporary yellow color in skin (not jaundice). Use with caution in patients with G6PD deficiency.
Quinidine	Gluconate: Tabs: 324 mg Vials: 80 mg/ml Sulfate: Tabs: 100, 200, 300 mg Extended Release Tabs: 300 mg Caps: 200, 300 mg Injection: 200 mg/ml	Test Dose: 2 mg/kg PO Therapeutic Dose: Children: IV: not recommended PO: 15-60 mg/kg/day Q6h Adults: IM: 400 mg/dose Q4-6h IV: 200-400 mg/dose PO: 100-600 mg/dose Q4-6h. Begin at 200 mg/dose and titrate to desired effect. Therapeutic levels: 3-7 µg/ml	Toxicity indicated by increase of QRS interval by >0.02 seconds (skip dose or stop drug). May cause GI symptoms, hypotension, tinnitus, blood dyscrasias. Can cause increase in digoxin levels if these drugs are used concomitantly.

Rabies Immune Globulin (RIG)	Injection: 150 IU/ml	20 IU/kg. Infiltrate 1/2 dose around wound if possible.	Local pain at injection site; urticaria, anaphylaxis.
Rabies Vaccine, Human diploid cell (HDCV)	Injection: Available from State Health Department	1 ml IM on days 0, 3, 7, 14, and 28, with antiserum (RIG) on day 0.	Infrequent local or mild systemic reactions. Collect serum for rabies titers on day 28.
Reserpine (Serpasil, Serpate)	Tabs: 0.1, 0.25 mg Amp: 2.5 mg/ml Vials: 2.5 mg/ml	General Use and Chronic Hypertension: 0.02 mg/kg/day PO ÷ Q12h Acute Hypertension: 0.07 mg/kg/dose IM repeat Q8-24h PRN (use with hydralazine if necessary). Due to hypersensitivity (marked hypotension) of some patients, 1/10 of dose should be given initially IM. (max. dose: 2.5 mg/day)	May cause CNS and respiratory depression in newborns of treated mothers. Discontinue 2 or more wks before elective surgery. Caution in patients with peptic ulcer.
Rifampin (Rimactane, Rifadin)	Caps: 150, 300 mg Liquid: 10 mg/ml (1%) can be made. See package insert	Antituberculosis: Children: 10-20 mg/kg/day QD Adults: 600 mg/day QD Meningococcal carriers or meningitis prophylaxis: 3-12 mos: 5 mg/kg/day QD x 2 days 1-2 yrs: 10 mg/kg/day QD x 2 days Adults: 600 mg BID x 2 days H. Flu Carriers or Prophylaxis: Children <4 yrs: 20 mg/kg/day ÷ bid x 4 days	Use with caution in liver dysfunction. May cause red color in body secretions (e.g. urine, saliva). GI irritation, CNS disturbance (ataxia, confusion, headache, fatigue), fever. Give 1 hr before or 2 hrs after meals. For child, mix contents of capsule in tablespoon of applesauce or have pharmacist make liquid preparation.

Salicylazo-sulfapyridine (Azulfidine, Sulfasalizine)	Tabs: 500 mg Enteric Coated Tabs: 500 mg Oral susp: 125 mg/5 ml	Initial: 75-150 mg/kg/day PO ÷ Q3-6h Maintenance: 40 mg/kg/day PO ÷ Q6h Max. adult dose: 6 gm/day	Orange-yellow discoloration of alkaline urine. Severe hypersensitivity reactions, blood dyscrasias, CNS changes, renal damage. Use with caution in G6PD deficiency.
Scopolamine hydrobromide, USP (hyoscine hydrobromide) (Transderm - scop)	Tabs: 400, 600 ug Injection: 0.3, 0.4, 0.5, 0.6, 0.8, 1.0 mg/ml Ophth. Sol'n: 0.25% Transderm 0.5 mg	6 ug/kg/dose PO or SC. Transdermal for children >12 yrs over 3 days only	See atropine. Contraindicated in urinary or GI obstruction and glaucoma. Transdermal reported to cause unilateral mydriasis.
Secobarbital (Seconal)	Caps: 50, 100 mg Supp: 30, 60, 120, 200 mg Injection: 50 mg/ml Elixir: 22 mg/5 ml Tabs: 50-100 mg Tabs (enteric coated): 50-100 mg	Sedation: Children: 6 mg/kg/day PO Q8h Adults: 20-40 mg PO BID-TID or 200-300 mg PO 2-3h pre-operatively	See amobarbital. T1/2 = 20-28 hrs.
Selenium Sulfide (Selsun)	2.5% Solution	Tinea versicolor: apply Q weekly x 4 weeks to affected areas. Lather and rinse from body areas after 5 min or from face after 10 min. Avoid eyes and genital area.	Local irritation, rare discoloration of hair, hair loss.

Sodium Polystyrene Sulfonate (Kayexalate)	Oral powder: 450 gm Susp: 2%, in Sorbitol Solution (4.1 mEq Na$^+$/gm)	Children: Practical Exchange Rate: 1 mEq K per 1 gm resin. Calculate dose according to desired exchange Q6h PO or Q2-6h PR. Usual dose: 1 gm/kg/dose Q6h PO or Q2-6h rectally Adults: 15-60 gm PO or 30-60 gm rectally Q6h	Use cautiously in presence of renal failure. (Na exchanged for K$^+$; may also cause hypomagnesemia and hypocalcemia). Do not administer with antacids or laxatives, containing Mg^{++} or Al^{+++}. Systemic alkalosis may result.
Spectinomycin (Trobicin)	Vials: 2 mg/5 ml, 4 mg/10 ml	Children: 40 mg/kg x 1 Adults: 2 gm IM as single dose. 4 gm if PCN resistant gonorrhea prevalent.	Not effective for syphilis. Vertigo, malaise, nausea, anorexia, chills, fever, urticaria.
Spironolactone (Aldactone)	Tabs: 25 mg	Children: 1.0-3.3 mg/kg/day BID-QID Adults: 25-100 mg/day BID-QID Max. dose: 200 mg/day	Contraindicated in acute renal failure. May potentiate ganglionic blocking agents and other antihypertensives. May cause hyperkalemia, GI distress.
Streptomycin sulfate	Vials: 500 mg/ml	Premature and Full Term: 20-30 mg/kg/day IM ÷ Q12h up to 10 days Children: 20-40 mg/kg/day IM ÷ Q8h up to 10 days Adults: 15-25 mg/kg/day IM Q12h x 7-10 days, then 1 gm/dose QD Tuberculosis: 20-50 mg/kg/day IM single dose (use higher dose for TB meningitis) Max. dose: 2 gm/day.	Reduce dose in presence of renal insufficiency. Follow auditory status. May cause CNS depression, other neurologic manifestations.

Succinylcholine (Anectine)	Vials: 20, 50, 100 mg/ml	**Neonates and Children:** <u>Initial:</u> 1-2 mg/kg/dose x 1 <u>Maintenance:</u> 0.3-0.6 mg/kg at intervals of 5-10 min PRN. **Adults:** <u>Initial:</u>0.6-1.1 mg/kg/dose x 1 <u>Maintenance:</u> 0.3-0.6 mg/kg at intervals of 5-10 min PRN; Continuous infusion: not recommended in children. Adults: 0.5-10 mg/min. (average dose 2.5 mg/min). Titrate dose to desired effect. Duration of action: 10 min.	Premedicate patient with atropine prior to administration. Must be able to intubate patient within 1 min. Side effects: bradycardia, hypotension, arrhythmia. Beware of prolonged depression in patients with liver disease, malnutrition, aminoglycoside Rx, hypothermia, hyperkalemia, pseudocholinesterase deficiency.
Sucralfate (Carafate)	Tabs: 1 gm	**Children:** Not approved for children <12 yr. **Adults:** 1 gm PO QID (1 hr AC and QHS)	Constipation, other GI complaints.
Sulfacetamide Sodium (Sulamyd)	Ophth Soln: 10%, 15%, 30% Ophth Ointment: 10%	Apply Q3-4h	See sulfisoxazole.
Sulfadiazine	Tabs: 60, 250, 300, 500 mg Tabs (chewable): 300 mg Susp.: 0.5 gm/5 ml	**Newborn:** Do not use. **Children** >2 mo old: <u>Loading:</u> 75 mg/kg/dose PO x 1 <u>Maintenance:</u> 150 mg/kg/day PO Q6h. Max. dose: 6 gm/day. **Adults:** <u>Loading:</u> 2-4 gm x 1 <u>Maintenance:</u> 1 gm Q4-6h. **Malaria:** Children: 100-200 mg/kg/day QID, to a max. of 2 gm/day x 5 days **Meningococcal prophylaxis:** <1 yr: 500 mg QD x 2 days 1-12 yr: 500 mg BID x 2 days >12 yr: 1 gm BID x 2 days	May cause crystalluria (keep urine output high and alkaline), fever, rash, hepatitis, vasculitis, bone marrow suppression. Hemolysis in patients with G6PD deficiency.

| Sulfisoxazole (Gantrisin) | Tabs: 500 mg, 1 gm; Susp: 500 mg/5 ml; Syrup: 500 mg/5 ml; Amp: 400 mg/ml; Ophth Sol'n: 40 mg/ml; Ophth ointment: 40 mg/gm | Initial: 75 mg/kg/dose PO, 50 mg/kg/dose IV. Maintenance: 150 mg/kg/day PO ÷ Q4-6h; 100 mg/kg/day IV ÷ Q6h. Maximum: 6 gm/day. Adults: Loading: 2-4 gm x 1. Maintenance: 4-8 gm/day Q4-6h. Rheumatic Fever Prophylaxis: <30 kg: 500 mg/day PO single dose. >30 kg: 1 gm/day PO single dose. Ophth Sol'n: 2-3 gtts Q4-8h. Ophth Ointment: 1-3 x daily. | Contraindicated in infants <2 mos, near-term pregnant or nursing mothers. Use cautiously in presence of renal or liver disease, or G6PD deficiency. Maintain adequate fluid intake. |
| Terbutaline (Brethine, Bricanyl) | Tabs: 2.5, 5 mg; Injection: 1 mg/ml | PO: <12 yr: Initial: 0.05 mg/kg/dose TID, increase as required. Max. dose: 0.10 mg/kg/dose TID or total of 5 mg/day. >12 yr - Adults: Initial: 2.5 mg/dose TID. Maintenance: Usually 5 mg or 0.075 mg/kg/dose TID. SC: <12 yr: 0.005-0.010 mg/kg/dose, max. of 0.25 mg/dose Q15-20 min. x 2. >12 yr - Adults: 0.25 mg/dose Q15-30 min. PRN x 1 only. Total of 0.5 mg is not to be exceeded within a 4 hr period. | Nervousness, tremor, headache, nausea, as with other sympathomimetic agents. |

Drug	Preparations	Dosage	Comments
Tetracycline HCL (many brand names)	Tabs: 250, 500 mg Caps: 100, 250, 500 mg Drops: 100 mg/ml (5 mg/gtt) Syrup: 25 mg/ml Vials: 100, 250, 500 mg OPHTH oint: 1%, 3% OPHTH susp: 1%	Older Infants and Children: PO: 25-50 mg/Kg/day ÷ Q6h IM: 15-25 mg/kg/day,÷ Q8-12h (not to exceed 250 mg/ injection) IV: 10-20 mg/kg/day ÷ Q12h Children >40 kg - Adults: PO: 1-2 gm/day Q6h IM: 250-300 mg/day Q8-12h IV: 250-500 mg/dose Q6-12h, depending on severity of illness	RECOMMENDED ONLY WHEN ANOTHER DRUG IS NOT SUITABLE. May cause increased intracranial pressure, tooth staining, decreased bone growth and GI reactions. Outdated drug may cause nephropathy. Not recommended in patients <8 yrs. PO doses 1 hr before meals. (Max. dose: 2 gm/day)
Theophylline	Many preparations See page 202. (Table of common oral theophylline preparations)	Children: 5-8 mg/kg/dose Q6h Neonatal apnea (PO): Usually 2-4 mg/kg/dose Q6h. Low dose: 2 mg/kg/day Q8h Max. PO theophylline doses to administer before determination of serum levels: Age (yrs.) — Dose (mg/kg/24h) 0-9 — 24 9-12 — 20 12-16 — 18 Adults — 13	Use with caution in cardiac, renal, hepatic, hyperthyroid, ulcer disease, and glaucoma. Most common side effects are GI disturbance (vomiting, nausea, anorexia, discomfort), nervousness, cardiac arrhythmias, seizures. Serum levels should be monitored. Therapeutic levels for asthma: 10-20 µg/ml. Therapeutic level for neonatal apnea: 7-13 µg/ml
Thiopental sodium (Pentothal)	Injection: 250, 400, 500 mg syringes 0.5, 1 gm vials	Cerebral edema: 1.5-3.0 mg/kg/ dose IV. Repeat PRN increased intracranial pressure General anesthesia: Children: 2 mg/kg x 1 IV Adults: 3-5 mg/kg x 1 IV Maintenance: Children: 1 mg/kg PRN Adults: 50-100 mg PRN	TI/2 is 3-8h in blood, but probably <30 seconds in brain. Toxicity: respiratory depression, hypotension, anaphylaxis, decreased cardiac output. Contraindicated in acute intermittent porphyria.

Drug	Forms	Dose	Comments
Thioridazine (Mellaril)	Tabs: 10, 15, 25, 50, 100, 150, 200 mg Concentrate: 30 mg/ml, 100 mg/ml Susp: 5, 20 mg/ml	Children (2-12 yrs): 1.0 mg/kg/day ÷ in 2-4 doses − increase gradually. Adult: Initially, 150-300 mg/day in 2-4 doses Max. dose: 800 mg/day	Drowsiness, extrapyramidal reactions, autonomic symptoms, paradoxical reactions, endocrine disturbances.
Thyroid USP	Tabs: 15, 30, 60, 125, 150, 180, 260, 325 mg	Initial: Infants: 15 mg/dose PO as single daily dose. Children: 30 mg/dose PO single daily dose. Usual Maintenance: 60-180 mg/day single daily dose. Increments: 15 mg/day at 1-2 week intervals	Follow and titrate with serum T₄ level. Decreases clotting functions, potentiates coumadin-type anticoagulants.
Ticarcillin (Ticar)	Vials: 1, 3, 6 gm	IM dose should not exceed 2 gm/injection. Adults: 200-300 mg/kg/day IV Q3-6h (higher dose for more severe infections). UTI: 150-200 mg/kg/day IV for complicated UTI or 1 gm (IM or IV) Q6h for uncomplicated UTI Children <40 kg: 200-300 mg/kg/day IV Q4-6h. UTI: 150-200 mg/kg/day IV Q4-6h (complicated UTI) or 50-100 mg/kg/day IM or IV Q6-8h (uncomplicated UTI) (CONTINUED)	Each gram contains 5.2 mEq Na. Activity similar to carbenicillin.

Ticarcillin (Ticar)	(CONTINUED)	Neonates: <u><2 kg:</u> Initial - 100 mg/kg. <u>age <7 days:</u> 150 mg/kg/day IV Q8h. <u>age >7 days:</u> 225 mg/kg/day IV Q8h <u>>2 kg:</u> Initial - 100 mg/kg <u>age <14 days:</u> 225 mg/kg/day IV Q8h <u>age >14 days:</u> 300 mg/kg/day IV Q8h	
Tobramycin (Nebcin)	Amp: 20 mg/2 ml, 80 mg/2 ml	Neonates: <u><1 wk:</u> 4-5 mg/kg/day ÷ Q12h <u>>1 wk:</u> 4-7.5 mg/kg/day ÷ Q8h <u>Children:</u> 7.5 mg/kg/day ÷ Q8h <u>Adults:</u> 3-5 mg/kg/day ÷ Q8h	Ototoxicity, nephrotoxicity. Activity similar to other aminoglycosides. Therapeutic levels: Peak: 6-10 µg/ml Troughs: <2 µg/ml
Tolazoline (Priscoline)	Vials: 25 mg/ml	1-2 mg/kg IV push test dose. Then: 1-2 mg/kg/hr constant IV infusion. Dissolve 50 mg/kg x wt (kg) in 50 ml D$_5$W. Then ml/hr = mg/kg/hr.	Monitor blood pressure, renal status and bone marrow status. GI and pulmonary hemorrhage have been observed.
Tolmetin Sodium (Tolectin)	Tabs: 200 mg Caps: 400 mg	Children: <u>Initial:</u> 15 mg/kg/day TID <u>Increment:</u> 5 mg/kg/day at 1 week intervals until therapeutic effect or adverse effects are observed. Max. dose: 30 mg/kg/day Adults: <u>Initial:</u> 400 mg TID <u>Maintenance:</u> Titrate to desired effect. Usually, 600-1800 mg/day TID	Not recommended for age <2 yrs. May cause GI irritation or bleeding.

Tolnaftate (Tinactin)	Cream: 1% Soln: 1% Powder: 1% Liquid, aerosol: 1% Powder, aerosol: 1%	Apply cream or 1-2 gtts of solution topically BID for 2-6 wks.	Persistent infection may require systemic therapy with griseofulvin.
Triamcinolone (Kenalog, Aristocort, Kenacort)	Injection, Repository: 40 mg/ml Injection, intra-lesional: 5, 25, 40 mg/ml Syrup: 2 mg, 4 mg/ml Tabs: 1, 2, 4, 8, 16 mg Topical preparation: 0.025%, 0.1%, 0.5%	Intralesional injection: 1 mg maximum/site at weekly or less frequent intervals Systemic use: 1/6 of dose recommended for cortisone Topical: Apply to affected areas BID-QID. Use least potent preparation which is effective	See section on Adrenocorticosteroids, page 205.
Trimethaphan (Arfonad)	Amp: 500 mg/10 ml	Dilute with D_5W and administer via IV infusion pump. Infusion Rate: Children: Begin at 0.1 mg/kg/min and titrate to maintain BP. Adults: Begin at 0.5-1 mg/min. Titrate as necessary to maintain BP.	Must monitor with arterial line. Produces profound hypotension and respiratory arrest if over-dosed. Histamine release and GI disturbance are side effects.

Trimethobenzamide HCL (Tigan)	Caps: 100, 250 mg Supp: 100, 200 mg Amp: 100 mg/ml	Children 15-40 kg: Oral: 100-200 mg TID-QID Rectal (not for use in neonates): <15 kg: 100 mg TID-QID >15 kg: 100-200 mg TID-QID Injectable not recommended for children Adults: Oral: 250 mg TID-QID Rectal: 200 mg TID-QID Injectable: 200 mg IM TID-QID	CNS disturbances are common in children (extrapyramidal symptoms, drowsiness, confusion, dizziness).
Trimethoprim Sulfamethoxazole (Bactrim, Septra; TMP-SMZ)	Tabs (reg. strength): 80 mg TMP/400 mg SMZ Tabs (double strength): 160 mg TMP/800 mg SMZ Susp: 40 mg TMP/200 mg SMZ per 5 ml	Children: Minor infections: UTI or Otitis Media: 8-10 mg/kg TMP or 40-50 mg/kg SMZ per day ÷ Q12h UTI prophylaxis: 2 mg/kg TMP as QD dose Severe infections: Pneumocystis carinii pneumonitis: 20 mg/kg/day TMP and 100 mg/kg/day SMZ ÷ Q6h x 14 days. Pneumocystis prophylaxis: 10 mg/kg/day TMP and 50 mg/kg/day SMZ BID. (CONTINUED)	See sulfisoxazole. Reduce dosage in renal impairment. Monitor hematologic status.

	(CONTINUED)		
Trimethoprim Sulfamethoxazole (Bactrim, Septra; TMP-SMZ)		Adults: Minor infections: UTI: 160 mg TMP + 800 mg SMZ BID Severe infections: septicemia: 160 mg TMP + 800 mg SMZ TID. Adults: Pneumocystis carinii: Prophylaxis: 10 mg TMP/kg/day + 50 mg SMZ/kg/day Q12h Treatment: 20 mg TMP/kg/day + 100 mg SMZ/kg/day Q6h Max. adult dose: 320 mg TMP and 1600 mg SMZ/day.	
Tripelennamine (Pyribenzamine)	Tabs: 25, 50 mg Long-acting tabs: 50, 100 mg Elixir: 37.5 mg/5 ml	Children: 5 mg/kg/day PO ÷ Q4-6h. (Max. dose: 300 mg/day) Adults: Tabs: 25-50 mg Q4-6h Sustained release tabs: 50-100 mg Q8-12h. (Max. dose: 600 mg/day)	Drowsiness and other side effects of antihistamines.
Valproic Acid (Depakene, Depakote).	Syrup: 250 mg/5 ml Caps: 250 mg Enteric coated tabs: 250, 500 mg	Initial: 10-15 mg/kg/day PO ÷ BID Increment: 5-10 mg/ kg/day at weekly intervals to max. of 60 mg/kg/day Maintenance: 30-60 mg/kg/day QD-TID. Therapeutic levels: 50-100 µg/ml	GI, liver and hematologic toxicity; weight gain, transient alopecia, pancreatitis. Drug interactions - increases phenobarbital levels by 30-40%. Transient decrease in phenytoin levels which revert to previous levels in several weeks.

Drug	Preparations	Dosage	Comments
Vancomycin (Vancocin)	Amp: 500 mg/10 ml Oral Sol'n: 500 mg/6 ml	Neonates: <7 days: 30 mg/kg/day IV ÷ Q12h Older Infants and Children: CNS infection: 60 mg/kg/day IV Q6h. Other infections: 40 mg/kg/day IV Q6h Adults: 40 mg/kg/day (max. dose: 2 gm/day) IV Q6h. Oral dose: 2 gm/1.73 M²/day Q6h	Ototoxicity, nephrotoxicity. Causes phlebitis.
Vasopressin (Pitressin)	Amp: 20 U/ml (aqueous) Amp: 5 U/ml (tannate in oil) Nose Drops: 50 U/ml (arginine vaso-pressin – Diapid)	Aqueous: 0.5-3 ml/day SC ÷ Q8h. Tannate in Oil: 0.25 ml/dose IM Q1-3 days PRN; may increase to 1-2 ml/dose. Nose Drops: 1-2 gtts in each nostril Q4-6h PRN. Titrate dose to achieve control of thirst and urination.	Side effects: tremor, sweating, vertigo, abdominal discomfort, nausea, vomiting, urticaria, anaphylaxis.
Verapamil (Isoptin, Calan)	Amps: 5 mg/2 ml	For IV use only: Initial dose: Administer IV over 2-3 min. 0-1 yr: 0.1-0.2 mg/kg (usually 0.75-2 mg) 1-15 yr: 0.1-0.3 mg/kg (usually 2-5 mg). Do not exceed 5 mg. Adult: 5-10 mg Repeat dose: Administer 30 min after first dose if necessary. 0-1 yr: 0.1-0.2 mg/kg. 1-15 yr: 0.1-0.3 mg/kg. Do not exceed 10 mg as a single dose. Adult: 10 mg (0.15 mg/kg)	Indicated for treatment of supraventricular tachyarrhythmias. Contraindicated in hypotension, shock, 2nd or 3rd degree AV block. IV beta adrenergic blocking agents should not be administered within a few hours of verapamil (both cause myocardial depression). Use only with continuous ECG monitoring.

Vidarabine (Adenine arabinoside, Ara-A, Vira-A)	Injection: 200 mg/ml Ophth oint: 3%	**Herpes simplex virus encephalitis and neonatal** HSV infection: 15 mg/kg/day given IV over 12 hrs x 10 days (add to standard IV fluids) Keratoconjunctivitis: Apply ointment to lower conjunctival sac Q3hrs, 5 x/day. Discontinue if not improved in 7 days.	Document HSV infection prior to therapy. Use with caution in renal and hepatic disease. Monitor hepatic and hematologic status. Do not dilute in biologic or colloid fluids.
Vitamin K₁ (Aqua-Mephyton, Konakion, Phytonadione)	Tabs: 5 mg Amp: 1 mg/0.5 ml (aqueous) Amp: 10 mg/ml (emulsion)	**Neonatal hemorrhagic disease:** Prophylaxis and treatment - 0.5-1.0 mg/dose IM, SC, or IV x 1. Oral anticoagulant overdose: Infants: 1-2 mg/dose IV Q4-8h Children and Adults: 5-10 mg/dose IV Liver disease or Malabsorption: 2.5-25 mg/day PO Vit. K deficiency: Infants and Children: 1-2 mg/dose IV x 1 or 2-5 mg/day PO. Adults: 5-25 mg/day PO	Follow protime. Use with caution in presence of severe hepatic disease. Large doses (>25 mg) in newborn may cause hyperbilirubinemia. IV injection not to exceed 3 mg/M²/min or 5 mg/min. IV doses may be associated with flushing, dizziness, hypotension, anaphylaxis.

Ref:

1. Package insert for products.

2. Benitz, WE and Tatro, DS: _The Pediatric Drug Handbook_, Year Book Medical Publishers, Inc., Chicago, IL, 1981.

3. Boyd, JR (editor-in-chief): _Facts and Comparisons_, J. P. Lippincott Co., St. Louis, MO, 1984.

4. Copyright 1984 PHYSICIANS'S DESK REFERENCE, Published by Medical Economics Co., Inc., Oradell, NJ 07649.

CANCER CHEMOTHERAPEUTIC AGENTS

Drug	Supplied	Remarks - Adverse Effects
Actinomycin-D (Dactinomycin, Cosmegen)	Vials: 0.5 mg (IV)	Cellulitis with extravasation, nausea, vomiting, alopecia, stomatitis, "radiation recall" effect, bone marrow suppression*.
L-Asparaginase (Elspar)	Vials: 10,000 U (refrigerate) (IV)	Fever, nausea, vomiting, hepatotoxicity, coagulation abnormalities, somnolence, tremors. Seizures*, hyperglycemia*, pancreatitis*, anaphylaxis/hypersensitivity reactions*.
BCNU (Carmustine)	Vials: 100 mg (refrigerate) (IV)	Nausea, vomiting, jaundice, facial flushing, phlebitis at IV site, local pain. Delayed (4-6 wks) leukopenia and thrombocytopenia*.
CCNU (Lomustine)	Caps: 10, 40, 100 mg (PO)	Nausea, stomatitis, neurologic dysfunction. Hepatotoxicity*, leukopenia*, thrombocytopenia*. Monitor hepatic, marrow status.
Cisplatinum (Cisplatin)	Vials: 10, 100 mg (IV)	Vomiting and nausea invariable. Significant nephrotoxicity and ototoxicity with long term use, myelosuppression.
Cyclophosphamide (Cytoxan)	Tabs: 25, 50 mg (PO) Vials: 100, 200, 500 mg (IV)	Vomiting, alopecia, hemorrhagic cystitis*, myelosuppression (esp. leukopenia)*, pulmonary fibrosis*, gonadal suppression, inappropriate ADH secretion with high doses.
Cytosine Arabinoside (AraC, Cytosar)	Vials: 100, 500 mg (IV)	Vomiting, fever, diarrhea, rash, oral lesions, hepatotoxicity. Bone marrow depression*.
Dacarbazine (DTIC)	Vials: 100, 200 mg (IV)	Vomiting, fevers, malaise, cellulitis on extravasation. Bone marrow depression*.
Daunorubicin (Daunomycin, Rubidomycin)	Vials: 20 mg (IV)	Cellulitis on extravasation, nausea, vomiting, alopecia, stomatitis, fever, rash, "red urine". Reduce dose in presence of hepatic insufficiency. Bone marrow suppression*; cardiac toxicity (cumulative dose 500 mg/M², may occur at lower cumulative dose—350 mg/M²—in presence of prior chest area radiotherapy or use of other antineoplastic agents)*.
Doxorubicin (Adriamycin)	Vials: 10, 50 mg (IV)	

*Dose limiting side effects.

196

Cancer Chemotherapeutic Agents (continued)

Drug	Form	Side effects
Fluorouracil (Efudex, 5-FU)	Vials: 500 mg (IV)	Nausea, photophobia, cerebellar signs, alopecia, rashes. Intractable vomiting*, diarrhea*, mucositis and GI ulceration*, bone marrow suppression*.
Hydroxyurea (Hydrea)	Caps: 500 mg (PO)	Rash, GI disturbances, nephrotoxicity, bone marrow depression*.
Leucovorin (Citrovorum Factor, Folinic Acid)	Amp: 3 mg/ml (PO, IM, IV) Vials: 10 mg/ml	Useful in preventing methotrexate toxicity and in treatment of other folic acid antagonist toxicity.
Mercaptopurine (6-MP, Purinethol)	Tabs: 50 mg (PO)	Vomiting, bone marrow depression*.
Methotrexate	Powder: 20, 50, 100 mg Amp: 2.5, 25 mg/ml Tabs: 2.5 mg	Mucositis, bone marrow depression* (esp. leukopenia), nausea, abdominal pain, GI bleeding, hepatitis*, rash.
Nitrogen mustard (HN₂)	Vials: 10 mg (IV)	Cellulitis with extravasation, nausea, vomiting, alopecia, rash, CNS toxicity. Bone marrow depression*.
Procarbazine (Matulane)	Caps: 50 mg (PO)	Nausea, vomiting, lethargy, CNS depression, alopecia, stomatitis, neuropathy. Bone marrow depression*.
Thioguanine (6-TG)	Tabs: 40 mg (PO)	Nausea, vomiting. Bone marrow depression*.
Thiotepa	Vials: 15 mg (IV)	Bone marrow depression*.
Vinblastine (Velban) Vincristine (Oncovin)	Vials: 10 mg (refrigerate) (IV) Vials: 1 mg, 5 mg (refrigerate) (IV)	Cellulitis on extravasation, peripheral neuropathy, areflexia, alopecia, ileus, constipation, stomatitis. Neurotoxicity*, bone marrow depression*, inappropriate ADH secretion.

*Dose limiting side effects.

DIGOXIN PREPARATIONS

PREPARATION	ROUTE OF ADMIN.	EFFECT Onset	EFFECT Max.	Duration	TOTAL EXCRETION	ORAL ABSORPTION	DOSE Digitalizing	DOSE Daily Maintenance	REMARKS
DIGOXIN (LANOXIN) Available in Tabs: 0.125 mg 0.25, 0.5 mg Elixir: 0.05 mg/ml Amp: 0.1, 0.25 mg/ml	IV IM PO	5-30 min 15-60 min 1-2 hrs	2-5 hrs 2-5 hrs 4-8 hrs	24 hrs	48-72 hrs	40-90%	Full-Term Newborn: TDD* 30-50 µg/kg IM or IV Premature: TDD* = 20 µg/kg IM or IV <2 yrs: TDD* = 60-80 µg/kg PO; 40-60 µg/kg IM or IV >2 yrs: TDD* = 40-60 µg/kg PO, 20-40 µg/kg IM or IV >10 yrs: TDD* = 0.75-1.25 mg PO or IV 1/2 dose stat; then 1/4 dose Q6-8h x 2	20-30% of TDD given in 2 divided doses/24 hr Parenteral = 75% of oral dose. Usual dose: 5-15 µg/kg PO QD Q12h, 4-12 µg/kg IM or IV divided Q12h. >10 yrs: 0.125-0.25 mg QD NOTE: Premature newborns will require a smaller dose.	Excreted via kidney. Use with caution in renal failure. Infants may not show digitalis effect on EKG. Adequate dose determined by clinical response. Serum levels do not correlate well with therapeutic effect and toxicity in infants and young children Symptoms of toxicity include nausea, vomiting, diarrhea, dizziness, headache, and visual symptoms. Various arrhythmias may occur, e.g. multiple ventricular extrasystoles. When symptoms or signs of toxicity occur, discontinue drug. K+ supplement may be indicated. Phenytoin often drug of choice in digitalis-induced arrhythmias.

* TDD = Total digitalizing dose

INTRAVENOUS ANTI-ARRHYTHMIA DRUGS

DRUG	DOSE	INDICATIONS	CAUTIONS
		TACHYARRHYTHMIAS	
Digoxin	See digoxin, page 197.	Supraventricular arrhythmias 1) PAT or PNT unresponsive to vagal stimulation. Also PAT in Wolff-Parkinson-White syndrome 2) Atrial flutter - fibrillation	Contraindicated in ventricular arrhythmias. May cause heart block and other arrhythmias. Monitor EKG.
Phenytoin (Dilantin)	See phenytoin, page 172.	1) Ventricular arrhythmias, especially ventricular tachycardia 2) Digitalis-induced arrhythmias, especially PAT with block	Bradycardia, hypertension. Monitor EKG.
Lidocaine (Xylocaine)	See lidocaine, page 156.	Ventricular arrhythmias	May cause hypotension, seizures, and cardiac or respiratory arrest. Monitor BP and EKG.
Phenylephrine HCl	See phenylephrine, page 171.	Supraventricular tachycardia	May cause tremor, paresthesias, chest pain, and ↓ blood flow to vital organs.
Propranolol	See propranolol, page 178.	Supraventricular tachycardia	See page 178.
Methoxamine (Vasoxyl)	See methoxamine, page 160.	Supraventricular tachycardia	May cause hypertension, headache, and nausea.

INTRAVENOUS ANTI-ARRHYTHMIA DRUGS (continued)

DRUG	DOSE	INDICATIONS	CAUTIONS
		TACHYARRHYTHMIAS (continued)	
Quinidine gluconate	See quinidine, page 180.	Ventricular arrhythmias, atrial flutter or fibrillation, and to prevent PAT in Wolff-Parkinson-White syndrome.	Use for atrial arrhythmias only in well-digitalized patient. May cause ventricular arrhythmias (increase in QRS by 0.02 sec or more) and hypotension. Monitor EKG and BP.
Verapamil	See verapamil, page 192.	Supraventricular tachycardia	Monitor ECG, BP. Contraindicated in 2nd or 3rd degree heart block.
		BRADYARRHYTHMIAS	
Atropine	See atropine, page 126.		
Epinephrine	See epinephrine, page 144.		Ventricular ectopic beats -- tachycardia. May be given via ET-tube.
Isoproterenol (Isuprel)	See isoproterenol, page 154.	Complete heart block or severe bradycardia	Use care in presence of congestive failure or ventricular irritability. Monitor EKG.

EMERGENCY MANAGEMENT OF HYPOXIC SPELLS
IN CYANOTIC HEART DISEASE (e.g. "Tetralogy Spells")

TREATMENT	RATIONALE
Knee-chest position	Decreases venous return and increases systemic resistance.
Morphine: 0.1-0.2 mg/kg IV or SC; may repeat in 1 hr	Decreases venous return.
Propranolol: Acute 0.15-0.25 mg/kg IV over 2-5 min; may repeat in 15 min x 1. Chronic - 1 mg/kg/dose PO divided Q6h. NOTE: DO NOT USE IF SURGERY IS PLANNED WITHIN SEVERAL DAYS.	Negative inotropic effect on (infundibular) myocardium.
Phenylephrine HCl: 0.1 mg/kg/ dose SC or IM Q1-2h PRN; 0.01 mg/kg IV	Increases systemic vascular resistance.
Methoxamine: 0.1 mg/kg IV	Increases systemic vascular resistance.
Sodium bicarbonate: 1-2 mEq/ kg/dose IV	Reduces metabolic acidosis.
Oxygen	Reduces hypoxemia (LIMITED VALUE).
NO digitalis preparations	Avoid positive inotropic effect on myocardium.
Correct anemia	Increases delivery of oxygen to tissues.
Correct pathological tachyarrhythmias	May abort hypoxic spell.

ANTI-CONVULSANTS FOR STATUS EPILEPTICUS

ANTICONVULSANT	DOSAGE AND ROUTE OF ADMINISTRATION	COMMENTS
Diazepam (Valium) Ampules: 5 mg/ml	IV: 0.2-0.5 mg/kg/dose given slowly. May repeat dose Q15 min x 2. Single dose not to exceed 5 mg for <5 yrs or 10 mg >5 yrs. Do not inject more rapidly than 5 mg/min. See page 138.	Hypotension and respiratory depression particularly following barbiturates or paraldehyde. NOTE: Do not dilute. Not good maintenance drug.
Phenobarbital 65 mg/ml 130 mg/ml	IV: 5-10 mg/kg/dose. Repeat in intervals of 20-30 min if necessary. Max. total dose 30-40 mg/kg. Do not exceed 600 mg/day. IM: 10 mg/kg Chronic Anticonvulsant: 4-6 mg/kg/day. PO Q12h starting dose. See page 170.	Monitor BP, respiration. Do not use with hepatic or renal disease, or porphyria. Action delayed when given IM (up to 2 hrs to obtain peak levels). Monitor blood levels with chronic use. Therapeutic range = 15-40 µg/ml.
Phenytoin (Dilantin) 50 mg/ml	IV: Loading dose - 15 mg/kg given in normal saline at rate not exceeding 50 mg/min. Maintenance: 4-7 mg/kg once daily. NOTE: Do not give IM. See page 172.	Monitor blood pressure and cardiac rate. Monitor blood levels with chronic use. Therapeutic range = 10-20 µg/ml.
Paraldehyde 1 gm/ml	IV: 5 ml per 100 ml normal saline at 2-3 mg/kg/hr (equals 0.1-0.15 ml/kg/hr paraldehyde) Rectal: 0.3 ml/kg. Repeat Q4-6h DEEP IM: 0.15 ml/kg Q4-6h. Adult max. dose: 4-10 ml See page 167.	Do not allow solution to stand in plastic bags. Action delayed 1 hr. Sterile abscesses may occur with IM injection.

SOME COMMON ORAL THEOPHYLLINE PREPARATIONS

NAME	GENERIC NAME	PREPARATION	ANHYDROUS THEOPHYLLINE EQUIVALENT	% ALCOHOL (if liquid)
		SHORT ACTING (Q6h doses)		
Aminophyllin	Aminophylline	Tabs: 100, 200 mg Vials: 250 mg/10 ml	79%	– 0%
Elixophyllin	Theophylline	Caps: 100, 200 mg Elixir: 80 mg/15 ml	100%	– 20%
Slo-phyllin	Theophylline	Tabs: 100, 200 mg Syrup: 80 mg/15 ml	100%	– 0%
Somophyllin	Aminophylline	Liquid: 105 mg/5 ml	86%	0%
Somophyllin-T	Theophylline	Caps: 100, 200, 250 mg	100%	–
Theophyl	Theophylline	Chewable tab: 100 mg	100%	–
Theophyl-225	Theophylline	Tabs: 225 mg Elixir: 225 mg/30 ml	100%	– 5%
		SUSTAINED RELEASE (Q8-12h doses)		
Elixophyllin-SR	Theophylline	Sustained Action Caps: 125, 250 mg	100%	–
Slo-phyllin Gyrocaps	Theophylline	Timed Released Caps: 60, 125, 250 mg	100%	–
Somophyllin-CRT	Theophylline	Time Released Caps: 50, 100, 200, 250, 300 mg	100%	–
Theo-Dur	Theophylline	Sustained Action Tabs: 100, 200, 300 mg	100%	–
Theo-dur Sprinkle	Theophylline	Sustained Action Caps: 50, 75, 125, 200 mg	100%	–
Theophyl-SR	Theophylline	Sustained Action Tabs: 125, 250 mg	100%	–

INSULIN

(NOTE: See DKA and subsequent insulin management pages 82-84.)

Dose determined by clinical situation

TYPE OF INSULIN	TIME AND ROUTE OF ADMINISTRATION	TIME OF ONSET (HR)	PEAK (HR)	DURATION OF ACTION (HR)	TIME WHEN GLYCOSURIA MOST APT TO OCCUR	TIME WHEN HYPO-GLYCEMIA MOST APT TO OCCUR
		Rapid Action – Short Duration				
*Crystalline Zinc (Regular)	IV (for ketoacidosis): 0.1 U/kg bolus, then 0.1 U/kg/hr as continuous IV infusion; 15-20 min before meals, SC.	1/2-1 hr	2-5	5-8	During night	10 AM to lunch
*Semi-Lente (Amorphous Zinc)	1/2-3/4 hr before breakfast; deep SC, never IV	1/2-1½ hr	5-10	12-16	During night	Before lunch
		Intermediate in Rapidity of Action – Relatively Long Duration				
Globin Zinc	1/2-1 hr before breakfast, SC	Intermediate – rapidity of onset increases with dose within 2-4 hrs	8-16	18-24 also increases with dose.	Before breakfast & before lunch	3 PM to dinner

* Contains no modifying protein, i.e. protamine or globin.

INSULIN (continued)

(NOTE: See DKA and subsequent insulin management pages 82-84.)

Dose determined by clinical situation

TYPE OF INSULIN	TIME AND ROUTE OF ADMINISTRATION	TIME OF ONSET (HR)	PEAK (HR)	DURATION OF ACTION (HR)	TIME WHEN GLYCOSURIA MOST APT TO OCCUR	TIME WHEN HYPOGLYCEMIA MOST APT TO OCCUR
*Lente (combination of 30% semi-lente & 70% ultra-lente)	1 hr before breakfast; deep SC; never IV	Intermediate - within 1-2½ hrs.	7-15	24	Before lunch	3 PM to dinner
NPH (Neutral-Protamine-Hagedorn) or Isophane	1 hr before breakfast; SC	Intermediate - within 1-1½ hrs.	8-12	18-24	Before lunch	3 PM to dinner
Delayed Action - Long Duration						
Protamine Zinc (PZI)	1 hr before breakfast; SC	Slow-acting - within 4-8 hrs	14-20	24-36	Before lunch	2 AM to breakfast
*Ultra-lente	1 hr before breakfast; deep SC, never IV	Very slow - 4-8 hrs	10-30	36+		During night early morning

*Contains no modifying protein, i.e., protamine or globin.
NOTE: More highly purified preparations have recently been introduced. They may produce less subcutaneous atrophy than previously available products and may correct insulin lipoatrophy when injected in the margins of affected sites.

ADRENOCORTICOSTEROIDS

1. <u>Common</u> <u>Side</u> <u>Effects</u> <u>with</u> <u>Prolonged</u> <u>Usage</u>

   A. <u>Acute</u> <u>Withdrawal</u>: Fever, myalgia, arthralgia, malaise, hypotension, hypoglycemia, shock.

   B. <u>Complications</u> <u>of</u> <u>Prolonged</u> <u>Use</u>: Hypokalemic alkalosis, glycosuria, increased susceptibility to infection, exacerbation of peptic ulcers, myopathy, psychoses, osteoporosis and vertebral compression fractures, thromboembolic phenomena, Cushing's habitus, acne, hirsutism, cataracts, hypertension, and ecchymoses.

2. <u>Doses</u> <u>for</u> <u>Physiologic</u> <u>Replacement</u>

   A. <u>Glucocorticoid</u>

   Hydrocortisone* -
   12.5 mg/M²/day IM or IV, QD
   25.0 mg/M²/day PO, divided TID

   Cortisone Acetate -
   15-16 mg/M²/day IM or IV, QD
   30-32 mg/M²/day PO, divided TID

   *In congenital virilizing adrenal hyperlasia (CVAH), administer hydrocortisone 37 mg/M² IM Q3 days.

   B. <u>Mineralocorticoid</u>

   Deoxycorticosterone Acetate (DOCA) -
   1.0-2.0 mg/day IM (in oil), single dose

   9α-fluorocortisol (Florinef) -
   0.05-0.15 mg/day PO

3. <u>Equivalent</u> <u>Doses</u> <u>for</u> <u>Same</u> <u>Clinical</u> <u>Effects</u>

Drug	Glucocorticoid Anti-Inflammatory	Mineralo-corticoid
Cortisone	100 mg	100 mg
Hydrocortisone	80 mg	80 mg
Prednisone	20 mg	100 mg
Prednisolone	20 mg	100 mg
Methylprednisolone	16 mg	no effect
Triamcinolone	16 mg	no effect
9αFluorocortisol	5 mg	0.2 mg
Dexamethasone	2 mg	no effect
DOCA	no effect	2 mg

4. Duration of Action

Cortisone acetate:	6 hr PO and IV (1/2 life 60-90 min); 3 days IM
Hydrocortisone Na succinate:	4-6 hrs IV (1/2 life 60-90 min)
Triamcinolone:	8-12 hrs PO
Dexamethasone:	8-12 hrs PO
Prednisone:	6-8 hrs PO

5. Some Common Dermatologic Steroid Preparations

Lowest Potency
  0.25% Hydrocortisone
  0.25% Methylprednisolone acetate (Medrol)
  0.04% Dexamethasone † (Hexadrol)
  0.5% Hydrocortisone

Low Potency
  0.01% Fluocinolone acetonide† (Synalar, Fluonid)
  0.01% Betamethasone valerate† (Valisone)
  1.0% Hydrocortisone
  0.025% Triamcinolone acetonide† (Kenalog)

Intermediate Potency
  0.1% Betamethasone valerate† (Valisone)
  0.025% Fluocinolone acetonide† (Synalar, Fluonid)
  0.05% Flurandrelonide† (Cordran)
  2.5% Hydrocortisone
  0.1% Triamcinolone acetonide† (Kenalog)

Highest Potency
  0.05% Fluocinomide† (Lidex)
  0.5% Triamcinolone acetonide†
  0.2% Fluocinolone† (Synalar HP)

†Fluorinated preparation

   Fluorinated steroids may cause skin atrophy and telangiecta-
siae with chronic use (>2 wks). Most compounds above are available in creams and ointments. Most are dispensed in 15, 30, and
60 gram tubes (except Betamethasone valerate which is dispensed
in 45 gram tubes). One gram of topical cream or ointment covers
a 10 cm x 10 cm area. A 30 to 60 gram tube will cover the entire
body of an adult one time.

USE OF DRUGS IN RENAL FAILURE

To adjust maintenance dosage in patients with renal insufficiency, one may lengthen the intervals between individual doses, keeping the dosage size normal. This method is known as the "interval extension" method. Alternatively, one may reduce the size of individual doses, keeping the interval between doses normal. This "dose reduction" method is recommended especially for drugs in which a relatively constant blood level is desired. In the following tables after identification of the method used (D for dose reduction or I for interval extension) recommendations are given for various levels of renal function as estimated by glomerular filtration rate. In the dose reduction method, the percentage of the usual dose that should be given at the normal dose interval is shown, whereas for the interval extension method the number of hours between doses of normal size is given.

These dosage modifications are approximations only. The individual patient must be followed closely for signs of drug toxicity, serum levels of the drugs must be measured when available, and the dosage and interval modified accordingly.

In the following tables, the quantitative effects of hemodialysis (H) and peritoneal dialysis (P) on drug removal are shown. "Yes" refers to removal of enough drug to warrant a supplemental dosage for maintenance of adequate therapeutic blood levels. "No" indicates no need for dosage adjustment with dialysis. The designation "no" does not preclude the use of dialysis or hemoperfusion for drug overdose.

The data in these tables are adapted from Bennett, J, et al., Ann Int Med 93:62, 1980.

USE OF DRUGS IN RENAL FAILURE
(Antibiotics)

	PHARMACOKINETICS				ADJUSTMENTS IN RENAL FAILURE			
Drug	Route of Excretion	Normal Half-Life	Normal Dose Interval	Method	Creatinine Clearance (ml/min)			Removal by Dialysis
					>50	10–50	<10	
Amikacin	Ren	2–2.5 hr	Q8–12h	I	Q12–18h	Q24–36h	Q36–48h	Yes (HP)
Amoxicillin	Ren	0.9–2.3 hr	Q8h	I	Q8h	Q8–12h	Q12–16h	Yes (H)
Amphotericin B	NonRen	24 hr	Q24h	I	Q24h	Q24h	Q24h	No (H)
Ampicillin	Ren (Hep)	1.5 hr	Q6h	I	Q6h	Q6–12h	Q12–16h	No (P)
CarBenicillin	Ren (Hep)	1.5 hr	Q4h	I / D	Q8–12h / 75%	Q12–24h / 50%	Q24–48h / 25%	Yes (H) / Yes (P)
Cefamandole	Ren	1 hr	Q4–6h	D / I	100% / Q6h	25–50% / Q6–9h	25% / Q9h	Yes (H)
Cephalexin	Ren	0.9 hr	Q6h	I	Q6h	Q6h	Q6–12h	Yes (HP)
Cephalothin	Ren (Hep)	0.5–0.9 hr	Q6h	I	Q6h	Q6h	Q8–12h	Yes (HP)
Doxycycline	Ren (Hep)	14–25 hr	Q12h	I	Q12h	Q12–18h	Q18–24h	No (HP)
Ethambutol	Ren	4 hr	Q24h	I	Q24h	Q24–36h	Q48h	Yes (HP)
Flucytosine	Ren	3–6 hr	Q6h	I	Q6h	Q12–24h	Q24–48h	Yes (HP)
Gentamicin	Ren	2 hr	Q8h	D / I	75–100% / Q8–12h	50–75% / Q12–24h	25–50% / Q24–48h	Yes (HP)
Isoniazid	Hep (Ren)	2–4 hr (slow) 0.5–1.5 hr (fast)	Q24h	D	Un-changed	Un-changed	66–100%	Yes (HP)

USE OF DRUGS IN RENAL FAILURE (continued)
(Antibiotics)

| | PHARMACOKINETICS | | | | ADJUSTMENTS IN RENAL FAILURE | | | |
| Drug | Route of Excretion | Normal Half-Life | Normal Dose Interval | Method | Creatinine Clearance (ml/min) | | | Removal by Dialysis |
					>50	10-50	<10	
Kanamycin	Ren	2-3 hr	Q8h	I D	Q24h 75%	Q24-72h 50%	Q72-96h 25%	Yes (HP)
Methicillin	Ren (Hep)	0.5 hr	Q4h	I	Q4h	Q4h	Q8-12h	No (HP)
Metronidazole	Ren (Hep)	6-14 hr	Q8h	I	Q8h	Q12h	Q24h	
Penicillin G	Ren (Hep)	0.5 hr	Q6h	D I	100% Q6h	75% Q6h	25-50% Q9-12h	Yes (H) No (P)
Streptomycin	Ren	2.5 hr	Q12h	I	Q24h	Q24-72h	Q72-96h	Yes (H)
Sulfisoxazole	Ren	3-7 hr	Q6h	I	Q6h	Q8-12h	Q18-24h	Yes (HP)
† Ticarcillin	Ren	1-1.5 hr	Q4-6h	D I	75% Q8-12h	50% Q12-24h	25% Q24-48h	Yes (HP)
§ Tobramycin	Ren	2.5 hr	Q8h	D I	75-100% Q8-12h	50-75% Q12-24h	25-50% Q24-48h	Yes (HP)
Trimethoprim -	Ren	.8-15 hr	Q12h	I	Q12h	Q18h	Q24h	Yes (H)
Sulfamethoxazole		9-11 hr						
Vancomycin	Ren	6-8 hr	Q24h	I	Q24-72h	Q72-240h	Q240h	No (HP)

† May inactivate aminoglycosides in patients with renal impairment
§ May add 4-5 mg/L to peritoneal dialysate to obtain adequate serum levels

USE OF DRUGS IN RENAL FAILURE
(Non-Antibiotics)

| | PHARMACOKINETICS | | | ADJUSTMENTS IN RENAL FAILURE | | | | |
| | | | | | Creatinine Clearance (ml/min) | | | Removal by Dialysis |
Drug	Route of Excretion	Normal Half-Life	Normal Dose Interval	Method	>50	10-50	<10	
Allopurinol	Ren	0.7 hr	Q12-24h	D I	Unchanged Q8h	Unchanged Q8-12h	50% Q12-24h	?
Acetaminophen	Hep	1.3-3.5 hr	Q4h	I	Q4-6h	Q6h	Q8h	Yes (H) No (P)
†Acetylsalicylic acid	Ren (Hep)	2-4.5 hr	Q4h	I	Q4h	Q4-6h	Avoid	Yes (HP)
Cimetidine	Ren	1.5-2 hr	Q6h	D I	100% Q6h	75% Q8h	50% Q12h	Yes (H)
Cyclophosphamide	Hep (Ren)	5-6 hr	Q12h	I D	Q12h Unchanged	Q12h Unchanged	Q18-24h 50%	Yes (H)
Digitoxin	Hep (Ren)	60-390 hr	Q24h	D	Unchanged	Unchanged	50-75%	No (HP)
§Digoxin	Ren (NonRen 15-40%)	36-44 hr	Q24h	D	100%	25-75%	10-25%	No (HP)
Diphenhydramine	Hep (Ren <4%)	4-7 hr	Q6h	I	Q6h	Q6-9h	Q9-12h	?
††Hydralazine	Hep (GI, Ren)	2-4.5 hr	Q8h (fast) Q12h (slow)	I	Unchanged	Unchanged	Q8-16h (fast) Q12-24h (slow)	No (HP)

† TI/2 given for <500 mg dose. With large doses TI/2 prolonged up to 30 hrs.
§ Decrease loading dose in end stage renal disease because of decreased volume of distribution.
†† Dose interval varies for rapid and slow acetylators with normal and impaired renal function.

USE OF DRUGS IN RENAL FAILURE (continued)
(Non-Antibiotics)

| Drug | PHARMACOKINETICS | | | ADJUSTMENTS IN RENAL FAILURE | | | | | |
	Route of Excretion	Normal Half-Life	Normal Dose Interval	Method	>50	Creatinine Clearance (ml/min) 10-50	<10	Removal by Dialysis
Insulin	Hep (Ren)	CZI 2 hr NPH 8-12 hr	Variable	D	100%	75%*	50%*	?
Methotrexate	Ren	Triphasic 1,3,27 hr	Single treatment	D	Unchanged	75%	50%	Poor (HP)
Methyldopa	Ren (Hep)	Biphasic 1.4 hr 5-8 hr	Q6h	I	Unchanged	Q9-18h	Q12-24h	Yes (HP)
Phenobarbital	Hep (Ren 30%)	36-96 hr	Q8h	I	Q8h	Q8h	Q8-16h	Yes (HP)
Primidone	Hep (Ren <20%)	3-12 hr	Q8h	I	Q8h	Q8-12h	Q12-24h	Yes (H)
Spironolactone	Hep	Biphasic 0.2 hr 10-35 hr	Q6h	I	Q6-12h	Q12-24h**	Avoid	?
Thiazides	Ren	1-2 hr	Q12h	D	Unchanged	Unchanged	Avoid	?

* Dose dependent on blood sugar.
** Hyperkalemia common with GFR<30 ml/min.

DRUGS REQUIRING NO MODIFICATION OF DOSE
IN RENAL FAILURE
Antibiotics

Drug	Dialysis	Drug	Dialysis
Chloramphenicol	H	Isoniazid	H/P
Clindamycin	no	Nafcillin	no
Cloxacillin	no	Oxacillin	no
Doxycycline	no	Pyrimethamine	?
Erythromycin	no		

Non-Antibiotics

Drug	Dialysis	Drug	Dialysis
Adriamycin	?	Indomethacin	?
Amitriptyline	no	Lidocaine	?
Chlorpheniramine	?	Meperidine	?
Chlorpromazine	no	Morphine	?
Clonadine	?	Naloxone	?
Codeine	?	Nitroprusside	H/P
Corticosteroids (any)	--	Pentazocine	?H
cortisone	no	Pentobarbital	no
methylprednisolone	no	Phenytoin	no
all others	?	Prazosin	?
Cytosine Arabinoside	?	Propoxyphene	no
Diazepam	no	Propranolol	no
Diazoxide	H/P	Quinidine	H/P
5-Fluorouracil	H	Secobarbital	?
Flurazepam	?	Theophylline	H/P
Furosemide	no	Valproic Acid	?
Haloperidol	?	Vincristine	?
Heparin	no	Warfarin	?
Imipramine	no		

GUIDE FOR PREOPERATIVE MEDICATION
BEFORE GENERAL ANESTHESIA

Age in Months	Drugs Used*
0-6	Atropine only
6-12	Atropine and Pentobarbital
over 12	Atropine (or scopolamine) Pentobarbital Morphine (or meperidine)

*Dosages:

Atropine (or scopolamine): 0.01-0.02 mg/kg (min. 0.15 mg; max. 0.6 mg)

Glycopyrrolate: 0.015 mg/kg IM

Pentobarbital: 3.0-4.0 mg/kg (max. 120 mg)

Morphine: 0.05-0.10 mg/kg (max. 10 mg)

Meperidine: 1.0 mg/kg (max. 100 mg)

LYTIC COCKTAIL (DPT)

Drug	Usual Dose	Cardiac Catheterization	
		Acyanotic	Cyanotic
Demerol	2 mg/kg	1.2 mg/kg	0.6 mg/kg
Phenergan	1 mg/kg	0.3 mg/kg	0.15 mg/kg
Thorazine	1 mg/kg	0.3 mg/kg	0.15 mg/kg

Max. dose = 50 mg Demerol
Give in one syringe and give deep IM.
Narcotics should be used with caution in children, especially if
<1 yr. Use continuous monitoring of patient.

DRUGS AND CHEMICALS TO BE AVOIDED BY PERSONS WITH "REACTING" (PRIMAQUINE SENSITIVE) RED CELLS (G6PD DEFICIENCY)

Antimalarials

Primaquine

Sulfonamides

1. Sulfanilamide
2. Sulfisoxazole (Gantrisin)*
3. Salicylazosulfapyridine (Azulfidine)
4. Sulfacetamide (Sulamyd)
5. Trisulfapyrimidine (Sultrin)

Nitrofurans

1. Nitrofurantoin (Furadantin)
2. Furazolidone (Furoxone)

Antipyretics and Analgesics

1. Acetylsalicylic Acid*
2. Acetophenetidin (Phenacetin)*
3. Antipyrine
4. p-Aminosalicylic Acid

Others

1. Sulfoxone*
2. Naphthalene
3. Methylene Blue*
4. Probenecid
5. Fava Bean
6. Vitamin K - water soluble analogs only
7. Aniline dyes
8. Ascorbic acid§
9. Chloramphenicol†

* Only slightly hemolytic to G6PD A$^-$ patients in very large doses.
† Hemolytic in G6PD Mediterranean but not in G6PD A$^-$ or Canton.
§ In massive doses

NOTE: Many other compounds have been tested, but are free of hemolytic activity. Penicillin, the tetracyclines, and erythromycin, for example, will not cause hemolysis. Also, the incidence of allergic reaction in these individuals is not any greater than that observed in normals. Any drug, therefore, which is not included in the list known to cause hemolysis, may be given.

MATERNAL MEDICATIONS AND BREASTFEEDING

Most compounds ingested by a lactating mother are excreted in the milk, usually in low concentrations. There are very few drugs whose use is an absolute contraindication to breastfeeding; but ideally the lactating mother should take no medications. In instances where potential harm exists, carefully monitor the infant, and obtain drug levels in both infant and milk. Be aware that antibiotics may make evaluation of sepsis difficult.

This summary includes data on commonly-used drugs which might be taken by lactating women. Unless otherwise specified, excretion in breast milk is based on standard therapeutic doses of the drug in question. For more detailed information, consult the references cited.

Drug	Excretion in Human Milk	Possible Effect on Infant	Breastfeeding Acceptable	Breastfeeding Contraindicated	Data Inconclusive
Acetaminophen	-/+	-	X		
Acetylsalicylic Acid	+	? platelet dysfunction	X**		
Amantadine	+	Vomiting, rash, urinary retention	X		
Amitriptyline	+	May inhibit milk ejection reflex	X		
Amphetamines	?	-	X		
Ampicillin or Amoxicillin	+	See Penicillin	X		
Aminoglycosides	-/+	Changes bowel flora	X*		
Atropine	+	Anti-cholinergic signs	X*		
Barbiturates	+	Lethargy	X*		
Bromides	+	Drowsiness, rash		X	
Caffeine	+	? irritability	X**		

* Closely supervise drug use in mother and monitor infant for possible drug effects.
** In moderation

Drug	Excretion in Human Milk	Possible Effect on Infant	Breastfeeding Acceptable	Breastfeeding Contraindicated	Data Inconclusive
Captopril	+	–	X		
Carbamazepine	+	–	X		
Cephalosporins	+	See Penicillin	X		
Chloral hydrate	+	–	X		
Chloramphenicol	+	? myelosuppression	X		
Chloradiazepoxide	+	–	X		
Chlorpromazine	+	Galactorrhea	X		
Clindamycin	+	–	X		
Codeine	+	–	X	–	
Corticosteroids	+	–	X*		
DDT	+	?			X
Diazepam	+	Lethargy, jaundice	X		
Digoxin/Digitoxin	+	–	X		
Dihydrotachysterol	+	–		X	
Diphenhydramine	+	–	X		
Disopyramide	–	–	X		
Erythromycin	+	–			X
Ethanol	+	Sedation	X**		
Fluorides	+	–	X		
Folic Acid	+	–	X		
Furosemide	+	–	X		

* Closely supervise drug use in mother and monitor infant for possible drug effects.
** In moderation

Drug	Excretion in Human Milk	Possible Effect on Infant	Breastfeeding Acceptable	Breastfeeding Contraindicated	Data Inconclusive
Heparin	-	-	X		
Heroin	+	?	X		
Hexachlorophene	?	-	X		
Hydralazine	+	-	X		
Ibuprofen	-	-	X		
Imipramine	+	-	X		
Indomethacin	+	-	X*		
Iodides	+	Goiter		X	
Iron preparations	+	-	X		
Isoniazid	+	CNS, hepatic	X*		
Lithium	+	Li toxicity	X		
Meperidine	+	-	X		
Meprobamate	+	Drowsiness	X		
Methadone	+	-	X*		
α-Methyldopa	+	?	X		X
Metoprolol	+	-	X		
Metronidazole	+	High concentration in milk		X	
Naldolol	+	-	X		
Naproxen	+	-	X		
Nicotine	+	? tachycardia, GI disturbances	X**		

*   Closely supervise   drug use in mother and monitor infant for possible drug effects.
** In moderation

Drug	Excretion in Human Milk	Possible Effect on Infant	Breastfeeding Acceptable	Breastfeeding Contraindicated	Data Inconclusive
Nitrofurantoin	+	Caution with G6PD-deficient infants	X		
Oral Contraceptives	+	Decreased lactation	X*		
Oxazepam	+	-	X		
Penicillins	+	? allergic sensitivity, complicates sepsis eval.	X		
Pentazocine	?	-	X		
Phenobarbital	+	Drowsiness	X**		
Phenolphthalein	+	-		X	
Phenylbutazone	?	-	X		
Phenytoin	+	? hepatic enzyme induction	X		
Prazepam	+	-	X		
Primidone	+	Drowsiness	X*		
Propoxyphene	+	-	X*		
Propranolol	+	-	X*		
Propylthiouracil	+	Goiter, agranulocytosis		X	
Quinidine	+	-	X		
Radio-opaque contrast agents	+	-	X		
Radioactive diagnostic and therapeutic agents	+	?		X	

* Closely supervise drug use in mother and monitor infant for possible drug effects.
** In moderation

Drug	Excretion in Human Milk	Possible Effect on Infant	Breastfeeding Acceptable	Breastfeeding Contraindicated	Data Inconclusive
Reserpine	+	Diarrhea, lethargy congestion, galactorrhea	X*		
Spironolactone	?	-	X		
Streptomycin	+	-		X	
Sulfonamides	+	Hemolysis, rash, jaundice		X†	
Tetracyclines	+	-	X		
Tetrahydrocannabinol	+	?			X
Theophylline	+	Irritability	X*		
Thiamine	+	-	X		
Thiazides	+	? thrombocytopenia	X		
Thiopental	+	-	X		
Thioridazine	+	-	X		
Thyroxine	?	-	X*		
Tolbutamide	+	-	X		
Trimethoprim	+	-	X		
Valproic Acid	+	-	X		
Vitamin B12	+	-	X		
Vitamin K	+	-	X		
Warfarin	+	-	X		

* Closely supervise drug use in mother and monitor infant for possible drug effects.
** In moderation
† In neonates
Ref: Drugs in Pregnancy and Lactation, Briggs, et al, Williams and Wilkins, Baltimore, 1983.
Statement of American Academy of Pediatrics, Committee on Drugs, Pediatrics 72(3), 375, 1983.

PART III

THERAPEUTIC DATA

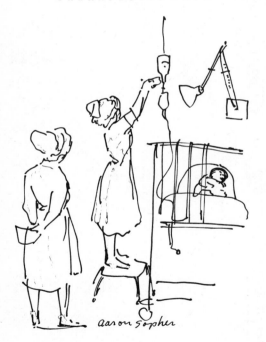

aaron gopher

FLUID AND
ELECTROLYTE THERAPY

1. ## General Considerations

   A. ### Atomic Weights

Aluminum (Al)	26.97	Lead (Pb)	207.21
Calcium (Ca)	40.08	Magnesium (Mg)	24.32
Carbon (C)	12.01	Manganese (Mn)	54.93
Chlorine (Cl)	35.46	Nitrogen (N)	14.01
Copper (Cu)	63.57	Oxygen (O)	16.00
Fluorine (F)	19.00	Phosphorus (P)	30.98
Gold (Au)	197.20	Potassium (K)	39.10
Hydrogen (H)	1.01	Sodium (Na)	23.00
Iodine (I)	126.92	Sulfur (S)	32.06
Iron (Fe)	55.85		

   B. ### Ion Calculations

   1) Moles:

   $$\text{Mole} = \text{molecular weight in grams}$$
   $$\text{Millimole} = \text{molecular weight in milligrams}$$

   Na 23
   Cl 35.5
   NaCl 58.5 gm = 1 mole
   58.5 mg = 1 mM

   2) Equivalents (number of electric charges per liter):

   Equivalent = atomic weight divided by valence
   mEq = equivalent weight in mg
   μEq = equivalent weight in μg

   For single valence ions 1 mM = mEq.
   For divalent ions 1mM = 2 mEq.

   3) Osmolality (number of particles per liter):

   Osmole = molecular weight divided by number of
   particles exerting osmotic pressure

   $$1 \text{ mM } Na^+ = 1 \text{ mOsm}$$
   $$1 \text{ mM NaCl} = 2 \text{ mOsm } (Na^+ + Cl^-)$$
   $$1 \text{ mM } Na_2SO_4 = 3 \text{ mOsm } (2Na^+ + SO_4^{--})$$

   Osmolality is the preferred term rather than osmolarity and represents solute concentration per unit solvent (water) rather than solution (serum).

   4) Approximate serum osmolality =
   $$2 \text{ (Na)} + \frac{\text{glucose (mg/dl)}}{18} + \frac{\text{BUN (mg/dl)}}{2.8}$$

2.   Calculation of Maintenance Requirements

   A.   Principle
        Water and electrolyte requirements are based on caloric
        expenditure.

   B.   Calculation of Caloric Expenditure for Maintenance Therapy
        1)   Standard basal calories:

STANDARD BASAL CALORIES		
Weight Kg	Calories/24 Hours Male and Female	
3	140	
5	270	
7	400	
9	500	
11	600	
13	650	
15	710	
17	780	
19	830	
21	880	
25	1020	960
29	1120	1040
33	1210	1120
37	1300	1190
41	1350	1260
45	1410	1320
49	1470	1380
53	1530	1440
57	1590	1500
61	1640	1560

        2)   Increment for temperature:
             Add 12% of above for each degree Centigrade (8%
             for each degree Fahrenheit) above rectal tempera-
             ture of 37.8°C (100°F).
        3)   Increment for activity:
             Add 0-30% of above for bed activity; e.g., coma or
             thrashing about.

   C.   Average Water and Electrolyte Expenditures Per 100
        Calories Metabolized Per 24 Hours

ROUTE	USUAL			RANGE		
	H_2O	Na*	K*	H_2O	Na*	K*
Lungs	15	0	0	10- 60	0	0
Skin	40	0.1	0.2	20-100	0.1- 3.0	0.2- 1.5
Stool	5	0.1	0.2	0- 50	0.1- 4.0	0.2- 3.0
Urine	65	3.0	2.0	0-400	0.2-30	0.4-30
TOTAL	125	3.2	2.4	30-610	0.4-37	0.8-34.5

*mEq/100 calories metabolized

1) In spite of 125 ml H_2O being lost for every 100 cal/24 hr, the usual H_2O requirement is 5-15 ml less (i.e., 110-120 ml) because of the production of endogenous H_2O through oxidation of carbohydrate, fat and protein.

2) Abnormally high values in above tables may be considered to represent abnormal losses.

D. Average Water and Electrolyte Requirements for Different Clinical States per 100 Calories per 24 Hours Based on data in preceding table.

	ml H_2O	mEq Na	mEq K
*Average patient receiving parenteral fluids	110-120	2-4	2-3
Anuria	45	0	0
Acute CNS infections and inflammation	80-90	2-4	2-3
Chronic renal disease with fixed specific gravity	140	variable	variable
Diabetes insipidus	Up to 400	variable	variable
Hyperventilation	120-210	2-4	2-3
Heat stress	120-240	variable	variable
High humidity environment	80-100	2-4	2-3
Paraoperative and post-operative patient	85	1-2	0

*Adequate maintenance solution
Na and Cl: 30 mEq/L
K: 20 mEq/L
Glucose: 5% or 10% as needed

This is provided by:

5 or 10% invert sugar or glucose in H_2O ....800 ml
Isotonic saline ....200 ml
Potassium chloride concentrate (Cutter) ....10 ml

OR

Dextrose 5% in 0.2% NaCl + 20 mEq/L KCl.

3. Deficit Therapy

A. Principles
1) Initial step: For shock or significant dehydration rapidly expand the extracellular volume in order to improve the circulation and renal function. Blood is used only for shock not responding to Ringer's lactate.
a) Ringer's lactate 20 ml/kg/1st hr.
b) Blood or plasma 10 ml/kg, if indicated.

2) Replace intracellular deficits slowly over 12-24 hrs. See table below for approximate magnitude of deficits.
3) Maintenance therapy for usual losses.
4) Replace continued abnormal losses.

B. Calculation of Deficits

PROBABLE DEFICITS OF WATER AND ELECTROLYTES IN INFANTS WITH SEVERE DEHYDRATION (10-12 PERCENT)

Condition	H_2O ml	Na mEq	K* mEq	Cl mEq
		Per Kg of Body Weight		
Fasting and thirsting	100-120	5- 7	1- 2	4- 6
Diarrhea				
Isotonic	100-120	8-10	8-10	8-10
Hypertonic	100-120	2- 4	0-4	-2- 6**
Hypotonic	100-120	10-12	8-10	10-12
Pyloric stenosis	100-120	8-10	10-12	10-12
Diabetic acidosis	100-120	8-10	5-7	6- 8

*Converted for breakdown of tissue cells:
  3 mEq K for each gram of nitrogen lost by catabolism
**Negative balance of chloride indicates excess at beginning of therapy.

C. Correction of Persistent Symptomatic Disturbances of Electrolyte Concentration

Formula: $(CD - CA)$ x fD x Wt* in kg = mEq required

CD= concentration desired (mEq/L)
CA= concentration present (mEq/L)
fD = apparent distribution factor as fraction of body weight
*Baseline weight prior to illness.

Electrolyte	Apparent Distribution Factor (fD)
Bicarbonate	0.4-0.5
Chloride	0.2-0.3
Sodium	0.6-0.7

4. <u>Replacement</u> <u>of</u> <u>Concurrent</u> <u>Losses</u> <u>in</u> <u>Addition</u> <u>to</u> <u>Maintenance</u>
   <u>Requirements</u>

COMPOSITION OF EXTERNAL ABNORMAL LOSSES*

Fluid	Na	K	Cl	Protein
		mEq/L		Gm%
Gastric	20- 80	5-20	100-150	----
Pancreatic	120-140	5-15	40- 80	----
Small intestine	100-140	5-15	90-130	----
Bile	120-140	5-15	80-120	----
Ileostomy	45-135	3-15	20-115	----
Diarrheal	10- 90	10-80	10-110	----

*These losses should be determined Q6h-Q8h.

5. <u>Water</u> <u>Requirements</u> <u>for</u> <u>Premature</u> <u>Infants</u>
   The following are guidelines only. Monitor and modify
   therapy according to urine output, serum sodium and weight.
   Requirements may be slightly lower during the first 24 hrs of
   life. Stool output is negligible in young prematures.

Weight	Environment	Fluids in ml/kg/hr			Total fluid in ml/kg/ 24 hrs
		Insensible	Urine	Total	
1000 gm	isolette	3.0	2.0	5.0	120
	warmer or phototherapy	4.5	2.0	6.5	150
1500 gm	isolette	2.0	2.0	4.0	100
	warmer or phototherapy	3.0	2.0	5.0	120
2000 gm	isolette	1.0	2.0	3.0	75
	warmer or phototherapy	2.0	2.0	4.0	100

Ref: Wu, P and Hodgman, J: <u>Pediatrics</u> <u>54</u>:704, 1974.

6. Hyponatremia - Diagnosis and Management
   Definition: Serum Na less than 130 mEq/L

Type	Na and H_2O Distribution	Disease States	Signs/ Symptoms	Therapy
I	ECF↓, Total Body Na↓, Weight ↓	Salt depletion diarrhea, Addison's CVAH, diuretic therapy	Tachycardia, poor skin turgor, decreased perfusion	Salt and water replacement.
II	ECF↑, Total Body Na-sl.↓, Weight↑	SIADH from many causes	May have neuromuscular irritability, seizures. No edema. Normal perfusion.	Water restriction. Hypertonic saline if symptomatic.
III	ECF↑, Total Body Na↑. Weight↑	Intractable heart failure, severe liver disease, acute and chronic renal failure	Those of underlying disease plus edema, ascites; decreased perfusion	Water restriction plus therapy of underlying disease.
IV	ECF↑, Total Body Na nl., Weight nl.	Hyperosmolarity, hyperglycemia*, Mannitol Rx, Glycerol Rx	May have CNS symptoms i.e., seizures, coma	Treat underlying disease.
V	"Pseudohyponatremia" ECF nl., Total Body Na nl., Weight nl.	Decrease in plasma water i.e., hyperlipemia, hyperproteinemia	None	Treat underlying disease.

* To correct serum Na for hyperglycemia: Serum Na decreases
  1.6 mEq/L for each increment of 100 mg/dl rise in serum glucose.

Ref: Katz, MA: New Engl J Med 289:843, 1973.

7. Anion Gap

   A. The anion gap represents the difference between
      unmeasured cations (UC) and unmeasured anions (UA).
      Clinically it is measured by:

   $$AG = UC - UA = Na - (Cl + HCO_3)$$
   Normal: 12 mEq/L ± 2 mEq/L

B.   Causes of Increased Anion Gap
   1) Decreased unmeasured cation: hypokalemia, hypo-
      calcemia, hypomagnesemia.
   2) Increased unmeasured anion:
      a) Organic anions: lactate, ketones.
      b) Inorganic anions: phosphate, sulfate.
      c) Proteins: hyperalbuminemia (transient).
      d) Exogenous anions: salicylate, formate,
         nitrate, penicillin, carbenicillin, etc.
      e) Incompletely identified: anion accumulating in
         paraldehyde, ethylene glycol, methanol and
         salicylate poisoning, uremia, hyperosmolar
         hyperglycemic nonketotic coma.
   3) Laboratory error:
      a) Falsely increased serum sodium.
      b) Falsely decreased serum chloride or bicarbonate.

C.   Causes of Decreased Anion Gap
   1) Increased unmeasured cation:
      a) Increased concentration of normally present
         cation: hyperkalemia, hypercalcemia, hyper-
         magnesemia.
      b) Retention of abnormal cation: IgG globulin,
         tromethamine (TRIS buffer), lithium.
   2) Decreased unmeasured anion: hypoalbuminemia.
   3) Laboratory error:
      a) Systematic error: hyponatremia due to viscous
         serum, hyperchloremia in bromide intoxication.
      b) Random error: falsely decreased serum sodium,
         falsely increased serum chloride or bicar-
         bonate.

Ref: Emmett, M and Narins, R: Medicine 56:38, 1977; Oh,
MS and Carroll, HJ: New Eng J Med 297:814, 1977.

COMPOSITION OF FREQUENTLY USED ORAL SOLUTIONS

Liquid	CHO gm/100 ml	Prot.* gm/100 ml	Cal/L	Na	K mEq/L++	Cl	HCO₃**	Ca mg/dl	P+
Apple juice	11.9	--	483	0.43	25	--	--	6	16
Coca Cola	10.0	--	400	3.6	--	--	13.4	3.0	16
Gatorade	4	--	170	23.5	2.5	17	--	23	--
Ginger ale	7.5	--	300	4.5	0.1	--	3.6	2.7	--
Grape juice	18.0	--	660	0.8	29.6	--	32	10.9	12
Jell-O water (1/2 strength)	9.7	0.8	404	5.5-16.5‡	0.1-0.2|	--	--	1	2.5
Kool-Aid## (sweetened)	10.0	--	416	0.2	0.1	--	--	1	18
Lytren	7.0	--	280	25	25	30	18	4	5
Milk (skim)	4.8	3.6	425	22	38	29	--	110	90
Milk (whole)	4.8	3.37	670	22	37.5	28	30	110	90
Orange juice (unsweetened)	11.0	--	451	0.35	51.2	--	50	10	18
Pedialyte	5.0	--	200	30	20	30	14	4	0
Pedialyte - RS	2.5	--	100	60	50	50	15	0	0
Pepsi-Cola	10.8	--	480	1.1	--	--	7.3	--	--
7-UP	10.0	--	411	0.5	--	--	--	--	--
Sprite	10.0	--	400	7.6	--	--	--	3	0
Water (Baltimore City)	--	--	--	3	0.5	4	--	--	6.8

* Protein or amino acid equivalent

** Actual or potential bicarbonate, such as lactate, citrate, or acetate

+ Calculated according to valence of 1.8

++ Approximate values: actual values may vary somewhat in various localities depending on electrolyte composition of water supply used to reconstitute solution.

‡ Depends on flavor (concord grape, black raspberry-lowest Na; wild cherry-highest Na)

Does not include electrolyte contribution from local water.

Adapted from: USDA Handbook #456 and JHA Diet Manual.

COMPOSITION OF FREQUENTLY USED PARENTERAL FLUIDS

Liquid	CHO	Prot.*	Cal/L	Na	K	Cl	HCO₃**	Ca	P+
	gm/100 ml			mEq/L++					mg/dl
D₅W	5	--	170	--	--	--	--	--	--
D₁₀W	10	--	340	--	--	--	--	--	--
Normal saline (0.9% NaCl)	--	--	--	154	--	154	--	--	--
1/2 Normal saline (0.45% NaCl)	--	--	--	77	--	77	--	--	--
D5 (0.2% NaCl)	5	--	170	34	--	34	--	--	--
3% Saline	--	--	--	513	--	513	--	--	--
8.4% Sodium Bicarbonate (1 mEq/ml)	--	--	--	1000	--	--	1000	--	--
Ringer's	0-10	--	0-340	147	4	155.5	--	4.5	--
Ringer's Lactate	0-10	--	0-340	130	4	109	28	3	--
Amino Acid 8.5% (Travasol)	--	8.5	340	3	--	34	52	--	--
Plasmanate	--	5	200	110	2	50	29	--	--
Albumin 25% (Salt Poor)	--	25	1000	100-160	<1	<120	--	--	--
Intralipid (Cutter)§	2.25	--	1100	2.5	0.5	4.0	--	--	0.8

* Protein or amino acid equivalent

** Bicarbonate or equivalent (citrate, acetate, lactate)

+ Approximate values: actual values may vary somewhat in various localities depending on electrolyte composition of water supply used to reconstitute solution

§ Values are approximate – may vary from lot to lot

P O I S O N I N G

1. The Unknown Poison (Partial Listing)

Sign or Symptom	Poison
EYES	
Pupillary dilatation	Belladonna alkaloids, atropine, meperidine, sympathomimetics, parasympatholytics, antihistamines, cocaine, camphor, benzene, botulinus toxin, cyanide, carbon monoxide, LSD, mescaline, thallium
Pupillary constriction	Opiates, sympatholytics, parasympathomimetics, barbiturates, cholinesterase inhibitors, chloral hydrate, phenothiazines, ethanol, organophosphate insecticides, phencyclidine
Nystagmus	Phenytoin, propoxyphene, PCP
Ptosis	Botulinus toxin, phenytoin, propoxyphene
Strabismus	Botulinus toxin, thallium
FACE AND SCALP	
Alopecia	Arsenic, radioactive agents, cancer chemotherapeutic agents, vitamin A, lead, boric acid, thallium
SKIN AND MUCOUS MEMBRANES	
Sweating	Cholinergics, arsenic, mercury, bismuth, organophosphate insecticides, fluoride, nicotine
Hot, dry skin	Atropine, belladonna alkaloids, botulinus toxin
Flushing	Sympathomimetics, anticholinergics, boric acid, carbon monoxide, alcohol, snake bites, atropine, antihistamines, phenothiazines
Salivation	Caustics, arsenic, mercury, bismuth, cholinergics, organophosphate insecticides, muscarine-containing mushrooms, salicylates, nicotine, fluoride
Dry mouth	Atropine, belladonna alkaloids, botulinus toxin, antihistamines, sympathomimetics, narcotics, anticholinergics
Burns	Corrosives, thallium, boric acid
Stomatitis	Cancer chemotherapeutic agents
Discoloration	Lead, mercury, thallium, bismuth, arsenic
gray color	Lead, phenacetin

cyanosis	Carbon monoxide, barbiturates, opiates, aniline dyes, methemoglobinemia
pink color	Cyanide
Jaundice	Arsenic, acetaminophen, mushroom toxins, naphthalene and other potentially hemolytic agents, carbon tetrachloride, phosphorus

NERVOUS SYSTEM

Ataxia	Lead, organophosphate insecticides, antihistamines, thallium, alcohol, phenytoin, propoxyphene, dextromethorphan
Obtundation and coma	Narcotics, barbiturates, phenothiazines, benzodiazepines, chloral hydrate, bromides, alcohols, lead, cyanide, carbon monoxide, nicotine, benzene, atropine, belladonna alkaloids, organophosphate insecticides, insulin, aniline dyes, mushrooms, salicylates, hydrocarbons, mercury, boric acid, antihistamines, arsenic, iron, digitalis, theophylline, phenytoin
Delirium	Atropine, belladonna alkaloids, cocaine, alcohol, lead, marijuana, arsenic, amphetamines, antihistamines, camphor, LSD, PCP, benzene, barbiturates, DDT, aniline dyes, theophylline, digitalis
Convulsions	Strychnine, camphor, cocaine, atropine, belladonna alkaloids, organophosphate insecticides, amphetamines, nicotine, lead, mushrooms, caffeine, theophylline, cyanides, tricyclic antidepressants, salicylates, narcotics, barbiturate withdrawal, boric acid, mercury, phenothiazines, antihistamines, arsenic, DDT, hydrocarbons, fluoride, digitalis, thallium, alcohols, PCP, propoxyphene, phenytoin
Headache	Atropine, organophosphate insecticides, carbon monoxide, benzene, anilines, lead, indomethacin
Muscle spasms	Atropine, strychnine, lead, spider and scorpion bites, phenothiazines, camphor, fluorides
Paresthesias, weakness, paralysis	Carbon monoxide, botulinus toxin, alcohols, curare, DDT, nicotine, cyanide, mercury, lead, arsenics, thallium, organophosphates, fluorides

GI TRACT

Nausea, vomiting, diarrhea, abdominal pain	Arsenic, iron, corrosives, lead, spider bites, boric acid, organophosphates, phosphorus, nicotine, fluorides, thallium, methanol, mushrooms, digitalis, opiates, DDT, botulinus toxin, cocaine, salicylates, theophylline, snake bites, food poisoning, mercury, naphthalene

Dysphagia	Caustics, botulinus toxin, camphor, iodine, arsenics
Hematemesis	Caustics, fluoride, iron, arsenic, salicylates, theophylline, warfarin, phosphorus

EAR

Tinnitus	Salicylates, quinine, quinidine, aminoglycosides, camphor, nicotine, methanol

RENAL

Proteinuria	Arsenic, mercury, phosphorus
Hematuria and/or hemoglobinuria	Arsenic, mercury, naphthalene, and other potential hemolytic oxidizers

HEMATOLOGIC

Anemia	Lead, naphthalene and other potentially hemolytic agents, snake venom
Hemorrhage	Warfarin, thallium
Methemoglobinemia	Nitrates, nitrites, anilines

RESPIRATORY

Respiratory depression and failure	Opiates, fluorides, cyanides, barbiturates, alcohols, snake venom, carbon monoxide, benzodiazepines, phenothiazines, organophosphates
Tachypnea and hyperpnea	Atropine, belladonna alkaloids, cocaine, amphetamines, strychnine, salicylates, camphor, hydrocarbons, snake venoms, cyanides, carbon monoxide, talc, caustics

CARDIOVASCULAR

Bradycardia	Digitalis, mushrooms, quinine, quinidine, lead, barbiturates, opiates, organophosphates
Tachycardia	Amphetamines, atropine, cocaine, sympathomimetics, caffeine, aminophylline
Hypertension	Amphetamines, sympathomimetics, lead, nicotine, mercury
Hypotension	Chloral hydrate, phenothiazines, iron
Cardiovascular collapse (shock)	Arsenic, boric acid, iron, phosphorus, food poisoning, lead, caustics
Arrhythmias	Digitalis, tricyclic antidepressants, theophylline, narcotics, amphetamines, phenothiazines, solvents

	BREATH ODOR
Alcoholic	Phenols, chloral hydrate, alcohol
Sweet	Chloroform, acetone, ether
Bitter almond	Cyanides
Pears	Chloral hydrate
Garlic	Phosphorus, arsenic, organophosphate insecticides
Wintergreen	Methyl salicylate
Violets	Turpentine
Pine	Pine oil

	GENERAL
Agitation	Caffeine, theophylline
Fever	Atropine, salicylates, food poisoning, antihistamines, phenothiazines, camphor, alcohols, theophylline, quinine, belladonna alkaloids

Adapted from: Arena, JM: Poisoning. Springfield, IL: Charles C. Thomas, 1979, pp 6-9.

Other General Ref: Skoutakis, VA: Clinical Toxicology of Drugs: Principles and Practice. Philadelphia: Lea and Febiger, 1982; Haddad, LM and Winchester, JF: Clinical Management of Poisoning and Drug Overdose. Philadelphia: W. B. Saunders, Co., 1983.

2. Prevention of Systemic Absorption

   A. Emesis
      1) For most ingestions, induce emesis. It removes up
          to 6 times more toxin than lavage. Contraindica-
          tions to emesis are:
          a) Stupor and coma
          b) Caustic ingestions
          c) Some hydrocarbon ingestions
          d) Hematemesis
          e) Seizures
      2) Syrup of Ipecac dosages:
          a) 9-12 months of age   - 10 ml
          b) 1-12 years of age   - 15 ml
          c) >12 years of age   - 30 ml
      3) Follow ipecac with 100-500 ml of clear fluids,
          according to age.
      4) If no emesis occurs in 20 min, repeat the dose only
          once and give more fluids.

   B. Gastric lavage
      1) Indications:
          a) Ipecac failure
          b) Infants <9 months of age
          c) Stuporous and comatose patients
          d) Post-ictal patients (emesis during a second sei-
              zure could be dangerous)
      2) Contraindications:
          a) Caustic ingestions
          b) Hydrocarbon ingestions (see Section H)
      3) Insertion and inflation of a cuffed endotracheal tube
          prior to gastric lavage protects against aspiration of
          gastric contents, especially in the patient with
          altered mental status or a depressed gag reflex.
      4) Method:
          a) Position patient on left side, with the head
              slightly lower than the body.
          b) Insert large-bore nasogastric or orogastric
              tube (12 French or larger in young children
              and infants).
          c) Lavage with 0.9% normal saline 50 ml per pass
              (up to 250-300 ml per pass in adolescents and
              adults), until gastric contents are clear. This
              may require several liters. Save initial pass
              for toxicologic examination. Add activated
              charcoal to the lavage solution to increase the
              amount of poison removed.

   C. Activated charcoal
      1) Indicated after emesis or lavage in all ingestions
          except caustics, hydrocarbons, alcohols, iron, boric
          acid, acetaminophen, or cyanide. (Do not give
          before emesis, as charcoal will inactivate ipecac.)

2) Effectively adsorbs and prevents systemic absorption of toxins.
3) <u>Dose:</u> 5 ml/kg PO or NG of a slurry containing 30 gm of charcoal per 250 ml of clear fluid.

D. <u>Cathartics</u>
1) Administer magnesium citrate in a dose of 1 ml/kg in younger children, up to 200 ml in the adolescent or adult. Magnesium sulfate or sodium sulfate are alternatives, both given in doses of 250 mg/kg as a 10% solution.
2) <u>Contraindications:</u> Major compromise of renal function.

<u>Ref:</u> Easom FJ, and Lovjoy, FH Jr.: <u>Ped Clin North Am</u> <u>26</u>:827-836, 1979.

E. <u>Dialysis</u>
1) Indicated in severe ingestions of dialysable substances, or when normal excretory pathways are compromised.
2) <u>Hemoperfusion</u> is useful for specific toxins.
3) Peritoneal dialysis is less efficient than hemodialysis, but more readily available.
4) To determine the potential efficacy of these various techniques in specific ingestions, refer to standard toxicology texts or to Winchester, JF: <u>Trans Am Soc Artif Intern Organs</u> 23:762, 1977; Papadopoulou, ZL and Novello, AC: <u>Ped Clin North Am</u> <u>29</u>:1039, 1982.

3. <u>Specific Poisonings</u>

A. <u>Salicylate Poisoning</u>
1) Symptoms: hyperpnea, hyperthermia, lethargy, dehydration, metabolic acidosis, coma
2) Establish the severity of ingestion
    a) The acute toxic dose (single-dose ingestion): 150 mg/kg
    b) Chronic overdosage can produce toxicity at much lower doses
    c) Preparations:
        (1) Children's aspirin: 1¼ grain (81 mg) tablets (36 tabs per bottle)
        (2) Adult aspirin: 5 grain (325 mg) tablets
        (3) Methyl salicylate (oil of wintergreen): 1.4 gm/ml
3) Test of salicylates
    a) Urine ferric chloride: Mix one ml of urine with one ml 10% $FeCl_3$ solution. Purple color change indicates a positive test. However, even an insignificant amount of salicylate will produce a positive test. Urinary ketones also will produce a false positive test; these can be removed by first boiling the urine.

b)   Phenistix: place one drop of serum on the test stick.
    (1)   tan color - serum level <40 mg/dl
    (2)   brown color - serum level 40-90 mg/dl
    (3)   purple color - serum level >90 mg/dl

c)   Serum salicylate level: therapy must be based upon quantitative serum level and not upon the above presumptive tests. At least two levels obtained several hours apart are necessary to determine the severity of ingestion, as continued slow absorption may increase the serum level for up to 24 hours.

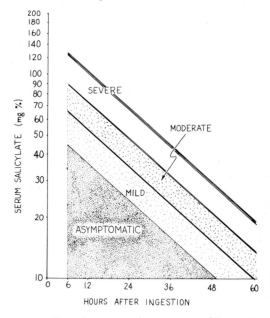

Done Nomogram: the nomogram relates serum salicylate and expected severity of intoxication at varying intervals following ingestion of a single dose of salicylate, starting six hours after the ingestion.

4) Treatment
   a) Institute therapy immediately. Do not wait for the salicylate level to return.
   b) Empty the stomach by emesis (preferably), or lavage with 0.9% normal saline. Administer activated charcoal and cathartic.
   c) Monitor serum electrolytes, calcium, arterial blood gases, glucose, urine pH and SG, and coagulation studies as needed.
   d) Treat fluid and solute deficits
      (1) replenish intravascular volume with D5 Ringer's Lactate at 20 ml/kg/hr for 1-2 hrs until adequate urine output is established.
      (2) then begin infusing D5 with 50 mEq Na HCO_3/L and 20-40 mEq K/L at rates of 3-6 L/ M^2/day (i.e., 2-4 times maintenance fluids). Aim for a urine output of 2 ml/kg/hr, as this will enhance salicylate excretion. Adjust concentrations of the electrolytes as needed to correct serum electrolyte abnormalities (esp. hypokalemia, which inhibits salicylate excretion), and to maintain a urinary pH >7.0.
      (3) In severe cases only, alkalinization of the urine can be accomplished by administering acetazolamide (5 mg/kg subcutaneously) immediately and repeated two more times at 5 hour intervals. Acetazolamide should never be given without concurrent bicarbonate. Ref: Finberg, L, et al.: Water and Electrolytes in Pediatrics. Philadelphia: W. B. Saunders Co., 1982, p. 203.
   e) Administer parenteral vitamin K as indicated by coagulation studies (especially in chronic intoxications).
   f) Continue fluid therapy until the patient is asymptomatic for several hours, regardless of the serum salicylate level.
   g) Proceed to hemodialysis in the presence of severe salicylism (levels >100), renal failure, pulmonary edema, coma or convulsions, or severe electrolyte abnormalities. Peritoneal dialysis with an albumin-containing solution can be initiated as arrangements are being made for hemodialysis.

Ref: Temple, AR: Pediatrics 62:873, 1978; Done, AK: Pediatrics 62:890, 1978; Pierce, AW: Pediatrics 54: 342, 1974.

B. <u>Acetaminophen Poisoning</u>

1) Symptoms: nausea, vomiting, and malaise for 24 hrs, improvement over the next 48 hrs, followed by clinical or laboratory evidence of hepatic dysfunction. Death can occur due to fulminant hepatic failure.

2) Evaluation

Likelihood of hepatic toxicity related to:

a) Dose: 140 mg/kg is considered toxic in adolescents and adults (but hepatic failure is uncommon in adults with ingestions <10 gm). No information is available on children, who may have less toxicity from the drug.

b) Plasma level: see nomogram. Draw level at 4 hrs post ingestion.

c) Delay in treatment: antidote is not effective if administered >10 hrs after ingestion.

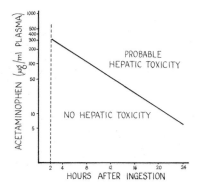

3) Therapy

a) Empty the stomach by emesis if within 1 hr of ingestion, thereafter by lavage (ipecac may interfere with toleration of oral acetylcysteine). Avoid charcoal - it adsorbs acetylcysteine.

b) For significant ingestions or ingestions of unknown amounts: ASAP administer acetylcysteine (Mucomyst) either IV or PO:

(1) <u>IV</u>: Use the sterile 20% Mucomyst commonly used for tracheobronchial instillation. Doses for adolescents and adults

(no recommendations available for children):

give 150 mg/kg in 200 ml of NS over 15 min.

then 50 mg/kg in 500 ml of NS over 4 hrs.

then 100 mg/kg in 1000 ml of NS over the next 16 hrs.

Ref: Prescott, LF, et al.: Brit Med J, 2:1097-1100, 1979.

    (2) PO or NG: Mucomyst diluted 1:4 in a carbonated beverage as a loading dose of 140 mg/kg, then 70 mg/kg Q4h for 5 doses (some recommend 18 doses).

c) The major error is to wait for the drug level to return. Treat immediately if you think it is a significant ingestion.

Ref: Rumack, BH, and Matthew, H: Pediatrics 55:871, 1975; Helliwell, M, et al.: Can Med Assoc J 125:827, 1981.

C. Hyperkalemia

  1) Diagnosis based on serum level and EKG abnormalities (see Cardiology section, page 66). Serum levels often do not correlate directly with EKG abnormalities.

  2) Treatment

    a) Serum level >6.0 mEq/L: discontinue all exogenous potassium sources and K^+ sparing diuretics.

    b) Significant EKG abnormalities: Begin continuous EKG monitoring and institute one or more of the following therapies either sequentially or concurrently and repeat them as necessary.

      (1) Administer 0.5 ml/kg of calcium gluconate 10% solution IV over 5-10 min, while monitoring for bradycardia and hypotension. Adult maximum dose is 10-20 ml.

      (2) Administer 1-2 mEq/kg sodium bicarbonate IV over 5-10 min.

NOTE: Sodium bicarbonate and calcium gluconate are incompatible solutions and will precipitate if given through the same IV line without flushing between doses.

      (3) Administer IV over 2 hrs: 0.5 gm/kg of glucose with 0.3 units regular insulin added per gram of glucose.

        c)   Administer Kayexalate (sodium polystyrene sulfonate resin) 1-2 gm/kg/day orally divided Q6h in 70% sorbitol solution (3 ml/gm resin) or as a retention enema in 20% sorbitol solution (5 ml/gm resin). One gram of Kayexalate per kg body weight should lower serum potassium approximately 1 mEq/L.

        d)   Proceed rapidly to dialysis if hyperkalemia appears imminently life-threatening. Arrhythmias which significantly compromise cardiac output may require temporary artificial pacing.

D.   Digoxin Intoxication

    1)   Symptoms: major manifestations are GI (anorexia, nausea, vomiting), CNS (headache, disorientation, somnolence, seizures), and CARDIAC (any new rhythm, esp. those combining increased automaticity of ectopic pacemakers and impaired conduction). Most cases result in GI symptoms with mild CNS and cardiac disturbances.

    2)   Evaluation

        a)   Doses of >0.07 mg/kg are associated with toxicity (or 2-3 mg in an adolescent).

        b)   Quinidine, amiodarone, or poor renal function will increase the digoxin level. Low K, Mg, or T_4 will increase the digoxin toxicity at a given level, as will high Ca.

        c)   Hyperkalemia correlates with a high digoxin level.

    3)   Treatment

        a)   Ipecac, charcoal (even several hours after ingestion), and cathartic.

        b)   Start continuous ECG monitoring.

        c)   In cardiac rhythm disturbances:

            (1) AV block: atropine alone 0.01 mg/kg IV may reverse sinus bradycardia or AV block. Repeated doses may be necessary. Avoid propranolol, quinidine, procainamide, or disopyramide if AV block is present.

                (a) Phenytoin improves AV conduction. Dose is 1-2 mg/kg, no faster than 50 mg/min. Repeat Q5 min until arrhythmia is controlled or maximum dose is reached.

                (b) Transvenous ventricular pacing is usually effective if atropine and phenytoin fail.

            (2) Ventricular tachycardia, PVCs: phenytoin and lidocaine are effective.

        d)   In severe poisonings, purified digoxin-specific Fab fragments rapidly reverse CNS depression, rhythm disturbances, and hyperkalemia; they can be life-saving. Continue CPR for prolonged periods if Fab fragments are available.

Ref: Smith, TW and Haber, E: New Engl J Med
289:1125, 1973; Smith, TW, et al.: New Engl J Med
307:1357, 1982; Zucker, AR, et al.: Pediatrics
70:468, 1982. Murphy, DJ, et al.: Pediatrics
70:472, 1982.

E. Iron Poisoning
    1) Diagnosis
        a) Symptoms
            (1) First phase: GI toxicity (30 min - 12 hrs
                 after ingestion) - nausea, vomiting, diar-
                 rhea, abdominal pain, hematemesis,
                 melena. Rarely - shock, seizures, coma.
            (2) Second phase: latent period (8-36 hrs
                 after ingestion) - improvement in clinical
                 symptoms.
            (3) Third phase: systemic toxicity (12-48 hrs
                 after ingestion) - hepatic injury or fail-
                 ure, hypoglycemia, metabolic acidosis,
                 bleeding, shock, coma, convulsions,
                 death.
            (4) Fourth phase: late complications (4-8
                 wks after ingestion) - pyloric or antral
                 stenosis, cirrhosis, CNS sequelae.
        b) Abdominal x-ray: iron containing tablets are
            radiopaque.
        c) Deferoxamine challenge test: give 2 gm IM
            deferoxamine. Presence of "vin rose" color to
            urine indicates a significant ingestion of iron.
        d) Serum iron level: Serum iron levels in excess
            of 300 μg/100 ml and/or serum iron levels
            exceeding serum iron-binding capacity by 50
            μg/100 ml or greater suggest severe iron poi-
            soning, if obtained within 4-6 hr after
            ingestion. Serum iron levels obtained beyond
            6 hrs after ingestion may not be elevated,
            even in the presence of severe poisoning.
    2) Treatment
        a) Induce emesis in all conscious patients with
            intact gag reflex.
        b) Lavage all patients (including after emesis)
            with 2 gm deferoxamine in 1 liter of H_2O buf-
            fered with $NaHCO_3$ to maintain gastric pH
            >5.0.
        c) After lavage, administer per NG tube 10 gm
            deferoxamine in 50 ml H_2O alkalinized with
            $NaHCO_3$ to maintain gastric pH >5.0. Do not
            administer activated charcoal.
        d) Obtain abdominal x-ray after lavage.
        e) Observe patient at least six hours after inges-
            tion.
        f) Treat patients with a history of iron ingestion
            who demonstrate GI or systemic symptoms, a
            positive deferoxamine challenge test, or evi-
            dence of iron tablets on abdominal x-ray, as
            follows:

        (1)   Treat shock and maintain urine output 1-2 ml/kg/hr.

        (2)   Begin continuous IV infusion of deferoxamine in 0.9% normal saline at 10-15 mg/kg/hr. (Rates >15 mg/kg/hr may induce hypotension.)

        (3)   Continue deferoxamine therapy until urine color is normal and patient is asymptomatic at least 24 hr.

    g)   Follow-up all patients for evidence of intestinal stricture and/or iron deficiency anemia.

Ref: Robotham, JL and Lietman, PS: *Am J Dis Child* 134:875, 1980.

F. Lead Poisoning

1) Diagnosis

    a)   Establish presumptive diagnosis with peripheral blood count and smear for basophilic stippling, long bone x-rays for "lead lines," and abdominal x-ray for radiopaque foreign matter.

    b)   Definitive diagnosis is based on blood lead and free erythrocyte protoporphyrin levels (FEP). Note that FEP may also be elevated in iron deficiency anemia.

        (1)   Class I (normal): blood lead <29 µg/100 ml whole blood, FEP <49 µg/100 ml whole blood.

        (2)   Class II (moderate risk): blood lead 30-49 µg/100 ml whole blood, FEP 50-109 µg/100 ml whole blood.

        (3)   Class III (high risk): blood lead 50-69 µg/100 ml whole blood, FEP 110-249 µg/100 ml whole blood.

        (4)   Class IV (urgent risk): asymptomatic patients with blood lead 70-100 µg/100 ml whole blood and/or FEP 250 µg/100 ml whole blood or greater.

        (5)   Class V (encephalopathy or impending encephalopathy): any symptomatic patient, or any patient with blood lead >100 µg/100 ml whole blood.

2) Treatment

    a)   Class I - none required

    b)   Class II

        (1)   Remove patient from lead sources.

        (2)   Reduce household dust with frequent wet-mopping and use of high phosphate detergents.

        (3)   Treat iron deficiency.

        (4)   Institute low-fat, lead-free diet, with adequate calcium, magnesium, zinc, copper, and iron.

c) Class III and IV
   (1) Remove patient from lead source and institute above diet.
   (2) Begin CaEDTA 1 gm/M²/day limited to 5 days, divided Q12h for Class III and Q6h for Class IV. Side-effects and relative contraindications to CaEDTA include hypercalcemia and impaired renal function. BAL (see below) may be used where CaEDTA is contraindicated.
   (3) At end of CaEDTA course, begin d-penicillamine not to exceed 500 mg/M²/day as one daily dose two hours before a meal (can be mixed in fruit or fruit juice). D-penicillamine is an investigational drug for lead chelation. It is contraindicated in, and can cause as side-effects, nephritis, proteinuria, neutropenia, and penicillin allergy. It can worsen plumbism if the patient continues to ingest lead; therefore, it should be used in an institutional setting only.
   (4) A shortened CaEDTA course of three days may be repeated at one week intervals as needed or where d-penicillamine is contraindicated.
   (5) Continue therapy until blood lead and/or FEP are in Class II range.

d) Class V
   (1) Avoid lumbar puncture unless required for differential diagnosis.
   (2) Establish urine output with 10-20 ml/kg IV 10% dextrose. Use mannitol 1-2 gm/kg IV if necessary. Then to minimize increased intracranial pressure, restrict fluids, but maintain normal serum electrolytes and a urine output of 0.5-1.0 ml/kg/hr.
   (3) Control seizures acutely with IV diazepam and paraldehyde. Phenobarbital and/or phenytoin are less useful for acute seizure control, but may be necessary for chronic seizure management.
   (4) Give BAL (British anti-Lewisite, Dimercaprol)
       (a) for symptomatic patient with blood lead 70-100 µg/100 ml, administer BAL 333 mg/M²/day IM Q4h for 2-3 days. Side-effects include vomiting, hypertension, and tachycardia. Keep patient NPO. BAL is contraindicated in patients with acute hepatocellular injury and in males with G6PD deficiency.

(b) for encephalopathic patient or patient with blood lead >100 µg/100 ml administer BAL 500 mg/M²/day IM Q4h for 3-5 days.

(5) Begin CaEDTA 1.5 gm/M²/day IM divided Q4h for 5 days with the second BAL dose. CaEDTA is contraindicated in the anuric patient.

(6) BAL and CaEDTA courses may be cautiously extended to 7 days if the patient remains symptomatic. Patients who rapidly become asymptomatic should have BAL discontinued and CaEDTA dose reduced to 1 gm/M²/day after 3 days.

(7) Further therapy with d-penicillamine and/ or repeated 3-day CaEDTA courses are as outlined under Class III and IV.

Ref: Chisolm, JJ and Barltrop, D: Arch Dis Child 54:249, 1979; Statement by CDC: J Pediatr 93:709, 1978; Charney, E, et al.: New Engl J Med 309:1089, 1983; Chisolm, JJ: J Pediatr 73:1, 1968; Chisolm, JJ: In Current Pediatric Therapy, 11th Edition, Gellis and Kagen (ed.), Philadelphia: W. B. Saunders Co., 1984 (in press).

G. Caustic Ingestions (Strong Acids and Alkalis)

1) All patients with a history of caustic ingestion should be hospitalized for endoscopy. Absence of oropharyngeal damage does not exclude esophageal burns.

2) Maintain patient NPO. Attempts to "neutralize" the burn are ineffective and obscure and delay endoscopy.

3) Begin intravenous fluid therapy.

4) Begin intravenous ampicillin 100-200 mg/kg/day.

5) Begin intravenous hydrocortisone sodium succinate 10-20 mg/kg/day.

6) Provide tetanus prophylaxis as indicated.

7) Obtain blood count, chest x-ray, blood type and crossmatch. Chest x-ray may demonstrate esophageal perforation.

8) Proceed to endoscopy. Do not pass NG tube. Discontinue endoscopy immediately if esophageal burn identified.

9) In the absence of esophageal burn, antibiotics and steroids may be discontinued. Provide care for local burns.

10) In the presence of esophageal burns, continue antibiotics for at least 5-7 days and steroids for 3 wks. Advance diet slowly after patient is able to handle own secretions well. Steroids may be changed to oral prednisone 2 mg/kg/day if tolerated. Taper prednisone slowly after full 3 wk course.

11) Provide close follow-up and further surgical therapy for esophageal or antral/pyloric strictures, as required.

Ref: Haller, JA, et al.: J Ped Surg 6:578, 1971.

H. Hydrocarbon Ingestions
1) Symptoms: Pulmonary: tachypnea, dyspnea, tachycardia, cyanosis, grunting, cough; CNS: lethargy, seizures, coma.
2) Evaluation:
    a) Aliphatic hydrocarbons have the greatest aspiration hazard and pulmonary toxicity. They include: gasoline, kerosene, mineral seal oil, lighter fluid, tar, mineral oil, lubricating oils.
    b) Aromatic hydrocarbons (benzene, toluene, xylene) and halogenated hydrocarbons (carbon tetrachloride) have mainly CNS and hepato-toxicity.
3) Therapy
    a) Removal of toxin
        (1) Avoid emesis or lavage if possible as these increase the risk of aspiration.
        (2) If the hydrocarbon contains a potentially toxic substance (insecticide, heavy metal, camphor) and a toxic amount has been ingested, induce emesis with ipecac in the fully conscious patient. In lethargic patients, intubate with a cuffed ETT then lavage.
        (3) Avoid charcoal. It does not bind aliphatics and will increase the risk of aspiration.
    b) Obtain CXR and arterial blood gases on patients with pulmonary symptoms.
    c) When to admit?
        (1) If the child is asymptomatic and remains so for 6 hrs, discharge home.
        (2) If symptomatic with a normal CXR, discharge home if symptoms resolve within 6 hrs; admit if symptoms persist.
        (3) If symptomatic with an abnormal CXR, admit.
    d) Treat pneumonitis with oxygen, PEEP. Antibiotics and steroids are not routinely warranted.

Ref: Anas, N, et al.: JAMA 246:840, 1981; Eade, NR, et al.: Pediatrics 54:351, 1974.

I. Theophylline Toxicity
1) Symptoms: GI: vomiting, hematemesis, bloody diarrhea; CV: tachycardia, arrhythmia, cardiac arrest; CNS: seizures, agitation, coma.

2) Evaluation:
   a) Obtain a theophylline level stat and again in 1-4 hours to see the pattern of absorption. Peak absorption has been reported to be delayed as long as 13-17 hrs after ingestion.
   b) Levels >20 mcg/ml associated with increasing toxicity; especially >40 mcg/ml.
   c) Levels >40 mcg/ml or patients with neurotoxicity require admission and careful monitoring.
   d) Hypokalemia may occur.

3) Therapy:
   a) Ipecac (preferably) or lavage.
   b) Charcoal followed by cathartic, regardless of the length of time after ingestion. Administration of charcoal at 2 hr intervals may enhance elimination.
   c) Establish IV access and treat dehydration.
   d) Charcoal hemoperfusion: an effective and safe method of rapidly lowering theophylline levels. Start hemoperfusion whenever signs of neurotoxicity (seizures, coma) are present. Whether a high theophylline level alone is an indication for hemoperfusion is controversial.

Ref: Gaudreault, R, et al.: J Pediatr 102:474, 1983; Sahney, S, et al.: Pediatrics 71:615, 1983.

J. Anticholinergic Toxicity
1) Agents: tricyclics, antihistamines, antiparkinsonians, scopolamine, belladonna, jimson weed, ophthalmic mydriatics, atropine.
2) Symptoms: "mad as a hatter, red as a beet, blind as a bat, hot as a hare, dry as a bone", oral dryness and burning, speech and swallowing difficulties, thirst, blurred vision, photophobia, mydriasis, skin flushing, tachycardia, fever, urinary urgency, delirium, hallucinations, cardiovascular collapse.
3) Treatment:
   a) Emesis or lavage, activated charcoal, and cathartic as above.
   b) Observation is all that is necessary in mild cases.
   c) In life-threatening emergencies (arrhythmias, hypertension, myoclonic seizures, severe hallucinations), physostigmine will reverse symptoms.

   NOTE: Neostigmine and pyridostigmine will not affect the CNS symptoms. Do not use physostigmine simply to maintain an alert state in an otherwise stable patient in coma.

    (1)   dose: in children <5 yrs, give physo-
stigmine 0.5 mg IV every 5 min until a
therapeutic effect is seen or a total dose
of 2.0 mg is achieved. In those >5
yrs, give 1-2 mg IV. Repeat in 10
min if ineffective. Max. dose = 4 mg in
30 min.

    (2)   rate: infuse at 1-2 mg/min. Faster rates
can cause seizures or precipitate a cholinergic crisis. Effective within 3-5 min.

    (3)   reversal: atropine should be available to
reverse cholinergic side effects, in
a dose of 0.5 mg for each 1 mg of physostigmine just given.

Ref: Rumack, BH: Pediatrics 52:449, 1973.

K.   Tricyclic Antidepressant Overdose
    1)   Symptoms: choreoathetosis, myoclonus, hypo- or
hypertension, arrhythmias, in addition to the symptoms of anticholinergic toxicity.
    2)   Evaluation:
        a)   Lethal dose varies from 10-30 mg/kg.
        b)   Plasma TCA levels >1000 ng/ml are associated
with severe toxicity.
        c)   A QRS duration of >100 msec correlates with
levels >1000 ng/ml.
    3)   Therapy:
        a)   Treat life-threatening symptoms (as in anti-
cholinergic toxicity). Treat seizures with
diazepam then phenytoin. For arrhythmias
refractory to physostigmine, give NaHCO$_3$ 1-2
mEq/kg to keep pH >7.4 (lessens risk of
arrhythmia), and phenytoin 1 mg/kg (increases
AV conduction). Phenytoin may be repeated
up to a maximum loading dose of 15-18 mg/kg.
        b)   Give charcoal and cathartic. In patients who
remain symptomatic, give charcoal Q6h for
24-48 hrs because of enterohepatic cycling.
        c)   Cardiac monitoring: once the level of con-
sciousness and QRS duration return to normal,
the risk of arrhythmia or sudden death is minimal.
        d)   Symptomatic and supportive care.

Ref: Burks, JS, et al.: JAMA 230:1405, 1974;
Biggs, JT, et al.: JAMA 238:135, 1977.

L.   Narcotics, Opiates, and Morphine Analogs
    1)   Suspect in any patient with depressed mental status
of unknown etiology.
    2)   Pupillary signs may be variable.

3) Administer IV nalaxone (Narcan) 0.01 mg/kg. If this is ineffective, administer 0.1 mg/kg. Improvement in mental status indicates a clinical response.

4) If clinical response occurs, continue to administer nalaxone as often and in as large a dose as required, until mental status remains improved and respirations are normal and stable.

5) Careful inpatient monitoring is required because of the short half-life of naloxone compared to most opiates.

Ref: Moore, R, et al.: Am J Dis Child 134:156, 1980.

BURNS

1. Initial Assessment

A. Vital signs
Assess and establish adequate airway, breathing, circulation. Intubation should be considered if evidence of inhalation injury is present--singed nares, cough, wheezes, hoarseness, facial burns, charring of lips, carbonaceous secretions, or history of fire in enclosed space--or if necessary for pulmonary toilet. (Inhalation injury mortality may be as high as 30%).

B. Serial ABG's is best method for monitoring pulmonary damage. CXR may not show changes for first 24-72 hours. Beware hypoxemia and carboxyhemoglobinemia.

C. Assess and begin treatment for any other injuries. Include EKG.

D. Begin fluid resuscitation with Ringer's Lactate 20 ml/kg/hr for 1-2 hours. Central lines for fluid therapy and CVP determination may be necessary.

E. Insert NG tube. Ileus usually seen with >20% burn.

F. Foley catheter may be needed for help with fluid monitoring (increased incidence of urethral strictures in preschool children).

G. Pain and anxiety may require IV analgesia.

2. Burn Assessment
Obtain weight and height to calculate surface area.

A. Surface area of burns (see charts)
   1) >10 yrs of age may approximate with the "Rule of Nines".
   2) <10 yrs of age use the Lund-Browder chart
   3) Degree of tissue damage with electrical burns may not be apparent.

B. Depth of burns
   1) 1st degree - only epidermis involved - painful and erythematous.
   2) 2nd degree - partial thickness - epidermis and dermis with sparing of dermal appendages -- painful, blistering, but may be indistinguishable from 3rd degree.
   3) 3rd degree - full thickness - epidermis and all of dermis, including dermal appendages -- whitish and painless.

ESTIMATION OF BODY SURFACE INVOLVED

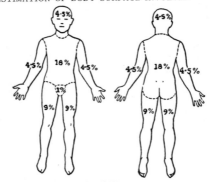

The Rule of Nines
(Not accurate for children <10 years of age.) The
percentage of body surface involved must be modified
according to age using the following chart.

Lund-Browder Chart

AGE - YEARS

AREA	0-1	1-4	4-9	10-15	ADULT	2°	3°	TOTAL
Head	19	17	13	10	7			
Neck	2	2	2	2	2			
Ant. Trunk	13	17	13	13	13			
Post. Trunk	13	13	13	13	13			
R. Buttock	2½	2½	2½	2½	2½			
L. Buttock	2½	2½	2½	2½	2½			
Genitalia	1	1	1	1	1			
R. U. Arm	4	4	4	4	4			
L. U. Arm	4	4	4	4	4			
R. L. Arm	3	3	3	3	3			
L. L. Arm	3	3	3	3	3			
R. Hand	2½	2½	2½	2½	2½			
L. Hand	2½	2½	2½	2½	2½			
R. Thigh	5½	6½	8½	8½	9½			
L. Thigh	5½	6½	8½	8½	9½			
R. Leg	5	5	5	6	7			
L. Leg	5	5	5	6	7			
R. Foot	3½	3½	3½	3½	3½			
L. Foot	3½	3½	3½	3½	3½			
				TOTAL				

3. Treatment

A. First-aid
   Clean towels soaked in cold water may prevent progression of burn. Do not use grease, butter, etc.

B. Triage
   May be treated as an outpatient if burn is less than 10-15% and no full thickness burns.
   1) Admission should be considered for any electrical burn (since underlying tissue damage is difficult to assess); for burns larger than above or involving critical areas such as face, hands, feet, perineum; or if child abuse or inadequate home situation is suspected.
   2) Burns in infants or in patients with chronic illness may require hospitalization.
   3) Burns of >20-30% body surface area, major hand, face, joint, or perineal burns, and electrical burns require transfer to a Burn Center after initial stabilization.

C. Outpatient
   1) Cleanse with betadine and water (1:4) solution or synthetic detergent removing exudate, necrotic skin, etc.
   2) Sulfadiazine (Silvadene) placed in thin layer over burn then covered with bulky gauze dressing.
   3) Follow patient every other day or daily.
   4) Home care - cleanse burn twice daily with mild soap followed with sulfadiazine and sterile dressing as above. Once epithelialization is underway, may be reduced to daily dressing change.
   5) Tetanus toxoid 0.05 ml IM if needed.

D. Inpatient
   1) Initial assessment and stabilization as previously detailed.
   2) Fluid resuscitation - goal is to provide sufficient fluid for prevention of shock and renal failure secondary to excessive fluid losses and third spacing. Formula is only a guideline and adequacy of perfusion should be assessed with urine output (>1 ml/kg/hr), BP, peripheral circulation, sensorium, CVP, and acidosis. Foley catheter may be placed to help monitor fluid status.
   3) Parkland formula - guideline for replacement of deficits and ongoing losses; for infants maintenance fluids have to be added to this:

   4 ml/kg/% burn of Ringer's Lactate (glucose may be added but beware stress hyperglycemia) over the first 24 hours; 1/2 of total given over the

first 8 hours <u>calculated</u> <u>from</u> <u>the</u> <u>time</u> <u>of</u> <u>injury</u>; the remaining half is given over the next 16 hours.

4) The second 24 hour fluid requirements average 50-75% of first day's requirement. Concentrations and rates best determined by monitoring weight, serum electrolytes, urine output, NG losses, etc.

5) Colloid may be added after 18-24 hours (1 gm/kg/ day albumin), to maintain serum albumin >2 gm/ 100 ml.

6) Withhold potassium generally for the first 48 hours because of large potassium release from damaged tissues.

7) Miscellaneous - maintain gastric pH >5 using antacids or cimetidine.

8) Tetanus toxoid as needed.

9) Surveillance cultures of urine, wounds, respiratory tract. Use of prophylactic antibiotics is controversial but a short course of penicillin (3-5 days) may reduce the incidence of early streptococcal wound infections. Typical pathogens to beware of - <u>Pseudomonas</u> <u>aeruginosa</u>, <u>Staph</u> <u>aureus</u>, <u>Candida</u> <u>albicans</u> and <u>Group</u> <u>A</u> <u>strep</u>.

10) Wound care - topical sulfadiazine cream, hydrotherapy, debridement daily.

11) Escharotomies for vascular, respiratory, or joint impairment.

12) Early physical therapy and splinting.

13) Allografting as needed to speed granulization and decrease risk of infection.

4. Nutrition

A. Marked catabolism in burn patients.

B. Daily caloric requirements approximate: <2 yrs -- 80 cal/kg plus 30 cal/% burn, 3-6 gm protein/kg/day; >2 yrs -- 60 cal/kg plus 30 cal/% burn, 2-8 gm protein/ kg/day.

C. Feeding may be met by enteral and/or parenteral hyperalimentation to promote healing, retard immune suppression, etc.

D. Zinc deficiency is common - supplement feeds with vitamins, Zn acetate, ascorbic acid, poly-vi-sol with Fe. Monitor weekly Ca, PO_4, total protein, albumin, transferrin, cholesterol, triglycerides, etc., as measure of sufficient nutrition.

E. Daily weights and electrolytes.

5. Prevention
    The best treatment is prevention! Measures include child-proofing the home, smoke detectors, turning hot water tap temperature down to 120-130°F (requires 5 min immersion at 120° to cause full-thickness burn versus 5 seconds at 140°).

6. Rehabilitation

    A. OT and PT consults early for range of motion, splinting, and exercises.

    B. Jobst garments for molding of maturing scar formation.

    C. Psychological consult for support of both victim and family.

Ref: Edelman, J, et al.: J Pediatr 75:509, 1969; Guzzetta and Randolph: Pediatrics in Review 4,(9): 271-278, 1983; Holder and Ashcroft: Pediatric Surgery. Philadelphia: W.B. Saunders, Co., 1980, pp. 123-137; Wilkinson, AW: J Pediatr Surg 8:103-116, 1973.

NEUROLOGY

1. Seizures

   A. Seizures are among the most common neurological disorders of childhood. One in 15 will have a seizure during the first 7 yrs of life. The majority end spontaneously to be followed by a post-ictal state.

   B. Drug Therapy Goal: eliminate seizures with minimal side effects:
      1) Identify seizure type; use the proper drug.
      2) Initiate therapy with a single drug, least toxic, increase dosage to tolerance or acceptable side effects before adding second or third drug.
      3) Loading dose - 2 to 3 times maintenance dose.
      4) Maintenance therapy alone requires 4-5 times the half-life of the drug to reach a steady state.
      5) Half-life guides to frequency of administration, e.g. - phenobarbital once a day, carbamazepine 2 or 3 times a day.
      6) Blood levels are useful guidelines to check compliance, determine changes in dosage, confirm suspected toxicity.
      7) Monitor acute, chronic adverse reactions; potential teratogenic effects.
      8) Be aware of drug interactions.
      9) Discontinue drugs after long-term use, over weeks to months, starting with one drug at a time.

   C. Caveats in Starting and Stopping Therapy
      1) A single non-febrile seizure incurs a 30% risk of recurrence. Therefore, not all patients with a single seizure need to be treated.
      2) A child who is seizure-free 2 years, with an improved or normal EEG, may be taken off anticonvulsants with a high rate of success.

Ref: Johnston, MV and Freeman, JM: Ped Clin North Am 28:170, 1981; Oppenheimer, EY and Rosman, NP: Emergency Clin N Am 1:125, 1983; Shinnar, S, et al: New Engl J Med, in press, 1984.

D. Commonly Used Drugs in the Control of Convulsive Disorders: (See formulary for specific dosages, $T\frac{1}{2}$, therapeutic range, and side effects)

Major Motor	Petit Mal	Complex Partial	Minor Motor	Focal Seizures
Carbamazepine	Ethosuximide	Carbamazepine	Valproic Acid	Phenobarbital
Phenobarbital	Valproic Acid	Phenytoin	Clonazepam	Phenytoin
Phenytoin	Clonazepam	Primidone	ACTH or Corticosteroids	Carbamazepine
Primidone			Ketogenic Diet	
Valproic Acid			Acetazolamide	

E. Drug Interaction
   Interference with the handling of antiepileptic drugs:
   1) Drugs which may <u>elevate</u> phenytoin levels:

Isoniazid	Dicoumarol
Chloramphenicol	Disulfiram
Methylphenidate	Phenobarbital

   2) Drugs which may <u>lower</u> phenytoin levels:

Diazepam	Carbamazepine
Chloridazepoxide	Ethanol
Clonazepam	Phenobarbital

   3) Drugs whose effects may be reduced by phenytoin
      therapy:

Griseofulvin	Nortriptyline
Warfarin and coumarins	Diazepam
Cortisol and dexamethasone	Doxycycline
Contraceptive pill	Digoxin
Vitamin D	Metyrapone
Carbamazepine	Theophylline

   Ref: Kutt, H: Epilepsia 16:393, 1975; Marquis, JF: <u>New</u>
   <u>Engl</u> J Med 307:1189, 1982.

F. Teratogenic
   The risk of all abnormalities in infants exposed to anti-
   convulsants during pregnancy is about 4% to 5%, approximately double the rate in the general population. Most
   common severe defects noted are cleft lip and palate and
   congenital heart lesions.

   Ref: American Academy of Pediatrics, Committee on Drugs.
   Pediatrics 63:331, 1979.

G. Status Epilepticus

Repeated seizures without regaining consciousness in between, or episodes of convulsive seizures lasting more than 30 min.

Guidelines for Management of Convulsive Status Epilepticus

I. Stabilization 0-10 min	Secure airway, blood pressure, nasal O_2, intubate if necessary.
	Blood for complete blood count, electrolytes, BUN, drug levels, calcium, magnesium, toxicology screen, glucose (serum Dextrostix).
	Start intravenous infusion with 5% dextrose in normal saline (if indicated use 25% dextrose, 1 ml/kg).
	Blood gas for O_2 + pH, if pH <7.1 give bicarbonate after adequate ventilation is established.
	Monitor respirations, blood pressure, and ECG.
II. Control seizures	
10-25 min	Diazepam, 0.3-0.5 mg/kg (10 mg maxium in 1 dose, to be given no faster than 2 mg/min), may repeat every 10 min for maximum of 3 doses.
	Be prepared to intubate patient.
	Phenytoin, start after 1st dose of diazepam; give 15-20 mg/kg, no faster than 50 mg/min; if bradycardia or hypotension occurs, slow infusion rate.
25-40 min	If seizures persist, intubate and then continue phenytoin infusion until seizures stop or to a maximum dose of 25 mg/kg.
40-60 min	If seizures continue, start infusion of phenobarbital, loading dose of 15 mg/kg, no faster than 30 mg/min; monitor respirations and blood pressure.
60-90 min	If seizures continue, start infusion of 4%-10% solution of paraldehyde diluted in normal saline; administer at rate fast enough to control seizures.
>90 min	If paraldehyde has not terminated seizures within 20 min from start of infusion, institute general anesthesia and neuromuscular blockade; EEG monitoring; keep EEG near flat for at least 2 hr then begin slow withdrawal of anesthesia.
III. Diagnostic Evaluation	Should coincide with control of seizures; detailed history, physical examination, and consideration of further diagnostic work-up with special consideration to treatable diseases (i.e., meningitis, encephalitis, metabolic disorders, overdoses, and mass lesions with cerebral edema).

Ref: Taken from Barbosa, E and Freeman, JM: Pediatrics in Review 4:185, 1982; adapted from: Delagado-Escueta, AV: New Engl J Med 306:1337, 1982.

H. Febrile Seizures
Brief, generalized seizures, associated with fever, occur between 3 months and 5 years without evidence of intracranial infection or defined cause. Distinguished from epilepsy (recurrent, non-febrile seizures). Anticonvulsant prophylaxis to prevent recurrent febrile seizures may be considered:
1) In the presence of an abnormal neurological exam.
2) After a prolonged (>15 min) or focal seizure.
3) Family history of non-febrile seizures.
With 2 of these factors, there is a 13% chance of epilepsy. While usually unnecessary, prevention of recurrent febrile seizures can be achieved if phenobarbital blood levels are maintained >15 μg/dl.

Ref: Consensus Development Conference on Febrile Seizures: Pediatrics 66:1009, 1980.

2. Head Trauma

A. Mild
Most head traumas in children are mild. Once evaluated by a physician, these patients can generally be observed at home. The following signs require the patient seek medical attention and re-evaluation:
1) Increased drowsiness.
2) Persistent emesis.
3) Pupil changes.
4) Gait disturbances.
5) Alterations in speech.
6) Worsening or persistent headache.
7) Post-traumatic seizures.

Skull x-rays are rarely helpful in mild trauma. Reserve for patients with high probability of skull fractures where knowledge of the fracture will change therapy.

Ref: Adapted in part from: Singer, HS and Freeman, JM: Pediatrics 62:819, 1978.

B. Severe Head Trauma
Team approach - pediatrician, general surgeon, neurosurgeon.
1) Initial stabilization: Immobilize neck, vital signs. ABC's of cardiopulmonary resuscitation. Circulation access. Brief history, assess level of consciousness, physical exam (changes requiring life-saving interventions), check for major trauma elsewhere.
2) Rule out neck injury: AP and lateral cervical spine x-rays. If no neck fracture is present and there is normal neck alignment, may proceed with safe manipulation of neck as needed.

3) Airway: May require bag and mask or endotracheal intubation. Hyperventilate if suspect elevated I.C.P. (see #8).

4) If necessary, additional IV catheter insertion. Bloods: Hct, electrolytes, BUN, creatinine, Ca++, glucose, type and crossmatch, ABG.

5) Exam:
   a) Periorbital hemorrhage: "raccoon eyes".
   b) Ecchymosis behind ears: "battle sign".
   c) Hemotympanum
   d) CSF otorrhea or rhinorrhea.

   a), b), c), d) - suggest basal skull fracture

   e) Cranial nerve abnormality.
   f) Motor system - posturing - decorticate (arms flexed), decerebrate (arms extended), asymmetry.

6) Skull trauma: x-rays (optional) - AP, lateral, inclined AP (Towne's view), facial trauma (Water's view), depressed skull fracture (tangential views).

7) Proceed to CAT scan after patient is stable.

8) Signs of increased intracranial pressure or impending herniation: consult neurosurgeon. (Suspect herniation with pupil asymmetry, non-reactive pupils, decorticate or decerebrate posturing.)
   a) Acute medical management. Hyperventilation (PaCO$_2$ <30 and >20 mmHg).
   b) Mannitol - 1/2 gm to 1 gm/kg or furosemide 1/2 to 1 mg/kg per dose.
   c) Restrict fluid after shock is corrected (1/2 to 3/4 maintenance).
   d) Steroids - Dexamethasone 1 to 2 mg/kg per loading dose (may be controversial).

9) Intracranial pressure monitoring: consult neurosurgeon, transfer to ICU.

10) Post traumatic seizures: treat status epilepticus or recurrent seizures. Prophylactic and long-term therapy is controversial.

Ref: Adapted in part from: Rosman, NP, et al.: Emergency Clin N Am 1:141, 1983.

3. Coma

A. Management
   1) Stabilize patient: Airway, breathing, circulation, IV access, EKG monitoring, support ventilation. Brief history if available, initial physical exam. Any evidence of trauma? Is patient post-ictal? Specific odor?
   2) Baseline electrolytes, glucose, serum Dextrostix, BUN, creatinine, Ca++, Mg++, Hct, and complete blood count: blood, urine, and gastric aspirate for toxicology; ABG, type, and cross match.

3) Give glucose, naloxone, other antidotes for specific intoxication, if known.

4) Suspect increased intracranial pressure. Treat as 2B, "Severe Head Trauma."

5) Persistent focal neurological deficit – proceed to CAT scan.

6) Meningitis: perform lumbar puncture for suspected meningitis, if increased intracranial pressure is not suspected and there is no evidence of a mass lesion.

7) Other studies: NH_4, hepatic, renal.

Ref: Adapted in part from: Packer, RJ and Berman, PM: In Textbook of Pediatric Emergency Medicine, Fleisher, G and Ludwig, S, (eds.). Baltimore: Williams and Wilkins, p. 87, 1983.

B. Glasgow "Coma or Responsiveness Scale"

1) May be useful following patients with coma, guiding management or predicting outcome.

2) Scale: min. 3; max. 15.

3) Eye opening:

Spontaneous	– 4
To speech	– 3
To pain	– 2
Nil	– 1

Best motor response:

Obeys	– 6
Localizes	– 5
Withdraws	– 4
Abnormal flexion	– 3
Extends	– 2
Nil	– 1

Best verbal response

Oriented	– 5
Confused orientation	– 4
Inappropriate words	– 3
Incomprehensible sounds	– 2
Nil	– 1

Ref: Taken from Jeannett, B and Teasdale, G: Lancet 1:878, 1977.

4. Acute Shunt Malfunction

"Anything that goes wrong with a person with shunted hydrocephalus is due to a shunt problem until proven otherwise."

Ref: Freeman, JM and D'Souza, B: Pediatrics 64:111, 1979.

A. Consult neurosurgeon, if you suspect obstruction or infection. If unavailable, or patient is deteriorating, any physician familiar with a shunt, may tap it.

> Procedure: <u>Sterile</u> preparation of site with betadine, alcohol. Insert 25 gauge needle into pumping device to measure pressure and remove CSF. If suspect blockage at ventricular end and patient is deteriorating, insert an LP needle through burr hole which admits shunt. Measure pressure with a manometer and send fluid for culture, cell count, differential, glucose, protein.

B. With suspicion of shunt malfunction or infection, admit patient for revision and therapy.

C. When a delay in revision is unavoidable, patient may be medically managed with hyperventilation and/or the following medication until surgery. Add antibiotics if infection is suspected.
   a) Isosorbide 1.5 or 2 gm/kg every 6 hrs, or
   b) Furosemide 1 mg/kg daily, or
   c) Diamox 60 to 100 mg/kg daily

P E R I N A T O L O G Y

1. Fetal Assessment

A. Assessment of Fetal Maturity by Ultrasonography
Measurement of fetal parameters by ultrasound can be
used to estimate gestational age. The accuracy of
ultrasonographic estimates decreases with advancing gestation. Repeated measurements improve accuracy. Fetal
crown-rump length in the first trimester is a good predictor of gestational age. In the second trimester, fetal
biparietal diameter is used. During the third trimester,
the rate of growth slows and isolated values of biparietal
diameter are much less accurate. Second trimester measurements of fetal limb length, particularly femur length,
correlate with gestational age. Standards for these measurements are available in the obstetric literature.

Ref: Robinson, M and Fleming, J: Br J Obstet Gynecol
82:702, 1975; Sabbagha, R, et al.: Obstet Gynecol 43:7,
1974; O'Brien G, et al.: Am J Obstet Gynecol 139:540, 1981.

B. Assessment of Fetal Maturity by Examination of Amniotic
Fluid
1) Amniotic fluid creatinine:
Creatinine concentration in amniotic fluid increases
through gestation, reflecting an increase in fetal
renal function as well as an increase in fetal muscle
mass.

Creatinine (mg/100 ml)	Weeks gestation
1.0 - 1.3	28-31
1.3 - 1.7	31-34
1.7 - 2.1	34-37
>2	>37

Ref: Doran, T, et al.: Am J Obstet Gynecol 119:829,
1974.

2) Amniotic fluid phospholipids:
Measurement of amniotic fluid phospholipids provides
a more direct analysis of lung surfactant and a
more accurate estimate of fetal lung maturity. The
lecithin to sphingomyelin ratio (L/S ratio) is the
most widely used index. An L/S ratio of 2.0 or
greater indicates fetal lung maturity in most cases*.
Measurement of other phospholipids, e.g. phosphotidyl inositol (PI) and phosphotidyl glycerol

*A notable exception is in diabetic pregnancies in
which there is a high incidence of false mature L/S
ratios and the appearance of PG is delayed.

Ref: Kulovich, M and Gluck, L: Am J Obstet
Gynecol 135:64, 1979.

(PG), provides further information about fetal lung development and improves reliability of the L/S ratio. PG is particularly useful since its presence correlates well with functionally mature lungs. The lung profile below graphically illustrates changes in the L/S ratio and concentrations of PI and PG with increasing gestational age and correlates this with lung maturity.

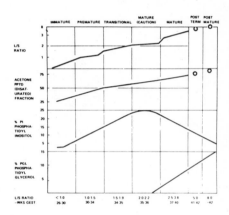

The form used to report the lung profile: The four determinations are plotted on the left. Weeks of gestation are plotted along the bottom and lung maturity at the top.

Adapted from: Kulovich, M, et al.: Am J Obstet Gynecol 135:57, 1979. Copyright 1977 by the Regents of the University of California.

C. Assessment of Fetal Well-Being Before Labor
   1) Fetal activity:
      The mother is asked to record each perceived fetal movement in a given period of time. A decrease or loss of fetal activity is a warning sign of possible fetal compromise or death.

   NOTE: Fetal activity should be used only as an adjunct to other determinations of fetal well-being. It is not a measure of placental function or reserve.

2) <u>Maternal urinary estriol excretion</u>:
Abnormalities involving the fetus, placenta or the mother can result in abnormally low estriol values. Because of day-to-day variability, single measurements are of little value. Serial estriol determinations provide a pattern of excretion that reflects the integrity of the feto-placental unit. Levels consistently over 12 mg/24h at term suggest an intact feto-placental unit, while levels below 4 mg/24h or a serial fall in estriol levels by 35% or more reflect a compromised fetus. Intermediate values of 4-12 mg/24h indicate a fetus at risk.

3) <u>Non-stress test (NST)</u>:
The fetal heart rate is continuously monitored with the mother at rest. A normal or reactive non-stress test requires that there be at least two accelerations in fetal heart rate >15 beats/min above baseline, lasting 15 sec or more, occurring within a 10 min period. An abnormal or nonreactive pattern is one that does not meet these criteria.

4) <u>Oxytocin challenge test (OCT)</u>:
Baseline fetal heart rate and uterine activity are monitored. Oxytocin is administered intravenously to the mother. The rate of infusion is increased every 15-20 min until there are 3 uterine contractions, each lasting at least 40 sec, within a 10 min period. If late decelerations occur, the OCT is positive and indicates possible decreased placental reserve. A negative OCT, the absence of late decelerations, is a good prognostic finding. Nipple stimulation, instead of oxytocin, can be used to induce uterine contractions for contraction stress testing.

D. <u>Assessment of Fetal Well-Being During Labor</u>

1) <u>Fetal heart rate (FHR) monitoring</u>:
   a) Normal baseline FHR is 120-160 beats per min. Isolated accelerations >160 b.p.m. suggest a good prognosis.
   b) There are normally short term fluctuations in FHR of 5-25 b.p.m. Loss of this beat-to-beat variability suggests fetal distress. Drugs, fetal sleep, prematurity, and other factors can also decrease variability.
   c) Early decelerations represent head compression and are benign.
   d) Variable decelerations represent umbilical cord compression. Isolated variable decelerations are of equivocal significance. Persistent, severe, variable decelerations are indication for fetal scalp pH sampling and further evaluation for fetal distress.

FETAL HEART RATE PATTERNS

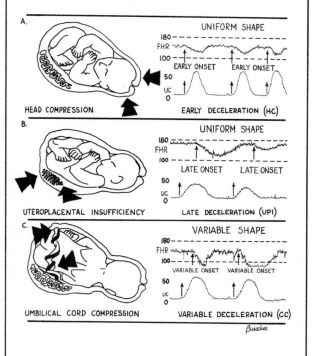

A. Early deceleration caused by compression of the fetal head.
B. Late deceleration caused by uteroplacental insufficiency.
C. Variable deceleration caused by umbilical cord compression.

Ref.: Clin. Perinatol. 1:149, 1974.

e) Late decelerations are caused by uteroplacental insufficiency and indicate fetal distress.

f) A sinusoidal or undulating FHR pattern has been considered a sign of severe fetal compromise and is associated with a high rate of perinatal loss.

Fetal heart rate patterns are illustrated on page 265.

2) Fetal scalp pH monitoring:
Normal fetal pH is 7.25-7.35, approximately 0.1 units lower than that of the mother. Normal fetal PCO_2 values are in the range of 40-45 mm Hg. Normal fetal PO_2 is 20-25 mm Hg. A fetal scalp pH of 7.20-7.25 may indicate fetal distress and is associated with an increased incidence of depression at delivery and lower 1 min Apgar scores. Fetal scalp pH <7.20 indicates significant fetal distress.

For references on fetal monitoring prior to and during delivery, see Petre, R (ed): <u>Clin Perinatology</u> <u>9</u> (2), 1982.

2. <u>Assessment</u> <u>of</u> <u>the</u> <u>Neonate</u>

A. <u>Apgar Scores</u>:
The infant is rapidly assessed on five criteria at 1 and 5 min after delivery. In the compromised infant, continued assessment is important and Apgar scores at 10 and 20 min are valuable.

APGAR SCORING			
SCORE	0	1	2
Heart Rate	Absent	< 100	> 100
Respiratory Effort	Absent	Slow Irregular	Good Crying
Muscle Tone	Limp	Some Flexion of Extremities	Active Motion
Reflex Irritability (nasal catheter)	No response	Grimace	Cough or sneeze
Color	Blue, pale	Extremities blue	Completely pink

Adapted from Apgar, V: <u>Anesth Analg</u> <u>32</u>:260, 1953.

NEUROLOGICAL SIGN	SCORE					
	0	1	2	3	4	5
POSTURE						
SQUARE WINDOW	90°	60°	45°	30°	0°	
ANKLE DORSIFLEXION	90°	75°	45°	20°	0°	
ARM RECOIL	180°	90-180°	<90°			
LEG RECOIL	180°	90-180°	<90°			
POPLITEAL ANGLE	180°	160°	130°	110°	90°	<90°
HEEL TO EAR						
SCARF SIGN						
HEAD LAG						
VENTRAL SUSPENSION						

(Redrawn from Dubowitz.)   See legend, next page.

TECHNIQUES OF ASSESSMENT OF
NEUROLOGIC CRITERIA (Modified from Dubowitz)

POSTURE: Observe infant quiet, supine. Score 0: arms, legs extended; 1: beginning flexion of hips and knees, arms extended; 2: stronger flexion legs, arms extended; 3: arms slightly flexed, legs flexed and abducted; 4: full flexion arms, legs.

SQUARE WINDOW: Flex hand on forearm enough to obtain fullest possible flexion without wrist rotation. Measure angle between the hypothenar eminence and the ventral aspect of the forearm.

ANKLE DORSIFLEXION: Foot is dorsiflexed as much as possible onto anterior aspect of the leg. Measure the angle between the dorsum of the foot and the anterior aspect of the leg.

ARM RECOIL: With infant supine, flex forearms for 5 sec, then fully extend by pulling on hands, then release. Score 2: arms return briskly to full flexion; 1: response is sluggish or incomplete; 0: arms remain extended.

LEG RECOIL: With infant supine, flex hips and knees for 5 sec, then extend by pulling on feet, and release. Score 2: maximal response - full flexion of hips and knees; 1: partial flexion; 0: minimal flexion.

POPLITEAL ANGLE: Hold infant supine with pelvis flat, thigh held in the knee-chest position. Extend leg by gentle pressure and measure popliteal angle.

HEEL TO EAR MANEUVER: With baby supine, draw foot as near to the head without forcing it. Observe distance between foot and head, and degree of extension at the knee. Knee is free and may be down alongside abdomen.

SCARF SIGN: With baby supine, pull infant's hand around the neck around the opposite shoulder. See how far the elbow will go across. Score 0: Elbow reaches opposite axillary line; 1: past midaxillary line; 2: past midline; 3: elbow unable to reach midline.

HEAD LAG: With baby supine, grasp the hands and pull slowly towards the sitting position. Observe the position of head in relation to trunk. In small infant, head may initially be supported by one hand. Score 0: Complete lag; 1: partial control; 2: head in line with body; 3: head anterior to body.

VENTRAL SUSPENSION: Suspend infant in prone position. Note back extension, extremity flexion, and head and trunk alignment. Grade according to diagrams.

2) Assessment of gestational age by physical criteria

External Sign	Score 0	1	2	3	4
Edema	Obvious edema of hands and feet; pitting over tibia	No obvious edema of hands and feet; pitting over tibia	No edema		
Skin texture	Very thin, gelatinous	Thin and smooth	Smooth; medium thickness. Rash or superficial peeling	Slight thickening. Superficial cracking and peeling especially of hands and feet	Thick and parchment-like; superficial or deep cracking
Skin color	Dark red	Uniformly pink	Pale pink; variable over body	Pale; only pink over ears, lips, palms, or soles	
Skin opacity (trunk)	Numerous veins, venules clearly seen, especially over abdomen	Veins and tributaries seen	A few large vessels clearly seen over abdomen	A few large vessels seen indistinctly over abdomen	No blood vessels seen
Lanugo (over back)	No lanugo	Abundant; long and thick over whole back	Hair thinning especially over lower back	Small amount of lanugo and bald area	At least 1/2 of back devoid of lanugo
Plantar creases	No skin creases	Faint red marks over anterior half of sole	Definite red marks over > anterior 1/2; indentations over < anterior 1/3	Indentations over > anterior 1/3	Definite deep indentations over > anterior 1/3

2) Assessment of gestational age by physical criteria (continued)

External Sign	0	1	2	3	4
Nipple formation	Nipple barely visible; no areola	Nipple well defined; areola smooth and flat, diameter <0.75 cm	Areola stippled, edge not raised, diameter <0.75 cm	Areola stippled, edge raised, diameter >0.75 cm	
Breast size	No breast tissue palpable	Breast tissue on one or both sides, <0.5 cm diameter	Breast tissue both sides; one or both 0.5 - 1.0 cm	Breast tissue both sides; one or both >1 cm	
Ear form	Pinna flat, and shapeless; little or no incurving of edge	Incurving of part of edge of pinna	Partial incurving whole of upper pinna	Well-defined incurving whole of upper pinna	
Ear firmness	Pinna soft, easily folded, no recoil	Pinna soft, easily folded, slow recoil	Cartilage to edge of pinna, but soft in places, ready recoil	Pinna firm, cartilage to edge; instant recoil	
Genitals Male	Neither testis in scrotum	At least one testis high in scrotum	At least one testis right down		
Female (with hips 1/2 abducted)	Labia majora widely separated, labia minora protruding	Labia majora almost cover labia minora	Labia majora completely cover labia minora		

3) <u>Dubowitz score and estimation of gestational age</u>
The total Dubowitz score is the sum of the scores
based on neurologic and physical criteria. Total
score is plotted against gestational age below
(redrawn from Dubowitz).

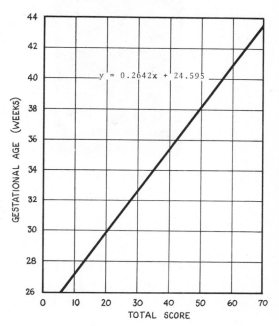

NOTE: Optimal timing for the Dubowitz exam is
within the first 24 hours of life, preferably between
12 and 24 hours of age.

From: Dubowitz, L, et al.: <u>J Pediatr</u> <u>77</u>:1, 1970.

4) <u>Assessment of gestational age by examination of anterior lens vessels</u>

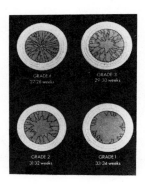

From: Hittner, H, et al.: <u>J Pediatr</u> <u>91</u>:455, 1977.

C. <u>Blood Pressure Measurement in the Premature Infant</u>
Range of the systolic blood pressure in mm Hg in healthy low birth weight infants in the first three hours of age. Blood pressures were measured by the Doppler method.

Body Weight, kg	Gestational Age, Weeks			
	27 – 30	31 – 34	35 – 37	38 – 40
0.80 – 1.0	43 – 46	45 – 48	47 – 50	49 – 51
1.10 – 1.30	46 – 49	48 – 51	50 – 52	51 – 54
1.40 – 1.60	48 – 51	50 – 53	52 – 55	54 – 56
1.70 – 1.90	51 – 54	52 – 56	55 – 57	56 – 59
2.00 – 2.20	53 – 56	55 – 58	57 – 60	59 – 61
2.30 – 2.40	55 – 58	57 – 60	59 – 61	61 – 63

Blood pressure normally rises over the first several days of life. To adjust for this rise, add the following increments in blood pressure according to post-natal age to the values above:

Hours of Age	BP Increments (mm Hg)
3 - 7	1
8 - 12	2
13 - 18	3
19 - 24	4
25 - 32	5
33 - 40	6
41 - 54	7
55 - 89	8
90 - 96	7

From: Bucci, G, et al.: _Acta Paed_ (Suppl) _229_:4, 1972.

D. Intrauterine Growth
    Length and Weight

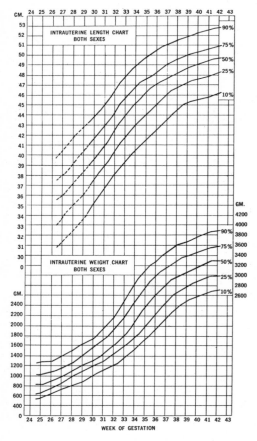

From: Lubchencho, L, et al.: Pediatrics 37:403, 1966.

D. Intrauterine Growth (continued)
    Head Circumference and Weight-Length Ratio

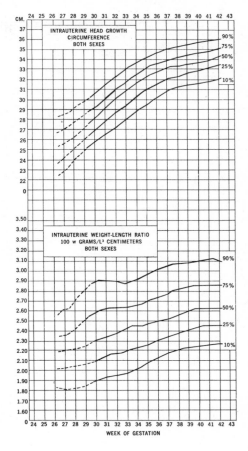

From: Lubchenco, L, et al.: Pediatrics 37:403, 1966.

E. <u>Premature</u> <u>Growth</u> <u>Chart</u>

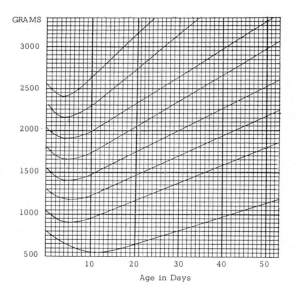

GRAMS

Age in Days

F.   Head Circumference in the Premature Infant

HEAD CIRCUMFERENCE OF PREMATURE INFANTS
FROM BIRTH TO 16 WEEKS

	Head Circumferences (cm)		
AGE	Gestation 30-33 wks (healthy)	Gestation 34-37 wks (healthy)	Gestation various (sick)
24 hrs	27.0 ± 0.7	32.0 ± 0.7	30.9 ± 0.9
1 wk	28.2 ± 0.7	32.7 ± 0.9	31.3 ± 1.0
2 wks	29.5 ± 0.8	33.8 ± 0.8	31.7 ± 0.8
3 wks	30.8 ± 0.8	35.0 ± 0.7	32.0 ± 0.8
4 wks	32.0 ± 0.9	35.8 ± 0.8	32.4 ± 0.7
6 wks	34.4 ± 0.7	37.1 ± 0.8	32.7 ± 0.8
8 wks	35.8 ± 0.8	38.5 ± 1.0	33.3 ± 0.9
12 wks	38.4 ± 1.1	40.3 ± 1.1	34.0 ± 0.9
16 wks	40.2 ± 1.0	41.8 ± 0.9	34.5 ± 0.9

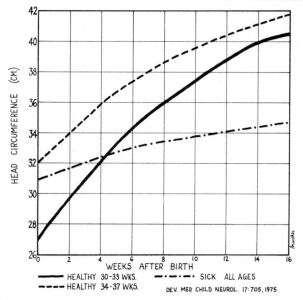

From Sher, P and Brown, S: Dev Med Child Neurol 17:705, 1975.

3. <u>Catheterization</u> of <u>the</u> <u>Umbilical</u> <u>Artery</u> <u>and</u> <u>Vein</u> Procedures
    for inserting umbilical catheters are found on page 10.

    A. <u>Placement of Umbilical Artery Catheter</u>
        1) Umbilical artery catheters can be placed at either of
            two positions: low position, at the level of lumbar
            vertebrae 3 to 4; high position, at the level of
            thoracic vertebrae 6 to 9. The length of the cathe-
            ter necessary to achieve either position is calculated
            from the graph below. Shoulder to umbilical length
            is measured as a perpendicular line dropped from
            the tip of the shoulder to a line extended from the
            umbilicus. A low line should be just above the
            bifurcation of the aorta. A high line should be
            above the diaphragm. Additional length must be
            added for the length of the umbilical stump.

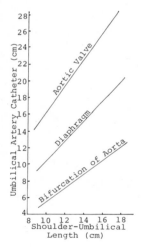

<u>Adapted</u> <u>from</u>: Dunn, P: <u>Arch</u> <u>Dis</u> <u>Child</u> <u>41</u>:69, 1966.

2)   Anatomic location of major branches of the aorta

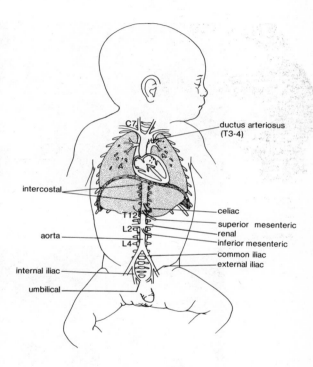

From: Fletcher, M, et al.: Atlas of Procedures in
Neonatology. Philadelphia: J.B. Lippincott, 1983.

3) Radiographic visualization of umbilical artery catheter position. AP and lateral radiographs showing
an umbilical artery catheter in the low position,
with the catheter tip at the level of the upper
margin of the fourth lumbar vertebra.

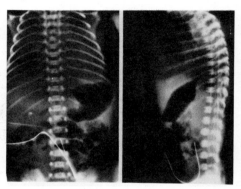

AP and lateral radiographs showing an umbilical
artery catheter in the high position, with the tip of
the catheter at the level of the ninth thoracic vertebra.

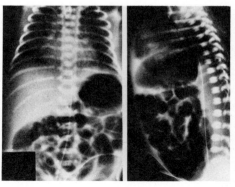

From: Fletcher, M, et al.: Atlas of Procedures in
Neonatology. Philadelphia: J. B. Lippincott,
1983.

B. Placement of Umbilical Vein Catheter
    1) An umbilical vein catheter should be placed in the
        inferior vena cava, above the level of the ductus
        venosis and the hepatic veins. The length of the
        catheter necessary to achieve this position is cal-
        culated from the graph below. Shoulder to
        umbilical length is measured as a perpendicular line
        dropped from the tip of the shoulder to a line
        extended from the umbilicus. The catheter tip
        should be placed between the levels of the dia-
        phragm and the left atrium. Additional length must
        be added for the length of the umbilical stump.

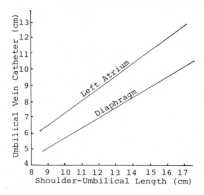

Adapted from: Dunn, P: Arch Dis Child 41:69,
1966.

2)   <u>Anatomic location of major tributaries of the inferior</u>
    <u>vena cava</u>.

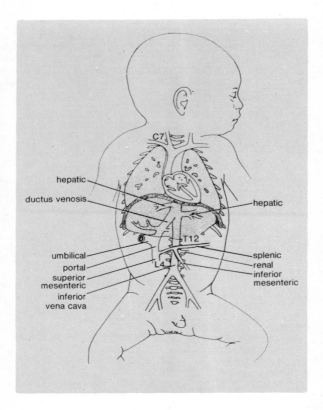

From: Fletcher, M, et al.: <u>Atlas of Procedures in</u>
<u>Neonatology</u>. Philadelphia: J. B. Lippincott, 1983.

3) <u>Radiographic visualization of umbilical vein catheter position.</u> AP and lateral radiographs showing the course and position of an umbilical venous catheter (black arrows) relative to an umbilical artery catheter (white arrows). The venous catheter runs anteriorly and to the infant's right of the arterial catheter. The umbilical artery catheter dips inferiorly and posteriorly toward the vertebral column as it enters the umbilicus.

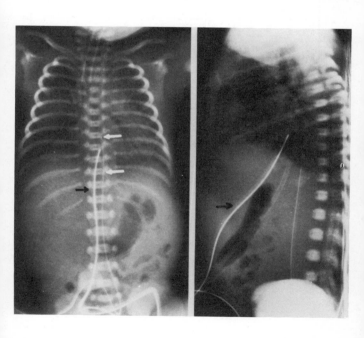

From: Fletcher, M, et al.: <u>Atlas of Procedures in Neonatology</u>. Philadelphia: J. B. Lippincott, 1983.

4. <u>Oxygen Dissociation Curves of Fetal and Adult Hemoglobins</u>

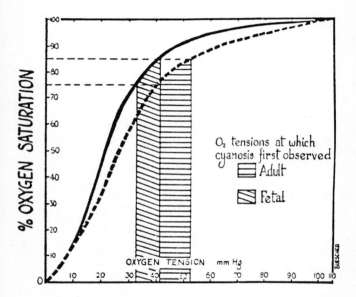

Oxygen dissociation curves of fetal and adult hemoglobins at pH of 7.40, 37°C. Cyanosis is observed at a saturation 75% - 85% which corresponds to different arterial tensions in the adult and the infant. Acidosis, ↑ PCO₂, ↑2,3-DPG cause the curve to shift to the right.

RESPIRATORY CARE AND PULMONARY FUNCTION

1. <u>Respiratory</u> <u>Rates</u> <u>of</u> <u>Normal</u> <u>Children</u> <u>of</u> <u>Both</u> <u>Sexes</u>, <u>Sleeping</u>
   <u>and</u> <u>Awake</u>

Age	Sleeping			Awake			Mean Difference Between Sleeping and Awake
	No.	Mean	Range	No.	Mean	Range	
6-12 mos	6	27	22-31	3	64	58-75	37
1-2 yrs	6	19	17-23	4	35	30-40	16
2-4 yrs	16	19	16-25	15	31	23-42	12
4-6 yrs	23	18	14-23	22	26	19-36	8
6-8 yrs	27	17	13-23	28	23	15-30	6
8-10 yrs	19	18	14-23	19	21	15-31	3
10-12 yrs	11	16	13-19	17	21	15-28	5
12-14 yrs	6	16	15-18	7	22	18-26	6

Ref: Kendig, EL and Chernick, V (eds.): <u>Disorders</u> <u>of</u> <u>the</u> <u>Res-</u>
<u>piratory</u> <u>Tract</u> <u>in</u> <u>Children</u>, Philadelphia: W. B. Saunders, Co.,
1983, p. 63.

2. <u>Lung</u> <u>Anatomy</u>

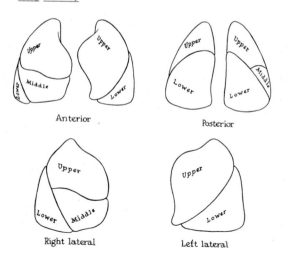

Anterior   Posterior

Right lateral   Left lateral

Ref: Kendig, EL and Chernick, V (eds.): <u>Disorders of the Respiratory Tract in Children</u>, Philadelphia: W. B. Saunders Co., 1983, p. 73.

3.   <u>Pulmonary Function Tests (PFT's)</u>

    A.   <u>Usefulness of PFT's</u>
        1)   To investigate pulmonary symptoms (such as cough, dyspnea, exercise tolerance).
        2)   To evaluate severity and follow progression of known pulmonary disorders (e.g. asthma, CF).
        3)   To follow and evaluate therapy of chronic pulmonary diseases.
        4)   For preoperative evaluation.

    B.   <u>The Routine Pulmonary Function Tests</u>
        (Interpretation of PFT's chart see page 291.)
        1)   Airway function measurements
            a)   Wright peak flow meter: to measure WPFR - good standards, but relatively insensitive.
            b)   Forced expiratory spirometer (with and without bronchodilators): to measure forced expiratory volume in one second (FEV_1), max. mid-expiratory flow (MMEF).
            c)   Inspiratory-expiratory flow volume loops:

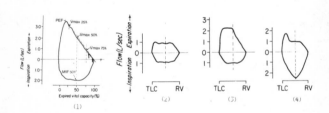

        (1)   normal flow volume loop
        (2)   fixed obstruction (e.g., postintubation tracheal stenosis) of the central airways (larynx, trachea, main stem bronchi)
        (3)   variable obstruction of the extrathoracic central airways
        (4)   variable obstructions of the intrathoracic central airways.

Ref: Ibid, p. 129.

2) Lung volume measurement
   a) static lung volume from spirometer:

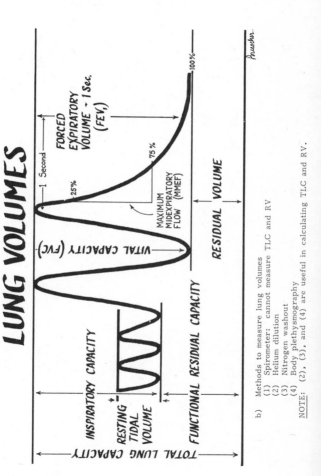

LUNG VOLUMES

Prueter.

b) Methods to measure lung volumes
   (1) Spirometer: cannot measure TLC and RV
   (2) Helium dilution
   (3) Nitrogen washout
   (4) Body plethysmography
   NOTE: (2), (3), and (4) are useful in calculating TLC and RV.

FORCED VITAL CAPACITY (FVC):
NORMAL VALUES

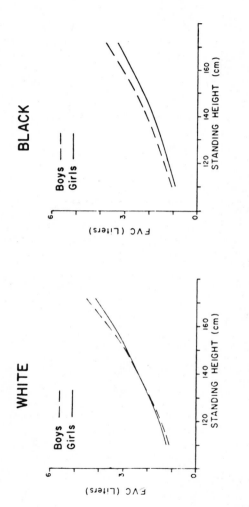

WHITE

SD ± 14% Female
± 13% Male

BLACK

SD ± 15% Female
± 17% Male

Ref: Hsu, KHK et al.: J Pediatr 95:14, 1979.

FORCED EXPIRATORY VOLUME IN ONE SECOND (FEV₁):
NORMAL VALUES

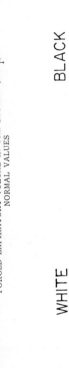

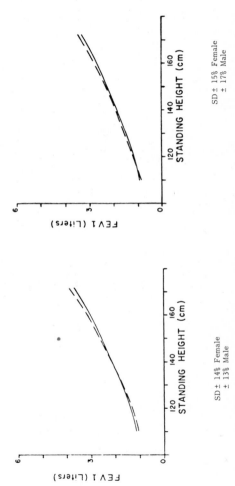

WHITE

SD ± 14% Female
± 13% Male

BLACK

SD ± 15% Female
± 17% Male

Ref: Hsu, KHK et al.: J Pediatr 95:14, 1979.

WRIGHT PEAK FLOW RATE (WPFR)
NORMAL VALUES

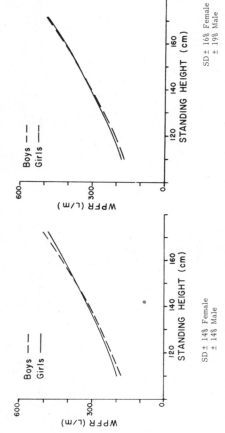

Ref: Hsu, KHK et al.: J Pediatr 95:14, 1979; J Pediatr 95:192, 1979.

INTERPRETATION OF PULMONARY FUNCTION TESTS

	OBSTRUCTIVE: e.g. asthma, cystic fibrosis	RESTRICTIVE: e.g. pleural disease, muscle weakness
Spirometry		
Forced vital capacity (FVC)*	normal or reduced	reduced
Forced expired volume in one second (FEV$_1$)*	reduced	reduced
FEV$_1$/FVC (%)**	reduced	normal ****
Maximal midexpiratory flow rate (MMFR)*	reduced	
Wright peak flow rate (WPFR)	normal or reduced	
Lung volumes		
Total lung capacity (TLC)*	normal or increased	reduced
Residual volume (RV)*	normal or increased	normal or increased
RV/TLC (%)***	normal or increased	
FRC*	normal or increased	normal

*Normal range: predicted ± 20%
**Predicted normal: >85%
***Predicted normal: 20 ± 10%
****Cannot diagnose restriction when there is obstruction by spirometry alone. In this case, lung volumes should be calculated by other methods (such as He dilution or N$_2$ washout). Lung volumes for blacks are lower than for whites (see charts on pages 288-290) when referenced to standing height.

3) Pulmonary gas exchange measurements
   a) Arterial blood gas

NORMAL VALUES	pH	PCO₂	HCO₃ (mEq/L)	CO₂
Child	7.35–7.45	35–45	24–26	25–28
Term Infant – birth	7.26–7.29	54.5		
– 1 hr	7.30	38.8		20.6
– 3 hr	7.34	38.3		21.9
– 1 to 3 d	7.38–7.41	34–35		21.4
Premature >1250 g – 1 to 3 d	7.38–7.39	38–39		
<1250 g – 1 to 3 d	7.35–7.36	37–44		

ABNORMAL VALUES	pH	PCO₂	HCO₃ (mEq/L)	CO₂
Metabolic Acidosis	↓	↓	↓	↓
Acute Respiratory Acidosis	↓	↑	←→	Sl.↑
Compensated Resp. Acidosis	←→ or Sl. ↓	↑	↑	↑
Metabolic Alkalosis	↑	Sl. ↑	↑	↑
Acute Resp. Alkalosis	↑	↓	←→	Sl.↓
Compensated Resp. Alkalosis	←→ or Sl. ↑	↓	↓	↓

   b) Diffusing capacity measurement using carbon
      monoxide (CO): (single breath method or
      steady state)

D_{LCO} in ml/min/mm Hg = amount of carbon
monoxide uptake by the lungs over a known
amount of pressure.

D_{LCO} is normal in asthma and bronchitis.

D_{LCO} is decreased in restrictive lung diseases
with thickened alveolar capillary membrane,
emphysema, anemia, lung resection, carbon
monoxide intoxication, pulmonary microembo-
lization.

D_{LCO} is increased in early left ventricular
failure, polycythemia.

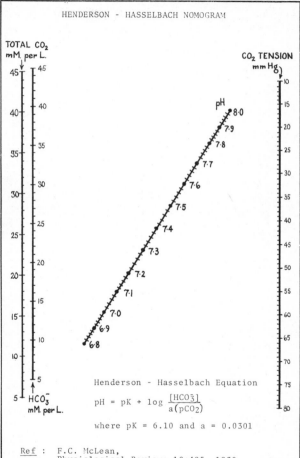

HENDERSON - HASSELBACH NOMOGRAM

TOTAL CO₂
mM. per L.

CO₂ TENSION
mm Hg

pH

HCO₃⁻
mM. per L.

Henderson - Hasselbach Equation

$$pH = pK + \log \frac{[HCO3]}{a(pCO_2)}$$

where pK = 6.10 and a = 0.0301

Ref : F.C. McLean,
       Physiological Reviews 18:495, 1938.

4. Intubation

A. Endoctracheal Tube Sizes

	Internal diameter (mm)
Premature infant	2.5 - 3.0 (see note 2)
Term infant	3.0 - 3.5
3 months - 1 year	4.0
2 years	4.5
2 - 15 years	$\frac{16 + \text{age (years)}}{4}$
Adult women	7.0 - 8.0 (average)
Adult men	8.0 - 9.0 (average)

Notes

1) Use ETT conforming to Z-79 standards (non-irritant).

2) Most premature neonates can accept a 3.0 ETT. 2.5 ETT's have increased airway resistance and are difficult to suction adequately.

3) The head should not be extended for placement of the ETT in newborns due to anatomic differences compared to adults.

4) Cuffed ETT's are used only in older patients (>10 years) secondary to the increased risk of subglottic stenosis. The subglottic region is the narrowest portion of the airway in young children, whereas the larynx is the narrowest portion in older children and adults.

5) If no leak is present, change to the next smaller tube.

Ref: Gregory, GA: Pediatric Anesthesia. New York: Churchill Livingston, 1983, p. 371; Fleisher, GR, et al. (eds.): Pediatric Emergency Medicine. Baltimore: Williams & Wilkins, 1983, p. 1251.

B. Laryngoscope Blades

Premature infant	Miller 0
Term - 1 year (2-5 kg)	Miller 1 or Wis-Hipple 1
1-1½ years (5-12 kg)	Wis-Hipple 1½
1.5-12 years	Miller 2 or
(12-30 kg)	Flagg child blade 2
(>30 kg)	Flagg adult blade 2
13 years + (>50 kg)	Macintosh 3 or Miller 3

Ref: Fleisher, GR, et al. (eds.): Pediatric Emergency Medicine. Baltimore: Williams & Wilkins, 1983 p. 1251; Scarpelli, EM, et al. (eds.): Pulmonary Disease of the Fetus, Newborn and Child. Philadelphia: Lea & Febiger, 1978, p. 106.

C. Drugs for Intubation:

NOTE: The dosage and frequency of administration of these agents is variable and should be individualized according to patient response. These agents should be used only by an experienced physician knowledgeable of their indications and effects.

	Dosage	Contraindications/Side Effects
Atropine	0.01-0.02 mg/kg Min 0.1 mg; Max 0.5 mg (can be injected intralingually if no IV access)	
Pavulon (defasciculating dose)	0.01 mg/kg	Not usually necessary in children <3 years
Thiopental Sodium (Pentothal)	Children: 2 mg/kg Adult: 3-5 mg/kg	Contraindicated in hemodynamically unstable patients secondary to hypotensive effects. The more ill the patient, the lower the dose which should be used.
OR Ketamine	1-2 mg/kg	Alternative to pentothal in hemodynamically unstable patients. Forbidden in head trauma secondary to its effect in increasing cerebral blood flow. Antidote to hallucinogenic effects = valium. Caution in use with propranolol and α-blockers.
Succinylcholine	1 mg/kg (lasts 3-10 min)	Dosage = 2 mg/kg in <1 year old. Hyperkalemia possible – contraindicated in burns, massive trauma, neuromuscular disease. Can cause bradycardia and cardiac arrhythmia (always give atropine first). Increases intraocular pressure – contraindicated in eye injuries.
OR Pavulon (paralyzing dose)	0.04-0.1 mg/kg	Reversal drugs: Atropine 0.02-0.03 mg/kg Neostigmine 0.04-0.08 mg/kg

Ref: Steward, DJ: Some Aspects of Paediatric Anaesthesia. Amsterdam: Excerpta Medica, 1982, p. 64-74; Gregory, GA, Pediatric Anesthesia. New York: Churchill Livingston, 1983, p. 467-470.

5. <u>Reference</u> <u>Data</u>

A. <u>Minute</u> <u>Ventilation</u> ($\dot{V}_E$) = respiratory rate x tidal volume

$\dot{V}_E$ X $P_A CO_2$ = constant

(TV)

TV = 10-15 ml/kg

B. <u>Alveolar</u> <u>Gas</u> <u>Equation</u>:

$$P_A O_2 = P_I O_2 - \frac{P_a CO_2}{R}$$

$$P_I O_2 = F_I O_2 \text{ X } (P_b - 47 \text{ mm Hg})$$

= 150 mm Hg at sea level in room air

R = respiratory exchange quotient

= 0.8 in most cases ($\uparrow$ with glucose intake, $\downarrow$ with fat)

P_b = 760 mm Hg

Ref: Kendig, EL and Chernick, V: <u>Disorders</u> <u>of</u> <u>the</u> <u>Respiratory</u> <u>Tract</u> in <u>Children</u>, Philadelphia: W. B. Saunders, Co., 1983, p. 27.

C. <u>Oxyhemoglobin</u> <u>Dissociation</u> <u>Curves</u>

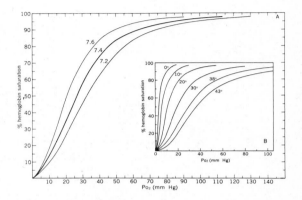

<u>Ref</u>: Lambertsen, CJ: Transport of oxygen, carbon dioxide, and inert gases by the blood, in Mountcastle VB (ed): <u>Medical Physiology</u>, <u>14th Edition</u> St. Louis: C.V. Mosby Co., 1980, p. 1725.

298

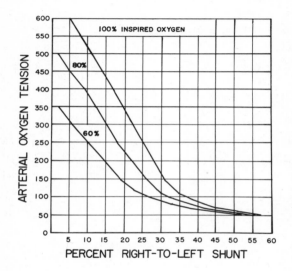

Calculations are based on an assumed hemoglobin of 16 gm%, an arteriovenous difference of 4 volumes per cent, a respiratory quotient of 0.8 and an arterial PCO_2 of 40 mmHg.

Ref: Avery, ME, et al.: <u>The Lung and Its Disorders in the Newborn Infant</u>, <u>4th Edition</u>, Philadelphia, W. B. Saunders Co., 1981, p. 69.

INFECTIOUS DISEASES

NOTE:

For more detailed and updated information on immunizations and isolation protocols, please refer to the current issues of Morbidity and Mortality World Report or the current edition of the "Red Book" - the Report of the Committee on Infectious Diseases of the American Academy of Pediatrics.

RECOMMENDED SCHEDULE FOR ACTIVE IMMUNIZATION OF INFANTS AND CHILDREN
1984

AGE	PREPARATION
2 months	DPT/TOPV
4 months	DPT/TOPV
6 months	DPT/TOPV*
12 months	Tuberculin Test**
15 months	Measles/Mumps/Rubella (MMR)
18 months	DPT/TOPV
4-6 years	DPT/TOPV
14-16 years	Td (and every 10 years thereafter)

RECOMMENDED SCHEDULE FOR PRIMARY IMMUNIZATION FOR CHILDREN NOT IMMUNIZED IN EARLY INFANCY

Under 6 Years of Age	
First Visit	DPT/TOPV/Tuberculin Test
Interval After First Visit	
1 month	MMR
2 months	DPT/TOPV
4 months	DPT/TOPV*
10-16 months or preschool	DPT/TOPV

*TOPV dose is optional. May be given in areas of high polio endemicity.

**Intradermal PPD (Mantoux) preferred. Tuberculin test may be given at 15 months (with MMR). Frequency of repeated tests depends on risk of exposure. Testing once every one to two years is generally recommended.

6 Years of Age and Over

First Visit	Td/TOPV/Tuberculin Test
Interval After First Visit	
1 month	MMR
2 months	Td/TOPV
8-14 months	Td/TOPV
Age 14-16 years	Td-repeat every 10 yrs

Interruption of immunizations does not require restarting of the series. The only restriction is that live virus vaccines (TOPV and MMR) be spaced at least 1 month apart. This timing requirement may be waived in certain unusual circumstances.

1. Active Immunization

    A. General Information
        1) No adverse effect has been reported in egg-sensitive children when vaccines are grown in chick fibroblast culture (e.g. mumps, measles).
        2) Care should be exercised in the administration of live virus vaccines in children with immunodeficiency or immunosuppressed states. Leukemics in remission who have not had chemotherapy for at least three months may receive live virus vaccines for infections to which they have not previously been immunized.
        3) Immunization of premature infants may be based on chronological age. However, if the child remains hospitalized, TOPV should not be initiated to prevent cross-infection in the nursery.
        4) Administration of live virus vaccines is contraindicated in individuals who have received gamma globulin within the previous three months because of possible interference with the desired immune response.
        5) Administration of all live virus vaccines is contraindicated in pregnant women.
        6) Defer immunizations in the presence of a febrile illness.

    B. Diphtheria/Pertussis/Tetanus (DPT)
        Adsorbed triple vaccine: usual dose is 0.5 ml. Injections should be given at least eight weeks apart.
        1) Precautions:
            a) Common side effects of pertussis vaccination include: redness, swelling or pain at site, and fever, and are not contraindications to further immunizations.
            b) There are few specific guidelines for immunizations in children with a history of febrile convulsion or other neurologic disorders. The

value of immunization must be weighed against the possibility of adverse reactions. Prophylactic antipyretics and anticonvulsants may be considered for children deemed to be at high risk for convulsions.

    c) Children with evolving neurologic disorders or severe reactions to DPT (fever >39°C, screaming, somnolence, shock, convulsions) should not receive further pertussis immunizations.

2) Special Situations:

    a) If a child under age 6 years has had proven pertussis, use DT only. (Parapertussis has no cross-immunity).

    b) Over the age of 6 years use Td antigen.

    c) In the face of a pertussis outbreak, give 0.25 ml pertussis vaccine, adsorbed, as a booster dose.

3) Guide to Tetanus Prophylaxis in Wound Management: (see page 309 also)

Previous Tetanus Immunization (Doses)	Clean, Minor Wounds		Tetanus-Prone Wounds	
	Toxoid (Td)	Tetanus Immune Globulin (TIG)	Toxoid (Td)	Tetanus Immune Globulin (TIG)
Uncertain	Yes	No	Yes	Yes
0 - 1	Yes	No	Yes	Yes
2	Yes	No	Yes	No*
3 or more	No**	No	No***	No

    *Unless wound is more than 24 hours old
   **Unless more than 10 years since last dose
 ***Unless more than 5 years since last dose

C. Hepatitis B

Recommendations are now under discussion for the use of hepatitis B vaccine. However, children at substantial risk of hepatitis B infection should be considered for vaccination on a case by case basis.

Those at risk include:

1) Clients of institutions for the mentally retarded
2) Hemodialysis patients
3) Homosexually active males
4) Illicit injectable drug abusers

5) Recipients of blood products with a high risk of hepatitis B transmission (Factor VIII, cryoprecipitate, prothrombin complex concentrate)
6) Household and sexual contact of HBV carriers
7) Infants of mothers who are hepatitis B chronic carriers

Dosage recommendations
Under 10 years of age: 3 doses of 0.5 ml IM (10 µg) at 0, 1, and 6 months. Over 10 years of age: 1.0 ml doses IM at 0, 1, and 6 months. HBIG and hepatitis vaccine may be given simultaneously to infants when transplacental transmission is likely. (See page 149 for HBIG.)

Typical profile of serological markers in patients with acute type-B hepatitis.

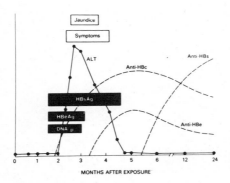

Ref: Schafer, DF and Hoofnagle, JH: Viewpoints on Digestive Diseases, 14:5, 1982, with permission.

Test Result			Interpretation
HBsAg	**anti-HBc IgM**	**anti-HAV IgM**	
–	–	+	Recent acute hepatitis A infection
+	+	–	Acute hepatitis B infection
+	–	–	Early acute hepatitis B infection or chronic hepatitis B
–	+	–	Confirms acute or recent infection with hepatitis B virus
–	–	–	Possible non-A, non-B hepatitis infection, other viral infection, or liver toxin.
+	+	+	Recent probable hepatitis A infection and superimposed acute hepatitis B infection; uncommon profile.

Key: + positive   – negative

Ref: Abbott Laboratories, <u>Perspectives</u> <u>on</u> <u>Viral</u> <u>Hepatitis</u>, North Chicago, IL, 1983, with permission.

D.   <u>Influenza</u>
Bivalent A and B vaccine is available, but the antigenic makeup of the vaccine varies from year to year, as do recommendations for its use.

<u>Indications</u>
Not routinely recommended for normal pediatric patients. Recommended for patients with significant heart disease, chronic bronchopulmonary disease, chronic renal disease, and metabolic disorders.   It has not been clearly established whether pregnant women should be vaccinated.   In epidemic years many other groups such as health and hospital workers may be candidates for immunization, depending on current opinion.

Administer split-virus (subvirion) vaccine in patients <12 years of age.

E.   <u>Measles</u>
Give live, attenuated measles virus vaccine 0.5 ml SQ into deltoid area.
1)   Contraindications
  a)   Febrile illness
  b)   Pregnancy
  c)   Leukemia or other malignancy
  d)   Defects of cell-mediated immunity
  e)   Immunosuppression
  f)   Untreated active tuberculosis
  g)   Administration of plasma or immune globulin in previous 8 weeks

2) Atypical measles

Cases of atypical measles (fever, headache, myalgias, a maculopapular eruption with peripheral edema, pneumonia, hilar adenopathy, and pleural effusion) may be seen in patients given only the killed virus measles vaccine which was administered from 1963-1967.

F. Mumps

Live attenuated virus is recommended for children 15 months and above and for adolescents and adults who have not had clinical disease. Give SQ only after excess antiseptic is cleaned off the skin.

Contraindications
1) Agammaglobulinemia
2) Malignancy, antimetabolite, or steroid therapy, immunodeficiency or immunosuppressed states
3) Pregnancy

G. Pneumococcal Polysaccharide Vaccine (0.5 ml SQ): Indicated in children >2 years old with sickle cell anemia, splenectomy, chronic nephrotic syndrome, chronic liver disease, malignancy, or primary immunodeficiency in an attempt to protect against systemic pneumococcal infections.

Contraindications:
1) Pregnant women (effect on fetus unkown)
2) Children <2 years old (inconsistent antibody responses).
Ref: Cowman, MJ, et al.: Pediatrics 62:721, 1976.

H. Poliomyelitis

The live vaccine is provided as a trivalent vaccine and administered orally. Storage and dose instructions vary with manufacturer. Oral polio vaccine virus is excreted by the vaccinee, so that it should not be used by household contacts of immunodeficient or immunosuppressed individuals. Injectable polio vaccine should be used instead.
1) Contraindications for live polio vaccine
   a) Immunodeficiency disease or immunosuppressive therapy
   b) Malignancy
2) Injectable polio vaccine (Salk) may be given to immunodeficient or immunosuppressed patients; response will be limited by underlying condition.

I. Rabies

The decision to treat for rabies must be based on whether the attack was provoked, the type of animal and its availability for observation, the immunization status of the animal, and the presence of rabies in the state or community.

After severe exposures to potentially rabid animals (particularly following bites around the head and neck), treatment consists of Rabies Immune Globulin (RIG) and immunization with Human Diploid Cell Vaccine (HDCV).

When available, Human Rabies Immune Globulin (HRIG) is the preferred serum. When HRIG is not available, use equine serum (RIG) if there is no history of hypersensitivity to horse serum, and if conjunctival and skin tests are negative.

If vaccine is used give 5 doses on day 1, 3, 7, 14, and 28 after exposure with HRIG also given on day 1. When HDCV is not available, one dose of RIG and 23 doses of duck embryo vaccine (DEV) should be administered (see package insert).

Postexposure Antirabies Treatment Guide

Species of Animal	Condition of Animal at Time of Attack	Treatment of Exposed Human

Wild:
  Skunk
  Fox
  Coyote
  Raccoon
  Bat
  Other carnivores
	Regard as rabid	(H)RIG + HDCV

Domestic:
  Dog
  Cat
	Healthy	None

	Unknown (escaped)	(H)RIG + HDCV Call Public Health Official
	Rabid or suspected rabid	(H)RIG + HDCV

Other:
  Livestock
  Rodents
  Lagomorphs
  (Rabbits
  and hares)
	Consider individually - see above discussion	

J.   Rubella
Live rubella vaccine is currently recommended by the American Academy of Pediatrics. It should be given at

15 months of age or before puberty, and should be given in a single subcutaneous dose of 0.5 ml. Antibody levels appear to have declined minimally over the 10 years the vaccine has been in use, but the duration of immunity is as yet uncertain.

Contraindications
1) Pregnancy
2) Immunosuppression, immunodeficiency or generalized malignancy
3) Hypersensitivity to the species from which a given vaccine is derived (see package insert)

K. Tuberculosis
    1) Guide to treating

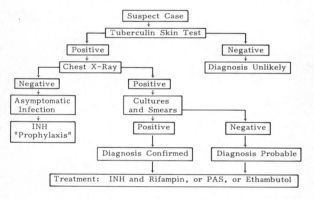

2) When the population of tubercle bacilli is large (e.g. miliary, extensive cavitary lesions, meningitis, or renal disease) or the patient is from an area where drug-resistant tuberculosis is prevalent, streptomycin should be included, but for no longer than 3 months.

3)   Newborn infants of mothers with tuberculosis:

Mother's Status	Infant	Other
Category I (TB exposure, no evidence of infection)	No therapy	PPD to mother and infant at 8 weeks post-partum
Category II (TB infection without disease, i.e. positive PPD reaction)	No therapy	-Chest x-ray of infant -Report to Public Health Department -Refer mother for therapy -Follow-up PPD, chest x-ray on infant at 8 weeks -Evaluate household contacts and clear home before discharge
	*BCG vaccine	If social-household evaluation hopeless, give infant BCG.
Category III (TB infection with disease)	INH preventive therapy	-Same as Category II above. -Isolate mother from infant until mother is not contagious. -If infant is non-reactive, repeat PPD on infant at 8 weeks.

*BCG (0.1 ml) is given SQ as superficially as possible over the right deltoid, or by the multiple puncture technique. If infant is non-reactive to PPD at 8 weeks, repeat BCG until reactive. Do not give BCG during INH administration, BCG organisms are inhibited by INH.

4)   Active disease should be considered in a person who received BCG if a PPD yields >10 mm induration or there is clinical evidence of TB. Infections with atypical mycobacteria may also give PPD reactions of 5-10 mm induration.

L.   Other
Cholera, yellow fever, plague, Rocky Mountain Spotted Fever, typhus, and smallpox vaccines are used only in foreign travel to affected countries and/or in other high risk situation.

2. Passive Immunization

    A. Hepatitis A
       Give 0.02 ml/kg of Immune Serum Globulin (ISG) to:
1) Anyone inoculated with a needle or who has had open lesions directly in contact with material (blood, serum, saliva or other body fluids) from a patient known to have hepatitis A.
2) Persons sharing common living quarters such as family members, roommates, sex partners, or individuals who dine regularly or use common plates or glasses with a patient with known hepatitis A.
3) Schoolmates in any class where more than one case of hepatitis A has been established.
4) Infants of mothers with HAAⵁ hepatitis.

       NOTE: For prolonged continuous exposure, give 0.06 ml/kg of ISG and repeat in 4-5 months. If no clinical evidence of disease has occurred in 10-12 months of intensive exposure, subclinical infection has probably occurred.

    B. Hepatitis B
       Hepatitis B Immune Globulin (HBIG) is the treatment of choice. ISG has had detectable anti-HBs after 1972 and may be used with variable effectiveness for passive immunization to hepatitis B when HBIG is not available.
1) Give 0.05-0.07 ml/kg HBIG to known susceptible persons or those shown to be HBsAb negative for needlestick or mucosal exposure to body fluids from a patient known to have hepatitis B as soon as possible within 7 days after exposure. Administer a second dose 25-30 days after the first. If HBIG is not available, use ISG in the same dosage schedule.
2) Infants born to mothers with known third trimester hepatitis B or who are HBsAg positive at delivery should receive HBIG 0.5 ml IM. This dose should be repeated at 3 and 6 months. If HBIG is not available, give ISG 0.6 ml/kg.

    C. Immunodeficiency Disorders
1) Intramuscular Immune Serum Globulin: 0.6-1.0 ml/kg IM every 2-4 weeks. A double dose is given at the onset of therapy. Indicated only for humoral immunodeficiency syndromes involving IgG. Dose and interval adjusted for each individual based on clinical response and IgG level.
2) Intravenous Immune Serum Globulin: please see package insert for dose.

       WARNING: The intravenous preparation only can be given IV, never use the IM preparation intravenously.

3) Plasma Therapy: 10-20 ml/kg IV, every 2-6 weeks. Continual plasmapheresis of one donor is essential to reduce the risk of hepatitis. If there is deficient T-cell function, the plasma should be irradiated (2000-3000 R) to avoid graft vs. host disease.

D. <u>Measles</u>
"Preventive" dose of Immune Serum Globulin is 0.25 ml/kg IM for otherwise normal unvaccinated infants and children.

For unvaccinated children with malignancies, immunodeficiency, or those on immunosuppressive therapy give 0.5 ml/kg (15 ml max.) IM.

E. <u>Pertussis</u>
Pertussis Immune Globulin is of no proven value and is not recommended.

F. <u>Rabies</u>
(see page 304 under Active Immunizations)

G. <u>Rubella</u>
The use of Immune Serum Globulin, 20 ml IM, may be considered for pregnant women exposed during the first trimester. It is of questionable benefit.

H. <u>Tetanus</u>
(See page 301 for recommendations for use of vaccine and globulin.) Use tetanus immune globulin (human) if the patient has had <2 previous doses of tetanus toxoid or if the wound is unattended for >24 hours. Use a dose of 250 to 500 units IM for susceptible wounds and 3,000 to 6,000 units IM (with some placed into the wound) for the clinical illness. If TIG is not available, use equine or bovine antitoxin after testing for hypersensitivity. Dosage is 3,000 to 5,000 units for those with susceptible wounds and 50,000 to 100,000 units (20,000 given IV, the rest IM) for clinical illness.

I. <u>Varicella-Zoster</u>
Zoster Immune Globulin (ZIG) is optimal therapy if given to immunocompromised patients within 72 hours of exposure. It is available from designated ZIG consultants (see 1982 Red Book, American Academy of Pediatrics or the American Red Cross).

Zoster Immune Plasma (ZIP) 10 ml/kg IV, may also be used; it carries the risk of hepatitis transmission.

Occasional lots of Immune Serum Globulin may have high VZ antibody titers (check with consultants). These may modify varicella when given in a dose of 0.6 to 1.2 ml/kg IM.

Ref: Stiehm, ER: Pediatrics 63:301, 1979.

3. Prophylaxis - Hemophilus Influenzae and Meningococcus
Although the efficacy of rifampin prophylaxis for H. influenza and meningococcal diseases is unknown, prophylaxis is currently recommended for household contacts, nursery school, and day care center contacts of the index case. The index case should also receive rifampin prophylaxis prior to discharge from the hospital, even after therapy with antibiotics. Rifampin is not recommended in pregnant women. (See page 181 for rifampin dosages.)

INCUBATION PERIODS AND ISOLATION PERIODS FOR SOME COMMON CONTAGIOUS DISEASES

Disease	Duration of Incubation Period	Isolation of Patient	Observation or Quarantine
Chickenpox (Varicella)	10-21 days	Until all vesicles are crusted (usually 7 days after onset); (communicable from two days before onset of rash)	7-21 days from first exposure
Diphtheria	2-6 days	Until two successive negative nose and throat cultures are obtained no less than 24 hours apart after cessation of antimicrobial therapy (communicable up to 4 weeks if untreated)	7 days from last contact or until negative culture is obtained. Contacts should receive a booster dose of DT or Td depending on age.
Hepatitis A	15-40 days (25 days avg)	Not clear. Enteric and blood precautions. Ideally, until 1 week after onset of jaundice. (Mainly enteric precautions.)	Observe for 6 weeks post-exposure
Hepatitis B	6 weeks to 6 months	Blood precautions. Isolate when HBsAg positive (late incubation period and during acute illness, and also in chronic carrier state). Enteric precautions unnecessary but secretion precautions advisable.	Up to 6 months, post-exposure
Hemophilus Influenza Meningitis	1-10 days	Respiratory isolation for the first 24 hours after beginning effective antibiotic therapy.	7 days from last exposure
Meningococcal Meningitis	Usually 1-7 days, may be longer	First 24 hours after beginning effective antibiotic therapy. (Respiratory isolation only.)	7 days from last exposure

INCUBATION PERIODS AND ISOLATION PERIODS FOR SOME COMMON CONTAGIOUS DISEASES (continued)

Disease	Duration of Incubation Period	Isolation of Patient	Observation or Quarantine
Mononucleosis	2-8 weeks	Avoid contact with saliva (cups, toothbrushes, etc.) for 3 months.	Observation only
Mumps	14-21 days	Duration of swelling or other manifestations; (communicable from 7 days before to 9 days after occurrence of swelling). Respiratory isolation for hospitalized patients.	14-21 days from first exposure
Pertussis	5-10 days (maximal, 21 days)	For 5-10 days (i.e., treatment period) (communicable for 4 weeks if untreated)	Two weeks from last exposure. Quarantine for those unvaccinated under 6 years; observe others.
Poliomyelitis	7-14 days (usual) 5-35 days (maximal)	Secretions--1 week Stools--up to 6 weeks	5 days for prodromal, minor illness
Rubella	14-21 days	Duration of catarrh and rash (communicable from 7 days before until 5 days after rash appears)	Observe 12-20 days from exposure
Rubeola	10-12 days	Until 5 days after appearance of rash; (communicable after 5th day incubation period)	14 days from exposure
Scarlet fever and Streptococcal pharyngitis	2-4 days (usual) ½-7 days (maximal)	Until 24 hours after antibiotics are begun	7 days from exposure

ISOLATION TECHNIQUES FOR VARIOUS ILLNESSES

Disease	Respiratory	Enteric	Wound and Skin	Strict	Protective
Disease	German Measles[1] Hemophilus influenza Meningitis[2] Meningococcemia Mumps Pertussis Tuberculosis	Cholera Diarrhea Enteropathic or enterotoxigenic E. coli Hepatitis (A&B)[3] Salmonella Shigella Staph enterocolitis Typhoid Fever Yersinia	Extensive wound Gas gangrene Localized zoster Melioidosis Plague Staph skin or wound Strep skin or wound	Cong. Rubella[4] Disseminated Zoster/ Varicella Extensive burn staph or strep Herpes simplex neonatorum Rabies Smallpox[5] Staph or strep pneumonia	Burns[6] Dermatitis – severe, extensive Hypersusceptibility to infection – agranulocytosis – leukemia – lymphoma
Handwashing	Upon entering and leaving room	Upon entering and leaving room	Upon entering and leaving room	Upon entering and leaving room	Upon entering and leaving room
Single Room	Yes, door closed	Desirable, esp. with incontinent children	Desirable	Yes, door closed	Yes, door closed
Gown	No	Yes	Yes with contact	Yes	Yes
Mask	Yes	No	Staph only	Yes	Yes
Gloves	No	Yes with contact	Yes with contact	Yes	Yes with contact
Excretions	No	Yes	No	Yes	No
Secretions	Yes	Hepatitis only	Yes	Yes	No

[1] Pregnant women should avoid contact.
[2] Until 24 hours after effective treatment is begun.
[3] Observe blood and secretion precautions, also.
[4] Requires gown, no gloves.
[5] Room not to be used by patients with eczema for one year
[6] Use sterile gowns and linen.

Ref: Report of the Committee on Infectious Diseases (Redbook).
Evanston, IL: American Academy of Pediatrics, 1982; Center for
Disease Control: MMWR 29:265-280, 1980; IBID, 31: 349-353, 1982;
IBID, 31: 317-328, 1982; IBID 32:1-17, 1983; Stiehm, ER:
Pediatrics 63:301, 1979; Cowman MJ, et al.: Pediatrics 62:721,
1976; Abbott Diagnostics Division: Perspectives on Viral
Hepatitis. Chicago: Abbott Laboratories, 1981.

KETOGENIC DIET

The ketogenic diet may be of value in the management of intractable grand mal or minor motor seizures. Best results are obtained in children 2-4 years of age. This diet is reserved for patients whose seizures are uncontrolled by usual anticonvulsant drugs. Adequate parental supervision and patient cooperation are essential.

1. Method of Starting Diet

    A. An initial period of starvation is necessary to establish adequate ketosis. This usually lasts 5-7 days. Follow dextrosticks and serum blood glucose closely during this time. Limit fluid intake to 400-800 ml per day unless adverse reactions occur. Begin the diet after the patient has lost 10% of body weight and the urinary ketones (Acetest or Keto Diastix) have been 4+ for several days. Terminate the starvation period before 10% weight loss if the patient's bicarbonate is <10 mEq/L or if Kussmaul respirations are present.

    B. Offer 1/3 of the calculated diet on the first day, then increase to 2/3, and finally to full rations on successive days, if ketosis is not appreciably lessened.

    C. Evaluate the patient both by clinical and laboratory means, including:
        1) Pulse and respirations Q4h
        2) Daily AM weights after voiding
        3) Urine specimens (ac, breakfast, and supper) for specific gravity and ketones.
        4) Fasting blood glucose, CO_2, K, and uric acid – follow PRN.

        NOTE: Treat symptomatic hypoglycemia and severe acidosis promptly.

    D. If anticonvulsant drugs are being given, try to taper them one at a time. Phenobarbital may be gradually eliminated during a two-week period after the first ketogenic meal. Other drugs may be reduced and discontinued during the starvation period. Do not administer drugs which contain a carbohydrate vehicle. Some patients will require anticonvulsant drugs in combination with the diet to control seizures.

2. Composition and Calculation of the 4:1 Diet

    A. The diet consists of 4 gm of fat (ketogenic), 1 gm of protein plus carbohydrate (antiketogenic).

    B. Method of Calculation
        1) The 4 gm of fat plus 1 gm of protein and CHO are considered a "dietary unit"; yield 40 calories.

    2)   Daily caloric requirement is 60-75 cal/kg/day, depending on age.

    3)   Determine number of "dietary units" required per day, i.e., total caloric requirement divided by 40.

    4)   Calculate gm of fat/day (number of "dietary units" x 4).

    5)   Calculate gm of protein/day (approximately 1 gm/kg/day).

    6)   Obtain gm of CHO by subtracting total gms of protein from total number of units (since 1 unit = 1 gm protein + CHO).

C.   Example (for a 5 year old weighing 18 kg)

    1)   Daily requirement: 18 kg x 70 cal/kg = 1260 cal/day.

    2)   Number of "dietary units": 1260 cal ÷ 40 cal/unit = 31.5 units

    3)   Number of gms of fat: 31.5 units x 4 gm fat/unit = 126 gm

    4)   Number of gms of protein: 1.0 gm/kg x 18 kg = 18 gms

    5)   Number of gms CHO: 31.5 gm (since protein + CHO = 1 gm/unit) - 18 gms = 13.5 gm

3.   Method of Discontinuing Diet

After 2 years on the 4:1 ratio, reduce to a 3:1 (ketogenic: antiketogenic) ratio for 3 months to 1 year and finally to a 2:1 ratio for another 3 months; then resume a normal diet.

NOTE: Urine should be checked daily for ketones while on diet; an abrupt decrease in ketosis may precipitate recurrence of seizures.

4.   Complications

A.   Hypoglycemia
B.   Urate nephropathy
C.   Severe acidosis

Ref: Gordon, N: Devel Med Child Neurol 19:535, 1977.

NOTE: The use of medium chain triglyceride (MCT) diet to induce ketosis has been advocated recently.

PART IV

REFERENCE DATA

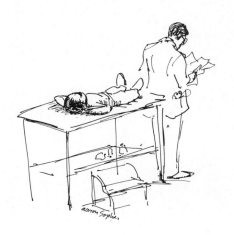

GIRLS
BIRTH TO 36 MONTHS
LENGTH AND WEIGHT

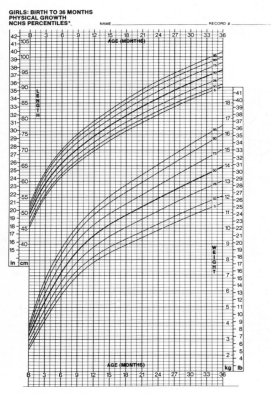

Adapted from National Center for Health Statistics data. Copyright
Ross Laboratories, 1976.

GIRLS
2 TO 18 YEARS
STATURE AND WEIGHT

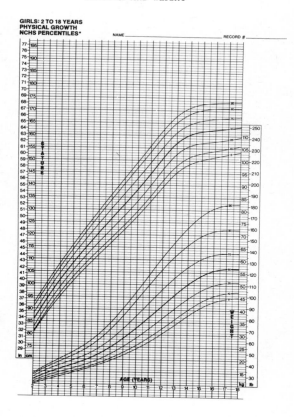

Adapted from National Center for Health Statistics data. Copyright
Ross Laboratories, 1976.

BOYS
BIRTH TO 36 MONTHS
LENGTH AND WEIGHT

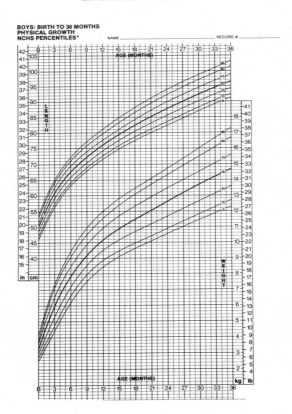

Adapted from National Center for Health Statistics data. Copyright Ross Laboratories, 1976.

BOYS
2 TO 18 YEARS
STATURE AND WEIGHT

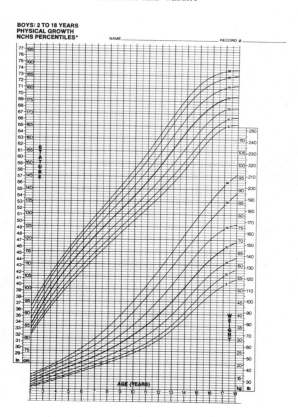

**BOYS: 2 TO 18 YEARS
PHYSICAL GROWTH
NCHS PERCENTILES***

Adapted from National Center for Health Statistics data. Copyright
Ross Laboratories, 1976.

HEAD CIRCUMFERENCE - GIRLS

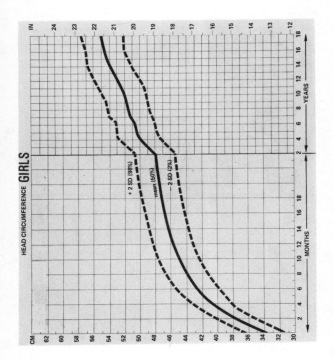

Ref: Nellhaus, G, Pediatrics 41:106, 1968.

HEAD CIRCUMFERENCE - BOYS

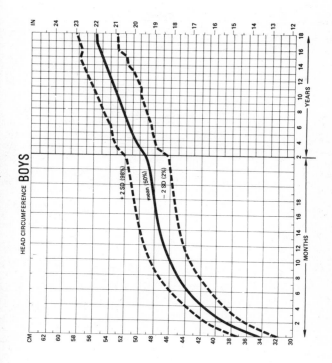

Ref: Nellhaus, G, *Pediatrics* 41: 106, 1968.

INCREMENTAL GROWTH CHARTS*
(GROWTH VELOCITY)

INSTRUCTIONS

1. Measure the child at the beginning and the end of a 6-month interval, if possible.

2. Subtract the initial measurement from the follow-up measurement to obtain the increment.

3. If the interval between measurements is not exactly 6 months (182 days), divide the increment by the interval in days and multiply by 182 to obtain the adjusted 6-month increment. The Table of Consecutively Numbered Days can be used to determine the interval between the measurements. If measurements are made in different years, add 365 to the day of the year for the follow-up measurement. Extrapolating increments from intervals of 3 months or less is not recommended.

4. Locate the intersection of the increment and the child's age at the **end** of the interval to determine the 6-month incremental percentile.

Interpretation: The accompanying charts permit definition of growth rate (growth velocity) relative to current reference data. Further investigation is indicated for children growing at rates markedly different from the 50th incremental percentile or for children whose incremental percentile changes rapidly.

Example 1 Girl at 5th NCHS* percentile at ages 6 and 12 months, aged 12 months at follow-up measurement

Measurement	Length	Date	Day**
Follow-up	69.8 cm	July 16, 1981	197
Initial	61.8 cm	January 15, 1981	15
Increment	8.0 cm	Interval	182

Her increment is 8.0 cm/6 months.
Her increment is between the 25th and 50th percentile.
She is short but growing at a normal rate.
* National Center for Health Statistics
** From Table of Consecutively Numbered Days

Example 2 Girl, aged 8 years at follow-up measurement

Measurement	Stature	Date	Day*
Follow-up	118.0 cm	April 22, 1981	477**
Initial	116.9 cm	November 21, 1980	325
Increment	1.1 cm	Interval	152

Her adjusted 6-month increment is $\frac{1.1 \text{ cm}}{152} \times 182 = 1.3$ cm.

Her increment is below the 3rd percentile.
Further investigation is indicated.
* From Table of Consecutively Numbered Days
** April 22 is day 112, to which 365 is added because follow-up measurement is in a different year (112 + 365 = 477).

Table of Consecutively Numbered Days

Day	JAN	FEB	MAR	APR	MAY	JUN	JUL	AUG	SEP	OCT	NOV	DEC	Day
1	1	32	60	91	121	152	182	213	244	274	305	335	1
2	2	33	61	92	122	153	183	214	245	275	306	336	2
3	3	34	62	93	123	154	184	215	246	276	307	337	3
4	4	35	63	94	124	155	185	216	247	277	308	338	4
5	5	36	64	95	125	156	186	217	248	278	309	339	5
6	6	37	65	96	126	157	187	218	249	279	310	340	6
7	7	38	66	97	127	158	188	219	250	280	311	341	7
8	8	39	67	98	128	159	189	220	251	281	312	342	8
9	9	40	68	99	129	160	190	221	252	282	313	343	9
10	10	41	69	100	130	161	191	222	253	283	314	344	10
11	11	42	70	101	131	162	192	223	254	284	315	345	11
12	12	43	71	102	132	163	193	224	255	285	316	346	12
13	13	44	72	103	133	164	194	225	256	286	317	347	13
14	14	45	73	104	134	165	195	226	257	287	318	348	14
15	15	46	74	105	135	166	196	227	258	288	319	349	15
16	16	47	75	106	136	167	197	228	259	289	320	350	16
17	17	48	76	107	137	168	198	229	260	290	321	351	17
18	18	49	77	108	138	169	199	230	261	291	322	352	18
19	19	50	78	109	139	170	200	231	262	292	323	353	19
20	20	51	79	110	140	171	201	232	263	293	324	354	20
21	21	52	80	111	141	172	202	233	264	294	325	355	21
22	22	53	81	112	142	173	203	234	265	295	326	356	22
23	23	54	82	113	143	174	204	235	266	296	327	357	23
24	24	55	83	114	144	175	205	236	267	297	328	358	24
25	25	56	84	115	145	176	206	237	268	298	329	359	25
26	26	57	85	116	146	177	207	238	269	299	330	360	26
27	27	58	86	117	147	178	208	239	270	300	331	361	27
28	28	59	87	118	148	179	209	240	271	301	332	362	28
29	29	—	88	119	149	180	210	241	272	302	333	363	29
30	30	—	89	120	150	181	211	242	273	303	334	364	30
31	31	—	90	—	151	—	212	243	—	304	—	365	31
Day	JAN	FEB	MAR	APR	MAY	JUN	JUL	AUG	SEP	OCT	NOV	DEC	

*Courtesy of Ross Laboratories, Columbus, OH, 43216, 1981.

INCREMENTAL HEAD CIRCUMFERENCE CHART
GIRLS: 0-36 MONTHS

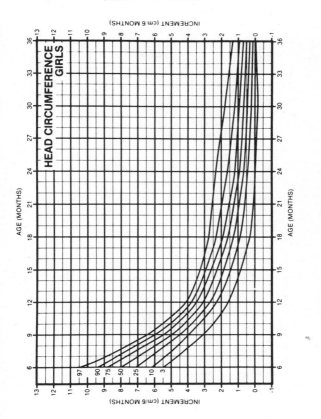

Adapted from the National Center for Health Statistics. Courtesy of
Ross Laboratories, Columbus, OH 43216, 1981.

INCREMENTAL HEAD CIRCUMFERENCE CHART
BOYS: 0-36 MONTHS

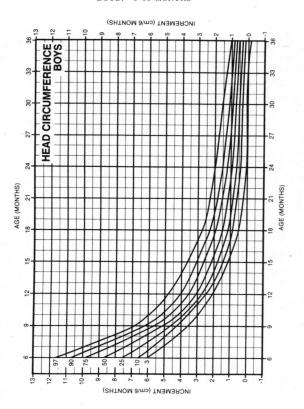

Adapted from the National Center for Health Statistics. Courtesy of
Ross Laboratories, Columbus, OH, 43216, 1981.

INCREMENTAL GROWTH CHARTS
GIRLS: 0-36 MONTHS

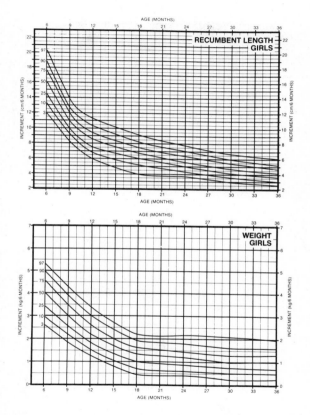

Adapted from the National Center for Health Statistics.   Courtesy of
Ross Laboratories, Columbus, OH, 43216, 1981.

INCREMENTAL GROWTH CHARTS
GIRLS: 2-18 YEARS

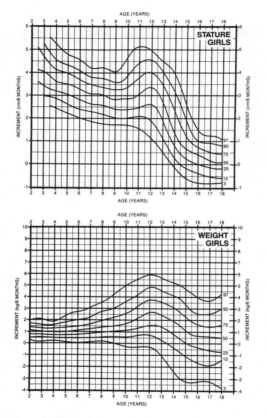

Adapted from the National Center for Health Statistics. Courtesy of Ross Laboratories, Columbus, OH, 43216, 1981.

INCREMENTAL GROWTH CHARTS
BOYS: 0-36 MONTHS

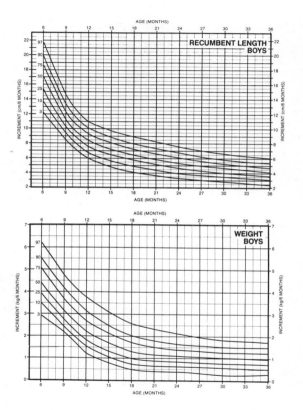

Adapted from the National Center for Health Statistics. Courtesy of Ross Laboratories, Columbus, OH, 43216, 1981.

INCREMENTAL GROWTH CHARTS
BOYS: 2-18 YEARS

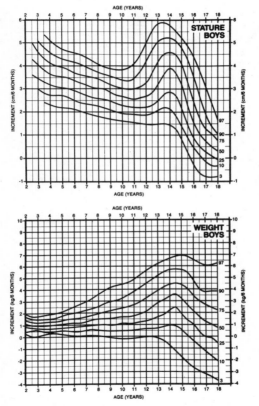

Adapted from the National Center for Health Statistics.   Courtesy of
Ross Laboratories, Columbus, OH, 43216, 1981.

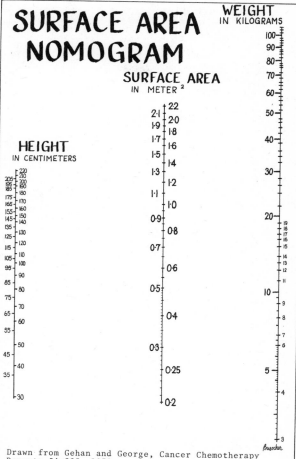

SURFACE AREA NOMOGRAM

WEIGHT IN KILOGRAMS

SURFACE AREA
IN METER²

HEIGHT
IN CENTIMETERS

Drawn from Gehan and George, Cancer Chemotherapy Reports 54:225, 1970.

BONE AGE

Age-at-Appearance Percentiles for Epiphyses and Round Bones

	Boys Percentiles			Girls Percentiles		
	5th	50th	95th	5th	50th	95th
Wrist						
Capitate	birth	3m	7m	birth	2m	7m
Hamate	2w	4m	10m	birth	2m	7m
Distal radius	6w	1y1m	2y4m	5m	10m	1y8m
Triquetral	1y6m	2y5m	5y6m	3m	1y8m	3y9m
Lunate	3y7m	4y1m	6y9m	1y1m	2y7m	5y8m
Scaphoid	3y6m	5y8m	7y10m	2y4m	4y1m	6y
Trapezium	3y1m	5y10m	9y	1y11m	4y1m	6y4m
Trapezoid	5y3m	6y3m	8y6m	2y5m	4y2m	6y
Distal Ulna		7y1m	9y1m	3y3m	5y4m	7y8m
Elbow						
Capitulum	3w	4m	1y1m	3w	3m	9m
Radial head	3y	5y3m	8y	2y3m	3y10m	6y3m
Medial epicondyle	4y3m	6y3m	8y5m	2y1m	3y5m	5y1m
Olecranon of ulna	7y9m	9y8m	11y11m	5y7m	8y	9y11m
Lateral epicondyle	9y3m	11y3m	13y8m	7y2m	9y3m	11y3m
Shoulder						
Head of humerus	37w*	2w	16w	37w*	2w	16w
Coronoid	birth		4m	birth		5m
Tubercle of humerus	3m	10m	2y4m	2m	6m	1y2m
Acromion of scapula	12y2m	13y9m	15y6m	10y4m	11y11m	15y4m
Acromion of clavicle	12y	14y	15y11m	10y10m	12y9m	15y4m

*Prenatal age

BONE AGE (continued)

Age-at-Appearance Percentiles for Epiphyses and Round Bones

	Boys Percentiles			Girls Percentiles		
	5th	50th	95th	5th	50th	95th
Hip						
Head of femur	3w	4m	8m	2w	4m	7m
Greater trochanter	1y11m	3y	4y4m	1y	1y10m	3y
Os Acetabulum	11y11m	13y6m	15y4m	9y7m	11y6m	13y5m
Iliac crest	12y	14y	15y11m	10y10m	12y9m	15y4m
Ischial tuberosity	13y7m	15y3m	17y1m	11y9m	13y11m	16y
Knee						
Distal femur	31w*		40w*	31w*		39w*
Proximal tibia	34w*		5w	34w*		2w
Proximal fibula	1y10m	3y6m	5y3m	1y4m	2y7m	3y11m
Patella	2y7m	4y	6y	1y6m	2y6m	4y
Tibial tubercle	9y11m	11y10m	13y5m	7y11m	10y3m	11y10m
Foot						
Calcaneus	22w*		25w*	22w*		25w*
Talus	25w*		31w*	25w*		31w*
Cuboid	37w*		16w	37w*		8w
Third cuneiform	3w	6m	1y7m	birth	3m	1y3m
Os calcis, apophysis	5y2m	7y7m	9y7m	3y6m	5y4m	7y4m

*Prenatal age

Modified from Garn, SM, Rohman, CG and Silverman, FN: Med Radiogr Photogr 43:45, 1967.

DENTAL DEVELOPMENT

| | DECIDUOUS TEETH | | PERMANENT TEETH | | | |
| | Eruption | | Shedding | | Eruption | |
	Maxillary	Mandibular	Maxillary	Mandibular	Maxillary	Mandibular
Central Incisors	6-8 mo	5-7 mo	7-8 yr	6-7 yr	7-8 yr	6-7 yr
Lateral Incisors	8-11 mo	7-10 mo	8-9 yr	7-8 yr	8-9 yr	7-8 yr
Cuspids	16-20 mo	16-20 mo	11-12 yr	9-11 yr	11-12 yr	9-11 yr
1st Premolar	–	–	–	–	10-11 yr	10-12 yr
2nd Premolar	–	–	–	–	10-12 yr	11-13 yr
1st Molars	10-16 mo	10-16 mo	10-11 yr	10-12 yr	6-7 yr	6-7 yr
2nd Molars	20-30 mo	20-30 mo	10-12 yr	11-13 yr	12-13 yr	12-13 yr
3rd Molars	–	–	–	–	17-22 yr	17-22 yr

NOTE: Sexes are combined although girls tend to be slightly advanced over boys. Averages are approximate values derived from various studies.

Ref: Vaughn, VC, et al (eds): Nelson's Textbook of Pediatrics. Philadelphia: W.B. Saunders, 1979, p. 32.

GIRLS
BLOOD PRESSURE PERCENTILES

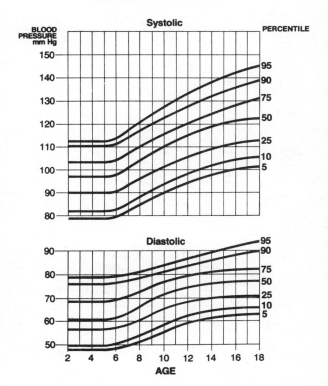

(right arm, seated)

With permission, Blumenthal, S, et al.: _Pediatrics_ 59:797 (Suppl.), 1977.

BOYS
BLOOD PRESSURE PERCENTILES

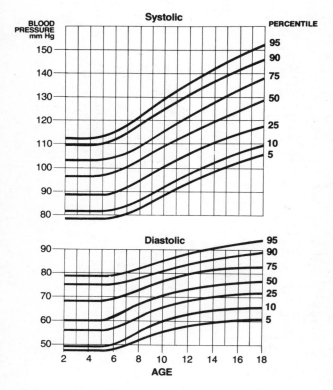

(right arm, seated)

With permission, Blumenthal, S, et al.: <u>Pediatrics</u> <u>59</u>:797 (Suppl.), 1977.

RECOMMENDED DAILY DIETARY ALLOWANCES

	Age	Wt	Ht	Energy	Prot.	Fat-Soluble Vitamins			Water-Soluble Vitamins				Minerals		
						Vit. A	Vit. D	Vit. E	Vit. C	Nia-cin	Ribo-flavin	Thia-min	Ca	P	Fe
	(yrs)	(kg)	(cm)	(kcal)	(g)	(µg RE)[1]	(µg)[2]	(mg αTE)[3]	(mg)	(mg)	(mg)	(mg)	(mg)	(mg)	(mg)
In-fants	0-½	6	60	kg × 115	kg × 2.2	420	10	3	35	6	0.4	0.3	360	240	10
	½-1	9	71	kg × 105	kg × 2.0	400	10	4	35	8	0.6	0.5	540	360	15
Chil-dren	1-3	13	90	kg × 100	23	400	10	5	45	9	0.8	0.7	800	800	15
	4-6	20	112	kg × 85	30	500	10	6	45	11	1.0	0.9	800	800	10
	7-10	28	132	kg × 85	34	700	10	7	45	16	1.4	1.2	800	800	10
Boys	11-14	45	157	kg × 60	45	1000	10	8	50	18	1.6	1.4	1200	1200	18
	15-18	66	176	kg × 45	56	1000	10	10	60	18	1.7	1.4	1200	1200	18
Girls	11-14	46	157	kg × 50	46	800	10	8	50	15	1.3	1.1	1200	1200	18
	15-18	55	163	kg × 40	46	800	10	8	60	14	1.3	1.1	1200	1200	18
Pregnant				+300[4]	+30	+200	+5	+2	+20	+2	+0.3	+0.4	+400	+400	
Lactating				+500	+20	+400	+5	+3	+40	+5	+0.5	+0.5	+400	+400	

[1] Retinol equivalents (1 µg retinol equivalent = 1 µg retinol or 6 µg carotene)
[2] As cholecalciferol (10 µg cholecalciferol = 400 IU vitamin D)
[3] αTocopherol equivalents (1 αTE = 1 mg d-α-tocopherol)
[4] + = in addition to normal recommended dietary allowances
Reproduced from "Recommended Dietary Allowances," 9th Edition, 1980 with permission of the National Academy of Sciences, Washington, DC.

COMPOSITION OF INFANT FORMULAS

Formula	Calories per oz.	per ml.	Percentage wt/vol (grams/100 ml) Protein *()	Fat *()	CHO *()	mEq/L Na	K	mg/L Ca	P	Ca/P ratio	mg/L Fe	Approx. Solute Load Renal Gi#	Gi#	Gi# (mOsm/L)
Cow's milk	20	.67	3.50(21)	3.70(50)	4.80(29)	22	40	1240	950	1.30/1	0.5-1.0	230		270
Enfamil 20**	20	.67	1.50(9)	3.80(50)	6.90(41)	9	17	530	445	1.20/1	1.5	100	250	296
Enfamil premature	20	.67	2.00(12)	3.40(45)	7.42(43)	12	19	790	398	2.00/1	1	180		220
Evaporated milk with karo syrup see page 340.	23	.77	3.12(16)	3.61(52)	7.89(32)	24	36	1161	946	1.23/1	1.8			
Human milk	21	.72	1.10(6)	4.50(56)	6.80(38)	7	13	340	140	2.40/1	1.5	75		273
Isomil	20	.67	2.00(12)	3.60(48)	6.80(40)	13	18	700	500	1.40/1	12	126	230	238
Isomil SF	20	.67	2.00(12)	3.60(48)	6.80(40)	13	18	700	500	1.40/1	12	126		136
Lofenalac	20	.67	2.20(13)	2.70(35)	8.80(52)	14	18	635	475	1.30/1	13	140		320
Nursoy	20	.67	2.10(13)	3.60(48)	6.90(40)	9	18	635	445	1.40/1	12	172		266
Nutramigen	20	.67	2.20(13)	2.60(35)	8.80(52)	14	18	635	475	1.30/1	13	130		430
Portagen	20	.67	2.40(14)	3.20(42)	7.80(44)	14	22	635	475	1.30/1	13	150	136	236
Pregestimil	20	.67	1.90(11)	2.70(35)	9.10(54)	14	19	635	425	1.50/1	13	130	311	326
Prosobee	20	.67	2.00(12)	3.50(48)	6.80(40)	13	21	635	500	1.30/1	13	130		180
RCF	***		2.00(20)	3.60(80)	0(0)	13	18	700	500	1.4/1	12	126		60

*() Percentage calories supplied by . . .
** also comes with Fe (12 mg/L)
*** varies with amount carbohydrate added
‡# vapor pressure method as determined by manufacturers method: Ernst, JA, et al: Pediatrics 72:350, 1983.
‡ freezing point depression
Ref: values listed were provided by manufacturers except when indicated otherwise.

COMPOSITION OF INFANT FORMULAS (continued)

Formula	Calories per oz.	Calories per ml.	Percentage wt/vol (grams/100 ml) Protein *()	Fat *()	CHO *()	mEq/L Na	K	mg/L Ca	P	Ca/P ratio	mg/L Fe	Approx. Solute Load (mOsm/L) Renal GI#	GI#	
Similac 20**	20	.67	1.55(9)	3.61(48)	7.20(43)	11	20	510	390	1.30/1	1.5	108	262	307
Similac 24 LBW	24	.80	2.20(11)	4.49(47)	8.49(42)	16	31	730	560	1.30/1	3.0	160	260	292
Similac PM 60/40	20	.67	1.58(9)	3.76(50)	6.88(41)	7	15	400	200	2.00/1	2.6	92	260	
Similac special care	20	.67	1.83(10)	3.67(47)	7.20(43)	13	21	1200	600	1.50/1	2.5	122	218	
Similac whey	20	.67	1.55(9)	3.61(48)	7.20(43)	10	19	400	300	1.33/1	12	104	270	
SMA 20	20	.67	1.50(9)	3.60(48)	7.20(43)	6.5	14	445	330	1.30/1	12.7	126	271	
SMA Preemie	24	.80	2.00(10)	4.40(50)	8.60(40)	14	19	750	400	1.88/1	3	175	235	

*() Percentage calories supplied by . . . .
** also comes with Fe (12 mg/L)
‡ vapor pressure method as determined by manufacturers method: Ernst, JA, et al: Pediatrics 72:350, 1983.
‡ freezing point depression
Ref: # values listed were provided by manufacturers except when indicated otherwise.

INGREDIENTS OF INFANT FORMULAS

Product	Protein	Fat	Carbohydrate	Comments
Cho-free	Soy protein	Soy oil	Add 12.8% dextrose	For carbohydrate and/or cow's milk protein intolerance
Cow's milk	80% casein, 20% lactalbumin	Butterfat	Lactose	
Enfamil	40% casein; 60% whey	80% soy, 20% coconut oils	Lactose	
Enfamil premature	40% casein; 60% lactalbumin	40% MCT oil, corn oil	Corn syrup solids, lactose	Premature infants
Evaporated milk based	80% casein; 20% lactalbumin	Butterfat	Lactose	Add 17 oz. water and 1 tablespoon Karo syrup to a 13 oz. can evaporated milk. Supplement with multivitamins and iron. Ref: C. DeAngelis, Pediatric Primary Care, 3 ed., Boston: Little, Brown, & Co., 1984.
Human milk	40% casein, 60% lactalbumin	Human milk fat	Lactose	
Isomil	Soy protein	Coconut and soy oils	*Corn syrup solids and sucrose	For cow's milk protein and/or lactose intolerance
Isomil SF	Soy protein	Coconut and soy oils	Corn syrup solids	For cow's milk protein, lactose, and/or sucrose intolerance
Lofenalac	Processed casein hydrolysate to remove phenylalanine	Corn oil	Corn syrup solids and modified tapioca starch	For phenylketonuria (PKU) - low in phenylalanine

*Corn syrup solids = dextrose, maltose, other glucose polymers

INGREDIENTS OF INFANT FORMULAS (continued)

Product	Protein	Fat	Carbohydrate	Comments
Neo-Mullsoy	Soy isolate and methionine	Soy oil	Sucrose	For cow's milk intolerance
Nursoy	Soy protein	Coconut, safflower and soybean oils	Sucrose	For cow's milk protein and/or lactose intolerance
Nutramigen	Casein hydrolysate	Corn oil	Sucrose, modified tapioca starch	Use for sensitivity to intact milk protein, or for lactose intolerance
Portagen	Sodium caseinate	88% MCT oil, 12% corn oil	Corn syrup solids, sucrose, 2% other CHO	Use in fat malabsorption states, lactose intolerance (liver disease)
Pregestimil	Casein hydrolysate with added L-cystine, L-tyrosine, L-tryptophan	60% corn oil, 40% MCT oil	85% corn syrup solids, 15% modified tapioca starch	Suitable for many malabsorption syndromes
Probana	Whole and non-fat cow's milk, banana powder, casein hydrolysate	Milkfat, corn oil	45% dextrose, banana powder*, lactose	High protein, low fat (fat malabsorption, celiac)
Prosobee	Soy protein isolate and methionine	80% soy oil, 20% coconut oil	100% corn syrup solids	Use for lactose and cow's milk protein intolerance; sucrose intolerance; galactosemia
Similac	Non-fat cow's milk	Coconut and soy oils	Lactose	

*Banana powder - sucrose, fructose, dextrins, starch

INGREDIENTS OF INFANT FORMULAS (continued)

Product	Protein	Fat	Carbohydrate	Comments
Similac 24 LBW	Non-fat cow's milk	MCT oil, coconut and soy oils	50% lactose and 50% corn syrup solids	Dilute initial feedings. For premature infants with fluid intolerance.
Similac PM 60/40	Casein and whey (60/40 ratio lactalbumin/casein)	Coconut and corn oils	Lactose	(Ca:P = 2:1) For those predisposed to hypocalcemia; low salt content
Similac special care	60% whey 40% casein	MCT oil, corn oil, coconut oil	50% lactose 50% corn syrup solids	Premature infants
SMA	non-fat cow's milk, demineralized whey	Coconut and safflower and soybean oil	Lactose	Low salt content

TUBE FEEDING FORMULAS - SUPPLEMENTAL FEEDINGS

PRODUCT	CHO SOURCE	PROTEIN SOURCE	FAT SOURCE	CHO gm/L	PROTEIN gm/L	FAT gm/L	mOsm/kg	Na/K+ mEq/L	RESIDUE	VITAMIN CONTENT	FEATURE	CAL/ML
AMIN-AID	Malto-dextrin sucrose	crystal-line essential amino acids	soy oil lecithin mono, digly-cerides	366	19	19	1095	14/<5	Low	Inade-quate	Low concentra-tion electro-lytes, essential amino acids only, lactose free	1.9
CRITI-CARE HN	Malto-dextrin corn starch	whey, soy, meat pro-tein hydro-lysate with essential amino acids	saf-flower oil	222	38	3	650	27/34	Low	Adequate >10 yr	Lactose free, absorbed in upper gut	1
ENSURE	Corn syrup, sucrose	Na and Ca caseinates, soy protein	Corn oil	145	37	37	450	32/32	Low	Adequate >10 yr	Supplemental feeding, lactose free; requires digestion	1
ENSURE PLUS	Corn syrup, sucrose	Na and Ca caseinates, soy protein	Corn oil	197	55	53	600*	46/48	Low	Adequate >10 yr	Same as ENSURE	1.5
FLEX-ICAL	Sucrose, dextrin	Casein hy-drolysate, amino acids	Soy oil, MCT oil	150	22	34	550*	15/38	Low	Adequate	Supplemental feeding, lactose free, absorbed in upper gut	1
FORMU-LA 2	Lactose, sucrose	Wheat, beef, egg, milk	Egg yolk, corn oil, beef fat	123	38	40	435-510	26/45	High	Adequate	Blenderized - requires absorp-tion and digestion	1

* Unflavored formulas. Flavored formulas add mOsm.

TUBE FEEDING FORMULAS - SUPPLEMENTAL FEEDINGS (continued)

PROD-UCT	CHO SOURCE	PROTEIN SOURCE	FAT SOURCE	CHO gm/L	PRO-TEIN gm/L	FAT gm/L	mOsm/Kg	Na/K+ mEq/L	RES-IDUE	VITAMIN CONTENT	FEATURE	CAL/ML
HEPATIC-AID	Malto-dextrin, sucrose	Crystalline amino acids	Soy bean oil, lecithin mono, digly-cerides	289	43	36	1158	14/5	Low	Inade-quate	High branch chain amino acid formula, low electrolytes, lactose free	1.6
ISOCAL	Glucose, oligo-saccha-rides	Na and Ca caseinates, soy protein	Soy oil, MCT oil	130	34	44	300	22/33	Low	Adequate >10 yr	Requires digestion, low Na, lactose free	1
NUTRI 1000	Sucrose, corn syrup	Skim milk	Corn oil	101	55	40	500	23/39	Med	Adequate >10 yr	Supplemental or tube feeding; requires func-tioning gut	1
OSMO-LITE	Hydro-lyzed corn starch	Ca-caseinate, soy protein	MCT, corn & soy oils	138	35	34	300	24/26	Low	Adequate >10 yr	Lactose free, low Na, requires digestion	1
PRECI-SION LR	Malto-dextrin, sucrose	Egg albumin	Soy oil, MCT oil	249	26	2	510*	30/22	Low	Adequate >10 yr	Lactose free, absorbed upper gut	1.1
PREC-ISION HN	Malto-dextrin, sucrose	Egg albumin	Soy oil	218	44	0.5	557*	42/23	Low	Adequate	Lactose free, high protein, absorbed upper gut	1

* Unflavored formulas. Flavored formulas add mOsm.

TUBE FEEDING FORMULAS - SUPPLEMENTAL FEEDINGS (continued)

PRODUCT	CHO SOURCE	PROTEIN SOURCE	FAT SOURCE	CHO gm/L	PRO-TEIN gm/L	FAT gm/L	mOsm/kg	Na/K+ mEq/L	RES-IDUE	VITAMIN CONTENT	FEATURE	CAL/ML
SUS-TACAL	Sucrose, lactose, corn syrup	Skim milk, caseinates, soy protein	Partially hydrogenated soy oil	138	60	23	625*	39/53	Med	Adequate >3 yr	High protein, requires digestion	1
TRAVA-SORB RENAL	Glucose, oligosaccharides, sucrose	Crystalline L-amino acids	Sunflower oils, MCT oil	271	23	18	590	0/0	Low	Inadequate	Electrolyte + lactose free, essential amino acids	1.3
VIVO-NEX	Glucose, oligosaccharides	L-amino acids	Safflower oil	226	21	1	550*	20/30	Low	Adequate ≥10 yr	Lactose free, no pancreatic stimulus, absorbed upper gut	1
VIVO-NEX HN	Glucose, oligosaccharides	L-amino acids	Safflower oil	210	42	1	810*	23/30	Low	Adequate ≥10 yr	Lactose free, absorbed upper gut, high protein	1
VITAL HN	Hydrolyzed corn starch, sucrose	Whey, soy and meat protein hydrolysate, and free essential amino acids	Safflower oil and MCT oil	185	41	10	460	17/30	Low	Adequate	Absorbed in upper gut, low Na, lactose free, 45% MCT	1

* Unflavored formulas. Flavored formulas add mOsm.

GUIDE FOR THE INTRODUCTION OF SOLIDS AND WHOLE COW'S MILK IN INFANCY

NOTE: Introduce foods one at a time, in small amounts at first.

FOOD GROUP	AGE	REASON	NOTES
JUICE	2-4 1/2 months	Vitamin C needed at 10 days of age unless breast fed, on vitamin drops, or vitamin C fortified formula	Vitaminized apple juice. Delay orange juice until 6 months - allergens in peel. Special commercial juices for baby are expensive and offer no advantages. Juices should not replace infant's milk intake.
CEREAL	3-4 months	Texture, B-Vitamins, minerals	Add formula to dry cereal and gradually thicken (Do not add to bottle). Begin with baby rice cereal, later soy, oatmeal, barley, then mixed. Baby cereals with fruit added are less nutritious and not recommended.
FRUIT	4-4 1/2 months	Vitamins, minerals, flavor, texture, prevents constipation	Use blended or strained (i.e. applesauce, apricots, bananas, peaches, pears, and plums). Commerical varieties contain sugar and tapioca. Avoid "desserts."
VEGETABLE	4-4 1/2 months	Vitamins, minerals, flavor, texture, prevents constipation	Use blended-at-home or store-bought strained asparagus, squash, wax beans, beets, carrots, creamed corn, peas, sweet potatoes, spinach, and green beans.
MEAT	5 months	Iron, protein, flavor, texture	Use blended or strained beef, chicken, lamb, liver, turkey, veal, and "meat dinners." Commercial varieties contain salt. Commercial "dinners" - less protein; should replace vegetables only.
EGGS	6 months	Protein, minerals vitamins	Egg white more allergenic. No need to use commercial egg yolk.

GUIDE FOR THE INTRODUCTION OF SOLIDS AND WHOLE COW'S MILK IN INFANCY (Continued)

FOOD GROUP	AGE	REASON	NOTES
POTATO	7 months	Minerals, vitamins	Mash, boil, or bake. Should not replace other vegetables.
TEXTURE FOODS	6-9 months or when teething begins	Texture, teething, encourages self-feeding (finger foods), chewing	Fruits, vegetables, and meats - more lumpy and less strained. Peeled apple, pudding, fish (no bones), mild cheese. Bread products - melba toast and Zwieback.
TABLE FOODS	1 year	Texture, to establish normal eating habits	Meats should be minced until child has enough teeth to chew. Mash other foods with fork.
WHOLE COW'S MILK	6 months	Protein, vitamins	An adequate substitution for breast milk or formula if child is receiving iron enriched cereals plus fruits and vegetables to provide vitamin C.

BLOOD CHEMISTRIES

These values are compiled from the published literature, <u>Pediatric Clinical Chemistry</u> and the Johns Hopkins Hospital Department of Laboratory Medicine. They are the most widely accepted normal values. Normal values, however, vary with the analytic method used. If any doubt exists, consult your laboratory for its analytical method and normal range of values. The values between the parentheses are normal values according to the International System (SI) of measurement.

Ref: Meites S (ed): <u>Pediatric Clinical Chemistry</u>, <u>2nd Edition</u>. The American Association for Clinical Chemistry, 1981.

Acid phosphatase:
Newborn	7.4-19.4 U/ml	(7.4-19.4 U/ml)
2-13 yrs	6.4-15.2 U/ml	(6.4-15.2 U/ml)
Adult	M: 0.5-11.0 U/ml	(0.5-11.0 U/ml)
	F: 0.2-9.5 U/ml	(0.2-9.5 U/ml)

Alanine Aminotransferase (ALT):
Infants	<54 U/L	(<54 U/L)
Children	1-30 U/L	(1-30 U/L)
Adults	M: 7-46 U/L	(7-46 U/L)
	F: 4-35 U/L	(4-35 U/L)

Aldolase:
Adult	< 8 U/L	(< 8 U/L)
Children	2x Adult Values	
Newborn	4x Adult Values	

Alkaline phosphatase:
Newborn	122-231 U/L	(122-231 U/L)
1 mo-1 yr	109-265 U/L	(109-265 U/L)
1-6 yrs	95-218 U/L	(95-218 U/L)
6-12 yrs	122-323 U/L	(122-323 U/L)
12-19 yrs	M: 55-367 U/L	(55-367 U/L)
	F: 27-221 U/L	(27-221 U/L)
>19 yrs	37-108 U/L	(37-108 U/L)

Alpha l-Antitrypsin: 2.1-5.0 gm/L
  PI type M (normal) >75% normal pool
  PI type MZ   55-75% normal pool
  PI type SZ   30-50% normal pool
  PI type Z or null   <40% normal pool

Alpha Fetoprotein: <10 mg/dl   (<0.1 gm/L)

Ammonia Nitrogen (Venous Sample): (Heparinized specimen in ice
  water and analyzed within 30 min)
  Newborn   90-150 µg/dl   (64-107 µmol/L)
  0-2 wks   70-129 µg/dl   (50-92 µmol/L)
  >1 mo   20-79 µg/dl   (14-56 µmol/L)
  Infant-child   29-80 µg/dl   (21-57 µmol/L)
  Adult   13-48 µg/dl   (9-34 µmol/L)

Amylase: Newborn: 5-65 U/L   (5-65 U/L)
       >1 yr: 25-125 U/L   (25-125 U/L)

Arsenic: <30 µg/dl   (<0.4 mmol/L)

Aspartate Aminotransferase (AST):
  Newborn   14-70 U/L   (14-70 U/L)
  6 wks-18 mos   13-64 U/L   (13-64 U/L)
  18 mos-5 yrs   16-46 U/L   (16-46 U/L)
  5 yrs-12 yrs   10-40 U/L   (10-40 U/L)
  12 yrs-16 yrs   15-35 U/L   (15-35 U/L)
  16 yrs-adult   10-27 U/L   (10-27 U/L)

Base Excess:
  Newborn   -10 to -2 mmol/L   (-10 to -2 mmol/L)
  2 mo-2 yrs   -6.6 to 0.2 mmol/L (-6.6 to 0.2 mmol/L)
  Child-adult   -2.3 to 2.3 mmol/L (-2.3 to 2.3 mmol/L)

Bicarbonate: 22-30 mEq/L   (22-30 mmol/L)
  Newborn:
    Premature   18-26 mEq/L   (18-26 mmol/L)
    Full Term   20-26 mEq/L   (20-26 mmol/L)
  12 yrs   20-25 mEq/L   (20-25 mmol/L)
  12 yrs-adult   22-26 mEq/L   (22-26 mmol/L)

Bilirubin (total):
  Cord   <1.8 mg/dl   (<30.6 µmol/L)
  24 hrs   Premature 1-6 mg/dl (17-103 µmol/L)
                Full term 2-6 mg/dl (34-103 µmol/L)
  48 hrs   Premature 6-8 mg/dl (103-137 µmol/L)
                Full term 6-7 mg/dl (103-120 µmol/L)
  3-5 days   Premature 10-12 mg/dl (171-205 µmol/L)
                Full term 4-12 mg/dl (68-205 µmol/L)
  1 mo-Adult   up to 1.5 mg/dl   (26 µmol/L)
  Conjugated: up to 0.5 mg/dl   (9 µmol/L)

Calcium (Total):

Premature <1 week	6-10 mg/dl	(1.5-2.5 mmol/L)
Full term <1 week	7.0-12.0 mg/dl	(1.75-3 mmol/L)
Child	8-11.0 mg/dl	(2-2.75 mmol/L)
Adult	8.5-11.0 mg/dl	(2.13-2.75 mmol/L)

Calcium (Ionized):   4.4-5.4 mg/dl   (0.1-1.35 mmol/L)

Carbon Dioxide (CO_2 content):

Cord blood	15-20 mmol/L	(15-20 mmol/L)
Child	18-27 mmol/L	(18-27 mmol/L)
Adult	24-35 mmol/L	(24-35 mmol/L)

Carbon Monoxide (carboxyhemoglobin):

Nonsmoker	<2% of total Hemoglobin
Smoker	<10% of total Hemoglobin
Lethal	>50% of total Hemoglobin

Carotenoids (Carotenes):

Birth	70 µg/dl	(1.31 µmol/L)
<1 yr	70-340 µg/dl	(1.31-6.38 µmol/L)
>3 yrs	100-150 µg/dl	(1.88-2.81 µmol/L)

Ceruloplasmin: 20-40 mg/dl   (1.32-2.64 µmol/L)
                        (280-570 units)

Chloride: 94-106 mEq/L   (94-106 mmol/L)

Cholesterol (Total):   (See Triglycerides table on page 354.)

Copper:

0-6 mos	<70 µg/dl	(<11 µmol/L)
6 mos-5 yrs	27-153 µg/dl	(4.2-24.1 µmol/L)
5-17 yrs	94-234 µg/dl	(14.2-36.8 µmol/L)
Adult	70-155 µg/dl	(11-24.4 µmol/L)

Creatine Kinase (Creatine Phosphokinase):

Age	Upper 95th percentile values, U/L	
	M	F
1 d	600	500
2-10 d	440	440
11-364 d	170	170
1.00-4.99 yr	109	100
5.00-6.99 yr	109	100
7.00-8.99 yr	103	85
9.00-10.99 yr	109	88
11.00-12.99 yr	108	85
13.00-14.99 yr	129	85
15.00-16.99 yr	247	74
17.00-18.99 yr	190	68

Creatinine (Serum):

Age, yr	Upper limits, mg/dl (μmol/L)	
	M	F
1	0.6 (53)	0.5 (44)
2-3	0.7 (62)	0.6 (53)
4-7	0.8 (71)	0.7 (62)
8-10	0.9 (80)	0.8 (71)
11-12	1.0 (88)	0.9 (80)
13-17	1.2 (106)	1.1 (97)
18-20	1.3 (115)	1.1 (97)

Adult, M & F: 0.5-1.2 (44-106); 0.5-1.4 (44-124)

1,25 Dihydroxyvitamin D (Calcitriol):

Newborn	21± 2 pg/ml	(50±4.8 nmol/L)
Child	43± 3 pg/ml	(103±7.2 nmol/L)
Adult	29± 2 pg/ml	(69.6±4.8 nmol/L)

Ferritin:

Children (6 mos-15 yrs)	7-144 ng/ml	(7-144 μg/dl)
Adult	F: 5-99 ng/ml	(5-99 μg/L)
	M: 10-273 ng/ml	(10-273 μg/L)

Fibrin Degradation Products:

Titer:	1:25=suspicious	1:50=positive

Fibrinogen: 200-400 mg/dl   (2-4 g/L)

Folic Acid (Folate):   1.9-14 ng/L (4.3-23.6 nmol/L)
                       (microbiological assay)

Galactose: 0-0.5 mg/dl   (0-0.03 mmol/L)

Gammaglutamyl Transferase (GGT):

Cord	19-270 U/L	(19-270 U/L)
Premature	56-233 U/L	(56-233 U/L)
0-3 wks	0-130 U/L	(0-130 U/L)
3 wks-3 mos	4-120 U/L	(4-120 U/L)
>3 mos	M: 5-65 U/L	(5-65 U/L)
	F: 5-35 U/L	(5-35 U/L)
1-15 yrs	0-23 U/L	(0-23 U/L)
16 yrs-Adult	0-35 U/L	(0-35 U/L)

Gastrin: <300 pg/ml   (<300 ng/L)

Glucose (Serum):

Premature	20-65 mg/dl	(1.1-3.6 mmol/L)
Full term	20-110 mg/dl	(1.1-6.4 mmol/L)
1 wk-16 yrs	60-105 mg/dl	(3.3-5.8 nmol/L)
>16 yrs	70-115 mg/dl	(3.9-6.4 mmol/L)

Haptoglobin:

Newborn	Detectable in only 10-20%
>1 yr	400-1800 mg of Hb bound/L (748-1118 μmol/L)

Iron (Iron binding capacity):

	Iron (μg/dl)	(μmol/L)	Iron Binding Capacity (μg/dl)	(μmol/L)	Approximate Percent Saturation (μg/dl)
Newborn	110-270	(19.7-48.3)	59-175	(10.6-31.3)	65%
4-10 mos	30-70	(5.4-12.5)	250-400	(45-72)	25%
3-10 yrs	53-119	(9.5-27.0)	250-400	(45-72)	30%
Adult	72-186	(12.9-33.3)	250-400	(45-72)	35%

Ketones:
    Qualitative: negative
    Quantitative: up to 3 mg%

Lactate:

Capillary blood		
(Newborn)	up to 30 mg/dl	(3.0 mmol/L)
(Child)	5-20 mg/dl	(0.56-2.25 mmol/L)
Venous	5-18 mg/dl	(0.5-2.0 mmol/L)
Arterial	3-7 mg/dl	(0.3-0.8 mmol/L)

Lactate Dehydrogenase (37°C):

Birth	upper limit = 3-9 x adult values	
1 d-1 mo	upper limit = 2-5 x adult values	
1 mo-2 yrs	upper limit = 2-3 x adult values	
2 yrs - 5 yrs	150-350 U/L	(150-350 U/L)
5 yrs - 12 yrs	150-300 U/L	(150-300 U/L)
12 yrs-16 yrs	130-280 U/L	(130-280 U/L)
16 yrs-Adult	110-200 U/L	(110-200 U/L)

Lactate Dehydrogenase Isoenzymes (% total):

LD_1 Heart	24-34%
LD_2 Heart, Erythrocytes	35-45%
LD_3 Muscle	15-25%
LD_4 Liver, trace muscle	4-10%
LD_5 Liver, muscle	1-9%

Lead (Whole Blood):   <40 μg/dl   (<1.93 μmol/L)

Lipase (Serum) (37°C): 20-180 U/L   (20-180 U/L)

Lipids (Total):   450-1000 mg/dl   (4.5-10.0 g/L)

Lipoproteins:

	Child-Adult	(g/L)	Newborn	(g/L)
Alpha	286-450 mg/dl	(2.86-4.5)	71-176 mg/dl	(0.71-1.76)
Pre-Beta	22-72 mg/dl	(0.22-0.72)	-	
Beta	276-438 mg/dl	(2.76-4.38)	51-158 mg/dl	(0.51-1.58)

Magnesium:
Newborn	1.52-2.33 mEq/L	(0.75-1.15 mmol/L)
	(2.1-2.2 mg/100 ml)	
Child	1.4-1.9 mEq/L	(0.70-0.95 mmol/L)
Adult	1.3-2.5 mEq/L	(0.65-1.25 mmol/L)
	(1.8-3 mg/100 ml)	

Manganese (Blood):
Newborn	2.4-9.6 µg/dl	(2.44-1.75 µmol/L)
2-18 yrs	0.8-2.1 µg/dl	(0.15-0.38 µmol/L)

Mercury (Urine):   <50 µg/24 hrs   (<250 nmol/24 hrs)

Metanephrine (Urine):
Child   0.02-0.16 µg/mg creatinine   (0.01-0.8 mmol/mol creatinine)

Methemoglobin: <0.3 g/dl or <3% of total Hb   (<46.5 µmol/L)

Normetanephrine (Urine):
Child   0.05-0.6 µg/mg creatinine   (0.03-0.3 mmol/mol creatinine)

5' Nucleotidase: 2.2-15.0 U/L   (2.2-15.0 U/L)

Osmolality: 285-295 mOsm/kg   (270-285 mOsm/L plasma)

Phenylalanine:
Newborn	<4 mg/dl	(<0.24 mmol/L)
Child	<3 mg/dl	(<0.18 mmol/L)

Phospholipids:
Cord blood	0.48-1.6 gms/L	(15-52 mmol/L)
2-13 yrs	1.66-2.47 gms/L	(54-80 mmol/L)
3-20 yrs	1.93-3.38 gms/L	(62-109 mmol/L)

Phosphorus (Inorganic):
Newborn	4.2-9.0 mg/dl	(1.36-2.91 mmol/L)
1 yr	3.8-6.2 mg/dl	(1.23-2.0 mmol/L)
2-5 yrs	3.5-6.8 mg/dl	(1.13-2.2 mmol/L)
Adult	3.0-4.5 mg/dl	(0.97-1.45 mmol/L)

Porcelain: 8-20 mEq/L

Porphyrins: <0.02 µmol/L   (<0.02 µmol/L)

Potassium:
<10 days of age	3.5-7.0 mEq/L	(3.5-7.0 mmol/L)
>10 days of age	3.5-5.5 mEq/L	(3.5-5.5 mmol/L)

Prolactin:

Age	ng/ml		µg/L
Newborn			
Premature	169		(169)
Full-term	280		(280)
4 wk	75		(75)
12 wks, full-term	adult range		
20 wks, premature	adult range		
Adult	0-30		(0-30)

Proteins Average (Range) in grams/dl:

Age	Total	Albumin	Globulin	Gamma Globulin
Premature	5.5	3.7	1.8	0.7
	(4.0-7.0)	(2.5-4.5)	(1.2-2.0)	(0.5-0.9)
FT Newborn	6.4	3.4	3.1	0.8
	(5.0-7.1)	(2.5-5.0)	(1.2-4.0)	(0.7-0.9)
1-3 mos	6.6	3.8	2.5	0.3
	(4.7-7.4)	(3.0-4.2)	(1.0-3.3)	(0.1-0.5)
3-12 mos	6.8	3.9	2.6	0.6
	(5.0-7.5)	(2.7-5.0)	(2.0-3.8)	(0.4-1.2)
1-15 yrs	7.4	4.0	3.1	0.9
	(6.5-8.6)	(3.2-5.0)	(2.0-4.0)	(0.6-1.2)

Pyruvate: 0.05-0.14 mEq/L   (50-140 mmol/L)

Sodium:

Premature	130-140 mEq/L	(130-140 mmol/L)
Older	135-145 mEq/L	(135-145 mmol/L)

Transaminase (SGOT): See AST (Aspartate Aminotransferase)

Transaminase (SGPT): See ALT (Alanine Aminotransferase)

Triglycerides:

	Normal Upper Limits Total Serum Cholesterol mg/dl (mmol/L)		Serum Triglycerides mg/dl (g/L)	
Age	Males	Females*	Males	Females*
0-4 yrs	203 (5.28)	200 (5.2)	99 (0.99)	112 (1.12)
5-9	203 (5.28)	205 (5.33)	101 (1.01)	105 (1.05)
10-14	202 (5.25)	201 (5.22)	125 (1.25)	131 (1.31)
15-19	197 (5.12)	200 (5.2)	148 (1.48)	124 (1.24)
20-24	218 (5.67)	216 (5.62)	201 (2.01)	131 (1.31)
25-29	244 (6.34)	222 (5.77)	249 (2.49)	144 (1.44)
30-34	254 (6.60)	230 (5.98)	266 (2.66)	150 (1.50)
35-39	270 (7.02)	242 (6.24)	321 (3.21)	176 (1.76)
40-44	268 (6.97)	252 (6.55)	320 (3.20)	191 (1.91)
45-49	276 (7.18)	265 (6.89)	327 (3.27)	214 (2.14)

*Use of oral contraceptives significantly raises both total serum cholesterol and serum triglyceride levels.

Urea Nitrogen: 5-25 mg/dl   (1.8-9.0 mmol/L)

Uric Acid:

Age, yr	mg/dl	(mmol/L)
0-2	2.0-7.0	(0.12-0.42)
2-12	2.0-6.5	(0.12-0.39)
12-14	2.0-7.0	(0.12-0.42)
14-adult, M	3.0-8.0	(0.18-0.48)
F	2.0-7.0	(0.12-0.42)

Vitamin A (Retinol):

0-1 yr	20-90 µg/dl	(0.7-3.14 µmol/L)
1-5 yrs	30-100 µg/dl	(1.05-3.50 µmol/L)
5-16 yrs	60-100 µg/dl	(2.09-3.50 µmol/L)
Adult	20-80 µg/dl	(0.70-2.79 µmol/L)

Vitamin B1 (Thiamine):
(Age unspecified)   5.3-7.9 µg/dl   (0.16-0.23 µmol/L)

Vitamin B2 (Riboflavin):
(Age unspecified)   3.7-13.7 µg/dl   (98-363 mmol/L)

Vitamin B12 (Cobalamin):
(Age unspecified)   130-785 pg/ml   (96-579 pmol/L)

Vitamin C (Ascorbic Acid):
                        0.2-2.0 mg/dl   (11.4-113.6 µmol/L)

Vitamin E:

Newborn	>0.3 µg/dl	(>0.7 µmol/L)
Child-Adult	0.5-1.2 µg/dl	(1.17-2.8 µmol/L)

Zinc:

0-1 yr	Range: 74-146 µg/dl	(11.3-22.3 µmol/L)
2-10 yrs	72-128 µg/dl	(11.0-19.6 µmol/L)
11-18 yrs	65-125 µg/dl	(9.9-19.1 µmol/L)
Adult	60-120 µg/dl	(9.2-18.4 µmol/L)

NORMAL SEROLOGIC REFERENCE VALUES

Anti-Streptolysin O Titer	
Preschool	<1:85
School ages and adults	<1:170
Older adults	<1:85

<u>NOTE</u>: Significant if rising titer can be demonstrated at weekly intervals.

Anti-Hyaluronidase	<1:256
Anti-Nuclear Antibody	<1:40
C-Reactive Protein	Negative
C'_3	70-176 mg/dl
C'_4	16-45 mg/dl
Carcinoembryonic Antigen (CEA)	<2.5 ng/ml
Febrile Agglutinins	<1:80 or <four fold rise in titer
Proteus OX-19 Agglutinins	<1:80 or <four fold rise in titer
Rheumatoid Factor-Latex	<20 negative 20-40 suggestive ≥80 positive
Tularemia Agglutinins	<1:80 or <four fold rise in titer
Waaler Rose Titer	1:10 Negative 1:20-1:40 Doubtful >1:80 Positive

Complement Fixation Tests should be negative or <1:8:
  Brucellosis
  Cytomegalic Inclusion Disease
  Eastern and Western Equine Encephalitis
  Epidemic Typhus
  Influenza Type A
  Influenza Type B
  Lymphocytic Choriomeningitis
  Lymphogranuloma Venereum
  Mumps
  Psittacosis
  Q Fever (American)
  Rickettsial Pox
  Rocky Mountain Spotted Fever
  St. Louis Encephalitis
  Toxoplasmosis
  Tularemia

LEVELS OF IMMUNOGLOBULINS

	IgG (MG/DL)	IgM (MG/DL)	IgA (MG/DL)	IgE (U/ML)
Serum				
Newborn	1031 ± 200*	11 ± 5	2 ± 3	0-7.5
6 mo	427 ± 186	43 ± 17	28 ± 18	–
12 mo	661 ± 219	54 ± 23	37 ± 18	–
24 mo	762 ± 209	58 ± 23	50 ± 24	137 ± 147
8 yr	923 ± 256	65 ± 25	124 ± 45	251 ± 167
16 yr	946 ± 124	59 ± 20	148 ± 63	330 ± 212
Adult	1158 ± 305	99 ± 27	200 ± 61	200†
Secretions				
Colostrum	10	61	1234	–
Stimulated parotid saliva	0.036	0.043	3.9	–
Unstimulated whole saliva	4.86	0.55	30.4	–
Jejunal fluid	34	70	–	–
Seminal fluid	510	90	116	–
Cerebrospinal fluid				
Normal	3 ± 1	0	0.4±0.5	–
Purulent infection	9	4	4	–
Viral infection	4	0.5	1	–

*Mean ± 1 standard deviation.
†Values up to 800 U/ml are normal.
Adapted from Nelson Textbook of Pediatrics, 1983, 12th Edition.

CEREBROSPINAL FLUID

Cell Count		% PMN's
Preterm mean	9.0 (0-25.4 WBC/mm³)	57%
Term mean	8.2 (0-22.4 WBC/mm³)	61%
>1 mo	0-7	0

Glucose		
Preterm	24-63 mg/dl	(mean 50)
Term	34-119 mg/dl	(mean 52)
Child	40-80 mg/dl	

CSF Glucose/Blood Glucose (%)
  Preterm   55-105
  Term   44-128
  Child   ˜50%

Lactic Acid Dehydrogenase: Mean 20 U/ml (range 5-30 U/ml)

Myelin Basic Protein: <4 ng/ml

Pressure: Inital L.P. (mm H_2O)
  Newborn   80-110(<110)
  Infant/Child   <200(lateral recumbent position)
  Respiratory movements   5-10

Protein		
Preterm	(mean 115)	65-150 mg/dl
Term	(mean 90)	20-170 mg/dl
Children	Ventricular	5-15 mg/dl
	Cisternal	5-25 mg/dl
	Lumbar	5-40 mg/dl

Ref: Sarff, LD et al: J Pediatr 88:473, 1976.

NORMAL VALUES - HEMATOLOGY

Age	Hgb (gm %)	Hct (%)	MCV (fl)	MCHC (gm/%RBC)	Retic (%)	WBC per mm³ x 100 range (avg)	% Neutrophils	Platelet (10³/mm³)
28 week gestation	14.5	45	120	31	5-10	--	--	275±60
32 week gestation	15.0	47	118	32	3-10	--	--	290±70
Full term								
1 day+	16.8-21.2	57-68	110-128	29.7-33.5	1.8- 4.6	7-35 (18)	45-85	310±68
1 week+	15.0-19.6	46-62	107-129	30.4-33.6	0.1- 0.9	4-20 (10)	30-50	
1 month+	11.1-14.3	31-41	93-109	33.3-36.5	0.1- 1.7	6-18 (10)	30-50	300±50
3-5 months	10.4-12.2	33	80- 96	31.8-36.2	0.4-1.0	6-17 (10)	30-50	
6-11 months	11.8	35	77	33	0.7- 2.3	6-16 (10)	30-50	
1 year	11.2	35	78	32	0.6- 1.7	6-15 (10)	30-50	
2-10 years	12.8	37	80	34	0.5- 1.0	7-13 (9)	35-60	
11-15 years	13.4	39	82	34	0.5- 1.0	5-12 (8.5)	40-60	
Adult								
Male	16.0±2.0	47±7	91 (82-101)	34 (31.5-36)	0.8- 2.5	4.3-10 (7)	25-62	300±50
Female	14.0±2.0	42±5			0.8- 4.1			

+Under 1 month of age, capillary Hgb exceeds venous: 1 hour - 3.6 gm difference
5 days - 2.2 gm difference
3 weeks - 1.1 gm difference

Absolute eosinophil count: avg 250/mm² (100-600/mm³)

Ref.: Adapted from Guest, GM and Brown, EW: Am J Dis Child 93:486, 1957; Matoth, Y, et al.: Acta Paed Scand 60:317, 1971; Wintrobe, Clinical Hematology 7th Edition, Philadelphia: Lea and Febiger, 1974; Mauer, AM: Pediatric Hematology. New York: McGraw Hill, 1961; Oski and Naiman, Hematologic Problems in the Newborn Infant. Philadelphia: W.B. Saunders, Co., 1972; Nathan, D and Oski, F: Hematology of Infancy and Childhood. Philadelphia: W. B. Saunders, Co. 1981.

NORMAL RANGES FOR HEMOGLOBIN AND MCV

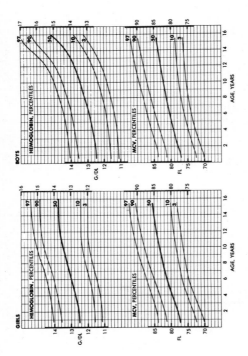

Ref: Dallman, PR and Siimes, MA: J Pediatr 94:26, 1979.

McLEAN, HASTINGS NOMOGRAM

Calcium more than 50% ionized / less than 50% ionized

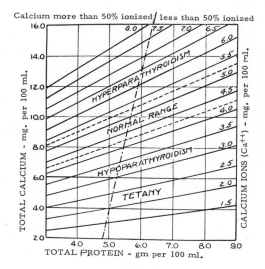

Ref: Harrison and Harrison, Disorders of Calcium and Phosphate Metabolism in Childhood and Adolescence, Saunders, 1979, p. 18.

TOTAL SERUM PROTEINS VS. TOTAL SERUM SOLIDS

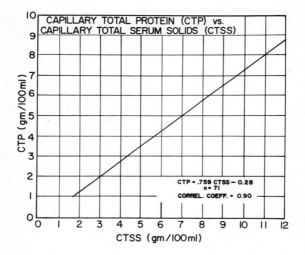

Ref: Thoene, JG, et al.: J Pediatr 71:413, 1967.

CONVERSION FORMULAS

Weight

Grams	Pounds
454	1.0
1000	2.2

To change pounds to grams, multiply by 454.

To change kilograms to pounds, multiply by 2.2.

Length

To convert inches to cms, multiply by 2.54.

Temperature

To convert degrees Celsius to degrees Fahrenheit: $(9/5 \times temperature) + 32$

To convert degrees Fahrenheit to degrees Celsius $(temperature - 32) \times 5/9$

TEMPERATURE EQUIVALENTS

Centigrade	Fahrenheit	Centigrade	Fahrenheit
34.0	93.2	38.6	101.4
34.2	93.6	38.8	101.8
34.4	93.9	39.0	102.2
34.6	94.3	39.2	102.5
34.8	94.6	39.4	102.9
35.0	95.0	39.6	103.2
35.2	95.4	39.8	103.6
35.4	95.7	40.0	104.0
35.6	96.1	40.2	104.3
35.8	96.4	40.4	104.7
36.0	96.8	40.6	105.1
36.2	97.1	40.8	105.4
36.4	97.5	41.0	105.8
36.6	97.8	41.2	106.1
36.8	98.2	41.4	106.5
37.0	98.6	41.6	106.8
37.2	98.9	41.8	107.2
37.4	99.3	42.0	107.6
37.6	99.6	42.2	108.0
37.8	100.0	42.4	108.3
38.0	100.4	42.6	108.7
38.2	100.7	42.8	109.0
38.4	101.1	43.0	109.4

CONVERSION OF POUNDS AND OUNCES TO GRAMS

Ounces	1 lb.	2 lb.	3 lb.	4 lb.	5 lb.	6 lb.	7 lb.	8 lb.
				GRAMS				
0	454	907	1,361	1,814	2,268	2,722	3,175	3,629
1	482	936	1,389	1,843	2,296	2,750	3,204	3,657
2	510	964	1,418	1,871	2,325	2,778	3,232	3,686
3	539	992	1,446	1,899	2,353	2,807	3,260	3,714
4	567	1,021	1,474	1,928	2,381	2,835	3,289	3,742
5	595	1,049	1,503	1,956	2,410	2,863	3,317	3,771
6	624	1,077	1,531	1,985	2,438	2,892	3,345	3,799
7	652	1,106	1,559	2,013	2,466	2,920	3,374	3,827
8	680	1,134	1,588	2,041	2,495	2,948	3,402	3,856
9	709	1,162	1,616	2,070	2,523	2,977	3,430	3,884
10	737	1,191	1,644	2,098	2,552	3,005	3,459	3,912
11	765	1,219	1,673	2,126	2,580	3,033	3,487	3,941
12	794	1,247	1,701	2,155	2,608	3,062	3,515	3,969
13	822	1,276	1,729	2,183	2,637	3,090	3,544	3,997
14	851	1,304	1,758	2,211	2,665	3,119	3,572	4,026
15	879	1,332	1,786	2,240	2,693	3,147	3,600	4,054

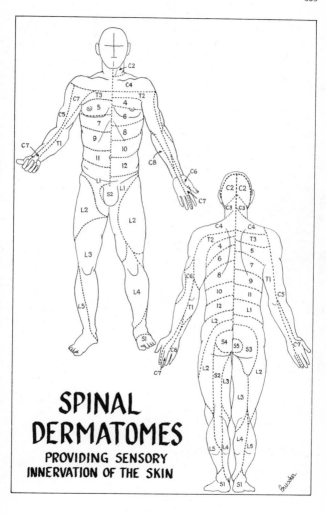

SPINAL
DERMATOMES
PROVIDING SENSORY
INNERVATION OF THE SKIN

INDEX